Understanding
Anaesthesia

Acquisitions editor: Melanie Tait
Development editor: Zoë A. Youd
Production controller: Chris Jarvis
Cover designer: Fred Rose

Understanding Anaesthesia

Fourth edition

Peter Simpson and Mansukh Popat

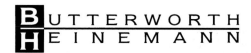
BUTTERWORTH HEINEMANN

OXFORD   AUCKLAND   BOSTON   JOHANNESBURG   MELBOURNE   NEW DELHI

Butterworth-Heinemann
Linacre House, Jordan Hill, Oxford OX2 8DP
225 Wildwood Avenue, Woburn, MA 01801-2041
A division of Reed Educational and Professional Publishing Ltd

℞ A member of the Reed Elsevier plc group

First published 1982
Second edition 1988
Third edition 1996
Fourth edition 2002

British Library Cataloguing in Publication Data
A catalogue record for this book is available from the British Library

Library of Congress Cataloguing in Publication Data
A catalogue record for this book is available from the Library of Congress

ISBN 0 7506 4853 8

For information on all Butterworth-Heinemann
publications visit our website at www.bh.com

Produced and typeset by Gray Publishing, Tunbridge Wells, Kent
Printed and bound by MPG Books, Bodmin, Cornwall

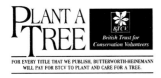

PLANT A TREE

British Trust for
Conservation Volunteers

FOR EVERY TITLE THAT WE PUBLISH, BUTTERWORTH-HEINEMANN
WILL PAY FOR BTCV TO PLANT AND CARE FOR A TREE.

3/28/04

Contents

Preface to Fourth Edition

There have been many changes in anaesthetic practice since the third edition of this book was published. New drugs, equipment and techniques are included in the appropriate chapters, all of which have been extensively reviewed and many new photographs and figures have been added. We have been careful in keeping to the original style of the book. We trust that this book will continue to be useful to all those hoping to gain an understanding of anaesthesia.

This new edition also marks the end of an era, since it is the first with which Dr Len Carrie is no longer actively involved. Dr Carrie was an inspiration behind *Understanding Anaesthesia* from the very beginning of the project. Without his enthusiasm, dedication and knowledge, the first let alone the subsequent editions, would never have come to fruition. We would wish to express our sincere thanks to him for all that he has contributed over many years.

Preface to First Edition

This introduction to the principles and practice of anaesthesia has been written primarily to cover the curricula of postgraduate nurses and operating department assistants,* both of which put considerable emphasis on a knowledge of physiology and pharmacology. At the same time, modern techniques of clinical measurement have been increasingly introduced into anaesthetic practice. We have therefore tried to include details of recent advances in anaesthesia in addition to the appropriate basic science teaching and the historical and practical aspects of the speciality

The early part of the book deals with the physiology and pharmacology relevant to anaesthesia, together with a general introduction to anaesthetic technique. Separate chapters deal with anaesthesia for particular surgical specialities and with regional anaesthetic techniques. The problems of intensive care, parenteral nutrition and chronic pain are also included to make the text as comprehensive as possible. Separate chapters towards the end of the book deal with varying aspects of clinical measurement and equipment related to anaesthesia, sterilisation of apparatus, theatre pollution and electrical safety.

The book has grown considerably in length from what was originally planned, but we found it difficult to shorten it if the subject matter was still to be fully covered. The format of a large number of short chapters with a precise of the contents placed under each chapter heading was chosen to make reference easy.

Although originally written for postgraduate nurses and ODAs, we hope that the text is likely to be of benefit to a wider audience including junior anaesthetists, medical students and nurses in intensive care.

---

*Joint Board of Clinical Nursing Studies (now English National Board), Course Number 182; City and Guilds Diploma Course for Operating Department Assistants.

Acknowledgements

We are indebted to Drs Rhys Evans and Simon Berg for contributing Chapters 35 and 37, respectively. We are also grateful to the Late Mr Richard Salt (formerly Principal Chief Technician in the Nuffield Department of Anaesthetics in the University of Oxford) and Mr Lawrence Hugill (formerly Sterile Services Manager of the Central Sterile Services Department at the Slade Hospital in Oxford) for invaluable assistance with Chapters 7 and 46 in the first edition of this book. We owe a special debt of gratitude to Miss Sue Crook who meticulously, but somehow always cheerfully, carried out (virtually single-handed) the formidable task of all the typing and secretarial work concerned with the first edition of this book.

1

Anaesthesia: History and Introduction

•History •Introduction

● HISTORY

Only a brief summary will be given here of some of the outstanding events in the history of anaesthesia; more detailed history is given in the relevant chapters.

Various dental extractions and operations had been carried out under nitrous oxide or ether anaesthesia in the few years before 1846, but modern anaesthesia is usually considered to date from 16 October 1846, when William T.G. Morton, a Boston dentist, successfully administered ether to a young man whose operation for a tumour on his neck was performed before an assembly of prominent medical men at the Massachusetts General Hospital.

Considering the slowness of communications in those days, the rate at which anaesthesia spread across the world was remarkable. By 19 December 1846 ether had been used in England for dental extractions, and by the following year John Snow, the first professional anaesthetist and one of the greatest names in early anaesthesia, had written a book about ether. Also in 1847, James Young Simpson, Professor of Midwifery in Edinburgh, introduced chloroform as an anaesthetic agent in obstetrics. Religious and other objections were finally overcome when Snow administered chloroform to Queen Victoria at the birth of Prince Leopold in 1853. Chloroform and ether were to remain the most popular anaesthetic agents for the next 100 years. Halothane was synthesised by Suckling in 1951 and its first use published in 1956.

There had been isolated instances of the successful use of nitrous oxide as an anaesthetic agent, but an unsuccessful demonstration of its use in 1845 by Wells at the Massachusetts General Hospital, its weakness as an agent and problems in devising equipment led to its virtual disappearance from the anaesthetic scene for some years. It began to regain popularity when Joseph Clover, another giant of early anaesthesia, used it as a relatively pleasant induction before ether anaesthesia.

Nitrous oxide was first used to relieve pain in childbirth by Klikovitch of St Petersburg in 1880, and became popular when Minnitt's nitrous oxide–air machine was introduced in 1934. These 'gas and air' mixtures are now obsolete and inhalational analgesia in labour is now usually provided by Entonox, premixed nitrous oxide and oxygen in one cylinder in the proportions 50 : 50, first described by Tunstall and produced by the British Oxygen Company (BOC) in 1961. The overall importance of nitrous oxide in anaesthesia has greatly increased since the introduction of muscle-relaxant drugs, because these agents provide excellent operating conditions under light, general anaesthesia.

Local analgesia dates from 1884 when Köller described the effect of cocaine applied topically to the eye. Spinal analgesia for a surgical operation was first carried out by Bier in 1899, and the first epidurals (which were in fact caudals) were carried out in 1901 independently by Sicard and Cathelin of France. The first time the lumbar approach to the epidural space was used was in 1921 by a Spanish military surgeon, Fidel Pagés. Although Dean of the London Hospital had used continuous spinal anaesthesia in 1907, real interest in continuous regional techniques dates from the 1940s, when Lemmon performed continuous spinal analgesia via a malleable needle. In 1945, Tuohy performed the first continuous spinal analgesia via a catheter introduced through a needle and the following year designed a needle with a tip specially designed for the purpose.

The first continuous lumbar epidurals were carried out by Hingson and Southworth of the United States also using malleable needles. In 1947, Curbelo of Havana was the first to carry out continuous epidural analgesia using a ureteric catheter, introduced with the help of a Tuohy needle.

Tracheal intubation, as a means of resuscitation using tubes made usually of metal or a wire spiral covered with leather, had been used since the late eighteenth century. It was not until 1880 that MacEwen of Glasgow first used a tracheal tube for administering an anaesthetic. Laryngoscopes were pioneered by Kirstein, Killian and Jackson in the late 1800s/early 1900s. The Macintosh laryngoscope was introduced in 1943. The use of rubber tubes for endotracheal anaesthesia developed from the work of Magill and Rowbotham, who used this technique to facilitate head and neck surgery on casualties of the First World War. Although John Logie Baird (of television fame) described fibreoptic image transmission in 1926, it was not until 1954 that the first flexible fibreoptic gastroscopy was performed by Hirchowitz in Michigan, USA. The first flexible fibreoptic guided tracheal intubation was described by Dr Peter Murphy in London in 1967 using a flexible choledochoscope. In 1983 a new era in airway management began with the introduction of the laryngeal mask airway (LMA) by Dr Archie Brain, a British anaesthetist.

One of the greatest advances in anaesthesia was the introduction of the neuromuscular-blocking agents to provide relaxation for surgical operations. Griffith and Johnson of Montreal in 1942 used the first agent, curare. Decamethonium, a long-acting depolarising muscle relaxant, was first used in 1949, and suxamethonium followed in 1951.

The glass syringe and needle were introduced by Pravaz of Lyons and popularised by a Scot, Alexander Wood, in 1854. In the first part of the twentieth century attempts were made to administer many agents (including chloroform and ether) intravenously. The first agent to make intravenous anaesthesia popular was hexobarbitone, introduced in 1932, and in 1934 Lundy of the Mayo Clinic introduced thiopentone into clinical use. Now, 70 years later, it still remains one of the most popular intravenous induction agents.

With the technical advances came the evolution of the professional anaesthetist. In the UK, the first examination for the Diploma in Anaesthetics was held in 1935 and Dr R.R. Macintosh was elected to the first chair of Anaesthesia in Oxford in 1937. Anaesthesia gained equal status with other specialities with the birth of the National Health Service in 1948.

● INTRODUCTION

The word 'anaesthesia' is derived from the Greek and means 'without feeling'. 'Analgesia', also from the Greek, means 'without pain'. There is widespread acceptance of the term general anaesthesia, but debate sometimes arises as to whether local anaesthesia or local analgesia is the correct term to apply to the effect produced by local anaesthetic or local analgesic drugs. Whatever the correct etymological derivation, these terms have become fairly freely interchangeable. The terms 'regional anaesthesia' and 'regional analgesia' are now commonly used to describe nerve-blocking techniques.

The 'Triad' of Anaesthesia

Any general anaesthetic can usually be divided into three components – narcosis (sleep), analgesia (pain relief), and relaxation (muscular relaxation). Different surgical operations require different proportions of the three components. Once a patient is unconscious it is not always clear how much analgesia an agent is providing. However, some agents undoubtedly provide more analgesia than others, and this is more obvious when the agents are used in subnarcotic concentrations. Hence nitrous oxide, an excellent analgesic, can be used in this way to provide pain relief in obstetrics. Halothane, a poor analgesic, is ineffective when so used.

In the same way, halothane when vaporised by a gas which has no analgesic properties (e.g. oxygen or air) tends to provide poor operating conditions for even minor operations unless fairly high concentrations are used. The addition of nitrous oxide to the halothane and oxygen, however, provides a versatile and popular anaesthetic mixture with good proportions of analgesia and narcosis.

In the early days of anaesthesia, when single agents were used (e.g. chloroform or ether), all the components of the triad had to be obtained from the single drug. The main problem was that muscular relaxation was provided by these single volatile agents only at the deeper levels of anaesthesia. The proportions of the narcotic and analgesic components were greatly in excess of those required for the operation; hence the patient sometimes took hours to regain full consciousness and often suffered from other distressing side-effects, in particular vomiting. The incidence of postoperative respiratory and venous thrombotic complications was high.

Modern anaesthetic agents allow the proportions of the three components of the triad to be more easily adjusted to individual requirements, with a corresponding improvement in the patient's operative and postoperative well-being. In particular, the introduction of muscle-relaxant drugs has meant that excellent relaxation may be obtained simply by an injection from a syringe, while the patient is only lightly anaesthetised – a great improvement on the profound and often prolonged anaesthesia required to provide similar operating conditions when a single anaesthetic agent was used.

Before each patient arrives in the anaesthetic room it is good practice for the anaesthetist and those who are helping him to decide which components of the triad will provide the best conditions for the operation and what combination of drugs can best be used to provide them. For example, for many operations where profound muscle relaxation is not required the induction of anaesthesia is most pleasantly and smoothly performed by an intravenous agent like propofol. Maintenance of anaesthesia may then be performed with nitrous oxide, oxygen, and a volatile agent like isoflurane or enflurane with the patient breathing spontaneously – the nitrous oxide providing more analgesia and the volatile agent more narcosis than that provided by the sleep dose of thiopentone or propofol. An alternative is to provide maintenance by an infusion of propofol and avoiding a volatile agent altogether.

For an operation where muscle relaxation is required, anaesthesia may still be induced intravenously and tracheal intubation carried out with the help of a muscle relaxant. Maintenance of anaesthesia can then be provided with nitrous oxide, oxygen and an adjuvant (volatile agent or infusion of propofol) with further increments of muscle relaxant as required. This sequence will also provide good operating conditions for thoracic surgery, where muscle relaxation is not so important but controlled ventilation is required to prevent the lung collapsing once the pleural cavity has been opened.

Despite the basic importance of the components of the triad of anaesthesia it should be realised that they are not the only factors affecting the decision about which anaesthetic agents to use. For example, even with modern agents it may be difficult after long operations to ensure that the patient will wake up quickly if a spontaneous respiration technique is employed. The rapid return of the patient's protective reflexes at the end of anaesthesia is always important and sometimes, for example, when recovery facilities are inadequate, may be vital to the patient's safety. For this reason an anaesthetist might use a muscle-relaxant technique even when relaxation is not particularly necessary.

Another example of other factors affecting the choice of anaesthetic technique could occur in the elderly patient, where adequate operating conditions with a spontaneous respiration technique might be provided only by an anaesthetic mixture of such strength that hypotension was unavoidable. Again, the anaesthetist might provide an anaesthetic that was safer for the patient if a muscle-relaxant technique were to be used.

This introduction indicates only some of the more important factors affecting the choice of anaesthetic technique. There are many others occurring in individual cases, but, with the wide choice of spontaneous respiration, controlled respiration and regional techniques available today, it should be possible to provide most patients with an anaesthetic which combines a high degree of safety with a low incidence of serious post-anaesthetic complications.

2

Applied Anatomy and Physiology in Anaesthesia

•Cardiovascular system •Respiratory system •Autonomic nervous system •Kidney •Fluid and acid–base balance

● CARDIOVASCULAR SYSTEM

Heart

The anatomical structure of the heart, as it lies in the thorax, is illustrated in Figure 2.1. The right and left sides of the heart are separate in normal circumstances, the blood flowing via the lungs to pass from the right side of the heart to the left. A small amount of blood either circulating through the bronchial as opposed to the pulmonary circulation, or draining from the coronary arteries into the coronary sinus and thence into the lumen

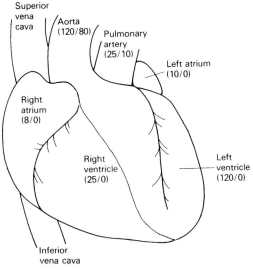

Figure 2.1 The heart (systolic and diastolic pressure indicated in mmHg).

of the ventricles, provides a 1–2% shunt of deoxygenated blood to the left side of the heart.

Normal Cardiac Contraction

Blood reaches the atria from the periphery via the superior and inferior venae cavae (SVC, IVC), flowing down a small pressure gradient. Venous return is enhanced both by the negative pressure created in the chest by active inspiration and by the peripheral muscle pump. Anaesthesia, involving intermittent positive pressure ventilation, may therefore diminish venous return and subsequently cardiac output. The atria act as a storage reservoir, allowing subsequent blood flow into the ventricles during diastole. Towards the end of diastole the atria themselves contract, providing an extra 10–20% of ventricular filling. Atrial contraction is not essential, but significantly improves ventricular filling and therefore cardiac output. This is evident when considering the relatively low cardiac output associated with atrial fibrillation or heart block. During systole the ventricles contract, forcing blood into the pulmonary artery and the aorta, and during this period the ventricular muscle is compressed and therefore little or no blood flows down the coronary arteries which supply oxygenated blood to the heart muscle. Coronary blood flow, and therefore myocardial oxygenation, only occurs during diastole. If the period of diastole is shortened by an increase in heart rate, myocardial oxygenation may be reduced, and if this tachycardia is accompanied by increased demands on the myocardium in the form of exercise or hypertension, in susceptible patients, angina may be precipitated by the relative imbalance of oxygen supply and demand.

Figure 2.1 also illustrates the pressures developed in the various chambers of the heart and the aorta. The atria are relatively low-pressure organs, while the ventricles generate a high systolic pressure equal to that in the aorta or pulmonary artery, but the end-diastolic pressure is only marginally above zero. The right ventricle pumps out the same quantity of blood as the left, but at a much lower pressure, the right side of the heart pumping against the pulmonary vascular bed. Pulmonary hypertension may therefore be caused by an increase in resistance of the pulmonary vasculature which, in turn, may be associated with lung disease or hypoxia.

Control of Heart Rate

The heart is formed from excitable tissue. Cardiac muscle differs only slightly from nervous tissue in its degree of excitability. It therefore possesses its own inherent rhythm, which will be apparent if the external influences on heart rate are removed. Normal conduction of the cardiac impulse originates in the sino-atrial node in the right atrium and proceeds across the atrium to the atrioventricular node and then down the bundle of His, which bifurcates to supply impulses to both the right and left ventricles. The normal heart rate generated from the sino-atrial node varies between 60 and 120 beats per minute in fit adults and young children, respectively. This beat is regular, varying only mildly with the respiratory cycle (sinus arrhythmia). The sino-atrial node, however, is influenced both from the brain via the vagus nerve, tending to slow the heart (bradycardia), and from sympathetic fibres or circulating catecholamines, both of which tend to produce an increase in heart rate (tachycardia). With normal conducting tissue this increase in heart rate is transmitted to the remainder of the atria and the ventricles. If a conduction defect exists, areas of the heart may produce their own inherent rhythm. If this develops from the atrioventricular node (nodal rhythm), the atrial rate may be maintained but efficient atrial contraction does not occur (Chapter 22). This may result in a relatively inefficient filling of the ventricles. If there is a complete heart block between the atria and the ventricles, the ventricles will beat with their own inherent rhythm at a rate of 40 beats per minute. This may allow extra beats from other excitable areas of the heart to interpose themselves, producing supraventricular or ventricular ectopic beats. All these disorders of cardiac rhythm tend to reduce the efficiency of heart filling and therefore cardiac output.

Cardiac Output

The volume of blood ejected from the heart in a fixed time is referred to as the cardiac output and is usually measured in litres per minute. This amount of blood is dependent both on the heart rate and on the volume of blood ejected from the left ventricle during each contraction. This last measurement is known as the stroke volume, the cardiac output being equal to the stroke volume multiplied by the heart rate. Cardiac output also influences the arterial blood pressure. The amount of blood ejected by the heart balanced against the resistance to flow offered by the peripheral circulation determines the pressure generated in the aorta and the major vessels. Arterial blood pressure, therefore, is equal to cardiac output multiplied by peripheral resistance.

Peripheral Resistance

The resistance in the peripheral circulation depends mainly on the degree of arteriolar vasodilatation or constriction. The veins act as capacitance vessels – i.e. a reservoir for blood – but are not capable of extreme contraction. The arterioles are under the control of the sympathetic nervous system (Chapter 13), arteriolar vasoconstriction occurring as a result of increased sympathetic activity. A reduction in sympathetic tone produces arteriolar vasodilatation. The parasympathetic system plays no part in vasodilatation which is effected simply by a reduction or abolition of sympathetic activity, as occurs when a patient faints.

The degree of peripheral vasodilatation is also affected by the release of local metabolites, which may be produced in excess as a result of reduced tissue oxygenation and by the production of lactic acid. Local acidosis or carbon dioxide release, together with accumulation of other metabolites, may produce arteriolar vasodilatation and therefore an increase in peripheral perfusion but a reduction in peripheral resistance.

Certain organs, such as the brain, the kidney and the coronary circulation, are able to control blood flow through their vascular beds, maintaining the flow at a constant level irrespective of fluctuations in arterial blood pressure. This phenomenon, known as autoregulation, is effected by local control of arteriolar diameter in response to tissue metabolism. In the case of the brain, for example, autoregulation means that cerebral perfusion pressure does not change between mean arterial blood pressures of 60 and 150 mmHg. Nevertheless, most vascular beds are capable of a degree of autoregulation.

By contrast, not all areas vasoconstrict at the same time. In sympathetic overactivity, when the subject needs to be ready to run away, vasoconstriction may be observed in the skin and splanchnic circulation; but vasodilatation will occur in the muscle beds to supply extra blood flow to this area.

Control of Blood Pressure

The baroceptor mechanism is responsible for controlling blood pressure. Baroceptors are situated in the arterial wall of the aortic arch and in the region of the common carotid arteries, and are sensitive to changes in pressure within the lumen of the vessel. As the pressure rises, the nerve-impulse activity, passing from these areas to the medulla of the brain, increases. If the pressure falls, activity decreases. This nervous activity controls the output of the vasomotor centre, the area of the brain responsible for control of blood vessel diameter.

Baroceptor activity inhibits the vasomotor centre. An increase in blood pressure, causing increased baroceptor activity, therefore inhibits the vasomotor centre producing vasodilatation and a fall in blood pressure. Conversely, a reduction in baroceptor activity causes increased vasomotor centre activity and vasoconstriction. The vasomotor centre is also influenced by hypoxia, hypercarbia and higher centres in the brain. The baroceptors also influence the cardiac centre in the brain controlling heart rate via the vagus nerve. Increased baroceptor activity resulting from an increase in blood pressure stimulates the vagus nerve, reducing heart rate and thereby lowering blood pressure. Hypovolaemia, conversely, is compensated for by peripheral vasoconstriction and an increase in heart rate.

● RESPIRATORY SYSTEM

The lungs lie in the thoracic cavity on either side of the mediastinum. They consist of conducting airways and lung tissue, whose function is to allow diffusion of gases from the air into the bloodstream across the alveolar-capillary membrane. Under ideal conditions this membrane is only two cells thick, allowing minimal interruption to gas diffusion. The alveoli themselves greatly increase the area available for gas exchange and so make this process more efficient.

The lungs are surrounded by two layers of a membrane, the pleura. The visceral pleura is closely applied to the lung surface and the parietal pleura lines the chest wall. Under normal conditions these two layers are closely applied to one another and there is only a potential space between them. The outward pull of the chest wall opposing the inward pull of the elastic recoil of the lung creates a negative pressure within the pleural space which is responsible for holding the lung in an expanded position.

Anatomy of the bronchial tree and its relevance to endobronchial intubation and one-lung anaesthesia for thoracotomy is discussed in Chapter 34.

Breathing

At the end of a normal, quiet expiration the lungs are in the resting respiratory position, their elastic recoil being opposed by the chest wall and the negative pressure in the intrapleural space. Inspiration is an active process initiated by the expansion of the thoracic cage, which inevitably draws the lungs outwards by negative pressure and, as a result, air flows down the bronchi. Initially, expansion of the thoracic cage is diaphragmatic, the intercostal muscles, which enlarge the thoracic cage itself, being used only when larger volumes of gas need to be exchanged as oxygen consumption rises in the body as a result of exercise. The diaphragm is supplied by the phrenic nerve from the third, fourth and fifth cervical nerves, while the individual intercostal nerves supply the various thoracic segments. For this reason a high thoracic extradural or spinal anaesthetic is unlikely to impair respiration seriously until it reaches the mid-cervical region. Patients with spinal cord transection are also able to breathe, provided that the level of cord damage is not above C3.

In contrast to inspiration, expiration is passive, depending solely on the elastic recoil of the lungs. Active expiration is possible by using extra muscles, such as those of the abdominal wall, to increase the upward movement of the diaphragm.

Normal Lung Volumes

The volumes of air contained in the lungs at different phases of the respiratory cycle are important in assessing lung function. These are illustrated in Figure 2.2, the most important being the tidal volume, i.e. the volume of air exchanged during normal quiet respiration, and the vital capacity which is the maximum amount of air that a patient is able to exchange.

An index of adequacy of lung function is obtained from a measurement of the volume of air which a patient is able to exhale forcibly (forced expiratory volume) in one second (FEV_1), expressed as a proportion of their vital capacity. This FEV_1 to vital capacity ratio is normally over 80%. At the end of maximal expiration a small amount of air, the residual volume, still remains in the lungs, this being air trapped in the alveoli at the end of a maximal expiration.

Compliance

The expression 'compliance' is used to indicate the degree of 'stiffness' of the lungs. A compliant organ is one which is easy to distend and therefore a lung with high compliance is relatively easy to distend, while low compliance implies that the lung is stiff as a result of acute or chronic disease, pulmonary oedema or infection. In lungs with low compliance a

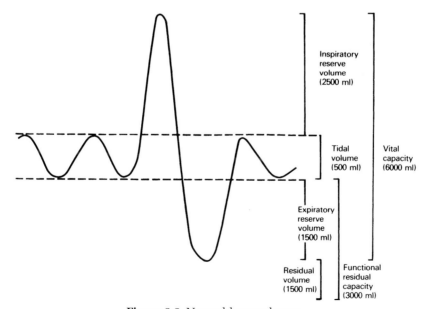

Figure 2.2 Normal lung volumes.

relatively large amount of energy may be needed to overcome the initial stiffness of the lungs when inspiration occurs, in the same way that a balloon is more difficult to blow up until it has begun to expand.

Gas Exchange

The volume of gas inspired in one minute is known as the minute volume. This is the product of the respiratory rate and the tidal volume and at rest is usually about 8 l/min in a 70 kg man. In extreme exercise this may increase by three to four times that amount. As the dead space in the lung (i.e. the volume of the airways not taking part in gaseous exchange) is a fixed portion of any breath (120–150 ml) an increase in respiratory rate will inevitably increase dead-space ventilation while an increase in tidal volume with no increase in respiratory rate will result in increased alveolar ventilation without any increased ventilation of the dead space. Deep breathing is therefore more advantageous to patients than rapid shallow respiration.

Once gas has reached the alveoli, oxygen and carbon dioxide are exchanged across the alveolar-capillary membrane to equilibrate with the blood concentrations of these gases. Other gases, such as anaesthetics and nitrogen, also diffuse freely across this membrane, although in the case of nitrogen, which is not consumed in the body, the overall net flow of gas from one side to the other is zero. Diffusion depends on the pressure exerted by each individual gas on either side of this membrane, the overall result being that gas diffuses down concentration gradients from an area of high concentration to a low one. In the lungs, therefore, oxygen flows from the alveoli into the bloodstream and carbon dioxide passes in the reverse direction.

As we live at atmospheric pressure, the total pressure exerted by all the gases present in room air must equal atmospheric pressure, that is 760 mmHg. Likewise, the overall pressure exerted by the gases in the alveoli or in the blood must also equal 760 mmHg. The composition of gases in these various compartments is illustrated in Table 2.1.

Carriage of Oxygen in the Blood

Oxygen is carried in the blood in two ways: (1) in combination with haemoglobin or (2) dissolved in the plasma. One gram of normal haemoglobin will combine with 1.38 ml oxygen so that, with a normal haemoglobin concentration of 14 g/100 ml blood, 20 ml oxygen will be carried in combination with haemoglobin in 100 ml blood. In this case the haemoglobin is said to be fully saturated with oxygen. The degree of saturation of haemoglobin and the amount of relative desaturation which occurs as the blood perfuses peripheral tissues and releases oxygen are dependent on the oxyhaemoglobin dissociation curve (Fig. 2.3).

Table 2.1 Physiological gas partial pressures (mmHg)

	Room air	Alveolar/arterial blood	Venous blood
Nitrogen	610	573	617
Oxygen	150	100	40
Carbon dioxide	–	40	46
Water vapour	–	47	47

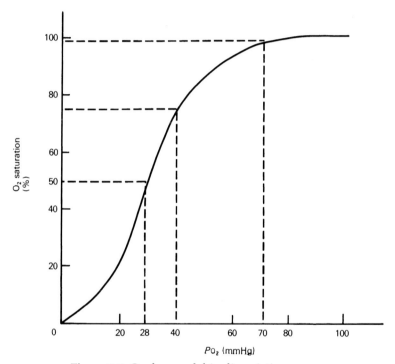

Figure 2.3 Oxyhaemoglobin dissociation curve.

Haemoglobin is fully saturated with oxygen when the arterial partial pressure of oxygen (P_{O_2}) is over 70 mmHg. Below this level, saturation falls rapidly for only a small fall in arterial P_{O_2} thus enabling the haemoglobin to release oxygen to the tissues while maintaining them at an adequate P_{O_2}. Certain factors tend to influence the readiness with which haemoglobin releases oxygen, such as temperature, acidosis and partial pressure of carbon dioxide (P_{CO_2}). This means that in certain conditions, when oxygen availability is at a premium, other factors in the body ensure adequate release from the haemoglobin.

Hypoxia

A lack of available oxygen within the body is known as hypoxia. Four main types are recognised, depending on the factors which cause them.

Hypoxic Hypoxia

This is due either to a lack of available oxygen in the inspired air or to difficulty in inspiration, both of which produce a low content of oxygen in the arterial blood.

Anaemic Hypoxia

This is due to a reduction in the available haemoglobin and therefore the oxygen carriage is reduced.

Stagnant Hypoxia

In cases of poor peripheral perfusion, when blood flow is sluggish through peripheral tissues as a result of vasoconstriction, hypoxia and cyanosis may occur as a result of excessive oxygen uptake from the available blood.

Histotoxic Hypoxia

This results from cellular damage, when the cells are unable to use the oxygen supplied to them.

Carbon Dioxide Transport

Carbon dioxide is carried in the blood in three ways:

In Solution in the Plasma

Carbon dioxide combines with water to form carbonic acid which, in turn, dissociates into hydrogen and bicarbonate ions:

$$CO_2 + H_2O \rightleftarrows H_2CO_3 \rightleftarrows H^+ + HCO_3^-$$

As Carbamino Compounds

Carbon dioxide combines with proteins to form carbamino compounds, but this is responsible for only a small amount of carbon dioxide carriage.

In the Form of Bicarbonate

Carbon dioxide in solution passes from plasma into the red cells while the blood is in the peripheral tissues. Carbonic acid, which is formed in the red cells under the influence of an enzyme, carbonic anhydrase, then dissociates into hydrogen and bicarbonate ions. The haemoglobin within the red cell combines with the free hydrogen ions, thereby neutralising them and preventing a change in pH. The free bicarbonate then diffuses out of the red cell in exchange for chloride ions moving into the red cell, the bicarbonate then being carried within the plasma. This exchange of bicarbonate with chloride is known as the chloride shift and occurs in the peripheral tissues. A reverse process occurs in the lungs when chloride leaves the red cell and bicarbonate enters it to re-form carbon dioxide, which is then excreted in the lungs (Fig. 2.4).

Venous blood contains a higher concentration of carbon dioxide than arterial blood (see Table 2.1) and on reaching the lungs gives off carbon dioxide which diffuses into the alveoli, thereby reducing the arterial CO_2 concentration. The influence of carbon dioxide carriage within the blood upon acid–base balance is dealt with on p. 30.

Control of Respiration

Although humans are able to increase and decrease their respiratory rate and depth at will, normal respiration is not under voluntary control. In normal man the respiratory centre in the medulla of the brain is sensitive

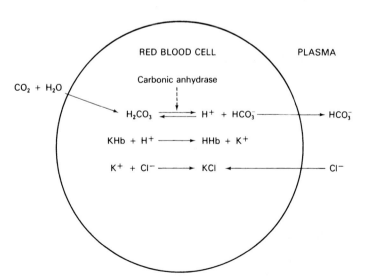

Figure 2.4 'The chloride shift' – red cell CO_2 transport.

to changes in the blood carbon dioxide concentration which, in turn, influences hydrogen and bicarbonate ions and the concentration of these within the cerebrospinal fluid (CSF). It is probably changes in CSF pH or bicarbonate concentration that influence the respiratory centre and alter respiratory rate. Normal breathing is therefore dependent on CO_2 concentration and not on hypoxia. The peripheral chemoreceptors situated in the aortic and carotid bodies are sensitive to oxygen lack, and severe hypoxia will stimulate the respiratory centre via the chemoreceptors. This, however, is an abnormal response and very few severely ill bronchitics regularly respond to a hypoxic respiratory drive.

AUTONOMIC NERVOUS SYSTEM

The autonomic nervous system is divided into the parasympathetic and sympathetic nervous systems and is concerned with the innervation of smooth muscle (e.g. gut, bronchi, bladder, blood vessels and eye), the heart and the secreting glands.

Sympathetic Nervous System

The sympathetic fibres rise in the lateral horn of the grey matter of the spinal cord in the thoracolumbar region from T1 to L2. The preganglionic sympathetic fibres (Fig. 2.5) synapse with the postganglionic fibres in the ganglia of the sympathetic chain running along the length of the spinal cord on the anterolateral bodies of the vertebrae. The postganglionic fibres then run in a mixed nerve to their point of action.

Parasympathetic Nervous System

The parasympathetic system has a cranio-sacral outflow, fibres being found in cranial nerves 3, 7, 9 and 10, and in the second, third and fourth sacral segments of the spinal cord. In contrast with the sympathetic system, where the postganglionic fibre tends to be long, the postganglionic parasympathetic fibre is often short. Hence the preganglionic fibres synapse in ganglia in the immediate vicinity of the effector organ. The parasympathetic activity in the cranial nerves may be summarised as follows:

- third nerve supplies the ciliary muscle and the iris of the eye
- seventh nerve supplies the submandibular and sublingual salivary glands
- ninth nerve supplies the parotid salivary gland
- tenth nerve (the vagus) supplies parasympathetic fibres to the thorax and abdomen affecting the heart, bronchi, gut and pancreas.

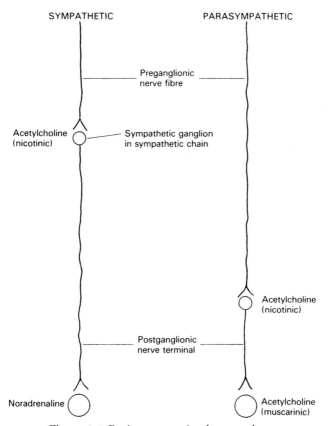

Figure 2.5 Basic autonomic pharmacology.

Transmission in the Autonomic Nervous System

The sites of action of the two main transmitting substances concerned, acetylcholine and noradrenaline, are indicated in Figure 2.5. The actions of acetylcholine are normally divided into muscarinic and nicotinic, the muscarinic being synonymous with parasympathetic activity and the nicotinic being those at the skeletal neuromuscular junction and the autonomic ganglia. These names are derived from the similarity of the individual actions of acetylcholine to those of the naturally occurring substances, muscarine and nicotine.

Actions of the Sympathetic Nervous System

These may be summarised in the 'fight and flight' reaction (Fig. 2.6), so that increased sympathetic activity produces the following effects: increased heart rate and blood pressure; vasoconstriction of skin and

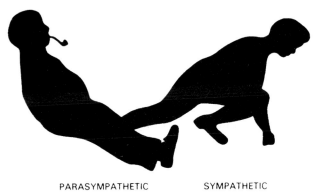

PARASYMPATHETIC   SYMPATHETIC

Figure 2.6 The autonomic nervous system.

vasodilatation in skeletal muscle; bronchial dilatation; and dilatation of the pupil of the eye. Gastrointestinal motility is inhibited and the sphincters constrict. The sweat glands and erector pilae muscles are also activated.

Actions of the Parasympathetic Nervous System

These may be likened to a fat man sitting down after a heavy meal (Fig. 2.6), so that there is a decrease in heart rate and an increase in gastrointestinal activity with the digestive tract sphincters relaxing and the bladder emptying. Bronchoconstriction occurs together with an increase in salivary, gastric and pancreatic glandular activity. The pupils constrict and the bladder sphincters relax.

The actions of both systems indicate some of the natural antagonism which occurs. In addition, however, certain autonomic activity – for example, vasoconstriction of the skin which is produced by increased sympathetic activity – is not counteracted by parasympathetic stimulation. Vasodilatation in skin is due simply to inhibition of sympathetic activity.

Acetylcholine Metabolism

Figure 2.5 indicates the sites at which acetylcholine acts as the transmitter substance, both in the synapse between pre- and postganglionic neurons and also, in the case of the parasympathetic system, at the nerve effector organ junction. In normal circumstances acetylcholine is metabolised by a naturally occurring enzyme, cholinesterase. An enzyme called plasma or pseudocholinesterase also exists, although its normal physiological function is uncertain. Acetylcholine is continually broken down by cholinesterase into choline and acetic acid. The amount of acetylcholine present may therefore be increased either by using an inhibitor of cholinesterase (i.e. an anticholinesterase, for example neostigmine or pyridostigmine) or by giving a drug that itself mimics the actions of acetylcholine.

The actions of acetylcholine may be broadly subdivided into muscarinic and nicotinic, the muscarinic being predominantly parasympathetic while the nicotinic actions are those at the skeletal neuromuscular junction and at the autonomic ganglia. The muscarinic (parasympathetic) effects of acetylcholine can be enhanced with drugs like carbachol or methacholine, both of which increase intestinal activity and bladder tone and increase exocrine secretions. Succinylcholine (suxamethonium chloride) resembles acetylcholine and for this reason acts in a similar way, first by stimulating the skeletal neuromuscular junction, causing fasciculation, and then by producing neuromuscular blockade as a result of excess stimulation. This effect can be mimicked by an excessive accumulation of acetylcholine, which may occur in patients given an overdose of anticholinesterase.

The effects of acetylcholine may be blocked by different drugs, depending on the site of action. The muscarinic effects of acetylcholine are blocked by atropine and hyoscine, and both these drugs therefore tend to produce a dry mouth, an increase in heart rate and a reduction in gastrointestinal motility. Other drugs also possess atropine-like actions, for example pethidine and the phenothiazine drugs as chlorpromazine and promethazine. The nicotinic actions of acetylcholine are stimulatory at the skeletal neuromuscular junction and at the autonomic ganglia. Of these, the neuromuscular effects are antagonised by the non-depolarising muscle relaxants, for example pancuronium, vecuronium and atracurium.

Adrenaline and Noradrenaline Metabolism

Noradrenaline is the main transmitter substance in the postganglionic sympathetic neuron. Figure 2.7 indicates the normal mechanisms of release, metabolism and reuptake of noradrenaline in this situation. After its release, noradrenaline may be taken up again into the adrenergic neurone and then either metabolised by monoamine oxidase or stored in granules ready for use again as a transmitter substance. Alternatively, it may be directly metabolised by catechol-*O*-methyl transferase, an enzyme which exists in the synaptic cleft between the neurone and the effector organ. Monoamine oxidase acts only on free noradrenaline in the nerve terminal and not on that stored in the vesicles. Noradrenaline is synthesised in the body from amino acids, an intermediary metabolite being dopamine.

Alpha and Beta Theory of Adrenergic Transmission

The effects of adrenaline at various sites in the body have been classified in terms of two groups of separate receptors, alpha (α) and beta (β), the main actions being summarised in Table 2.2.

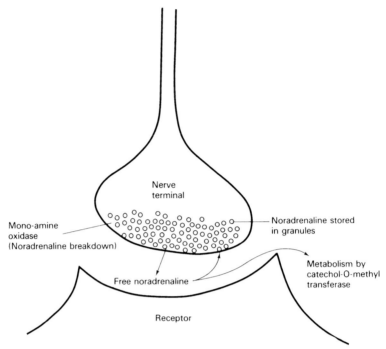

Figure 2.7 Adrenergic nerve terminal.

Table 2.2 Main actions of adrenaline in the body

Adrenaline	
α	β
Force of cardiac contraction	Heart rate (β_1)
Peripheral vasoconstriction	Bronchodilatation (β_2)
(skin + gut)	Muscle + kidney vasodilatation

While adrenaline itself possesses both α- and β-activity, other sympa-thomimetic amines possess relatively more of one or the other (Table 2.3). The β-effects are further subdivided into β_1 (effects on the heart) and β_2 (effects on the lung). The site of action of the α-effects has also been subdivided into α_1 and α_2.

In normal clinical situations, the α-effects of adrenaline most commonly observed are skin vasoconstriction causing an increase in blood pressure, while the β-effects are bronchodilatation and an increase in heart rate. These effects of adrenaline are also blocked by different drugs, for example, α-adrenoceptor blocking drugs, phentolamine, phenoxybenzamine and

Table 2.3 Drugs affecting α- and β-adrenergic receptors

α-Stimulants	Adrenaline
	Noradrenaline
	(Dopamine)
β-Stimulants	Isoprenaline (β_1 and β_2)
	Salbutamol (β_2)
	Dopamine (β_1)
	Dobutamine
α-Blockers	Phentolamine
	Phenoxybenzamine
β-Blockers	Propranolol
	Practolol (β_1)
	Oxprenolol (β_1)
	Atenolol (β_1)
	Sotalol (β_1)

tolazoline, and β-blocking drugs, for example, propranolol, atenolol and oxprenolol. Although labetalol possesses both α- and β-blocking activity, the β-blocking effects would appear to be both longer lasting and considerably greater than the α-blocking effects.

● KIDNEY

The kidneys are situated retroperitoneally on either side of the midline between T12 and L3. Together, at rest, they receive 25% of the cardiac output and serve several important functions. These are control of fluid and electrolyte concentrations within the body; regulation of blood pressure; and formation of red blood cells by secretion of the hormone erythropoietin.

The basic filtration unit of the kidney is the nephron, of which there are about one million in each kidney. Their structure is illustrated in Figure 2.8.

Basically, there are two distinct populations of nephrons, those whose Bowman's capsule is situated within the cortex itself and those whose capsule is near the renal medulla, the juxtamedullary group of nephrons.

The cortical nephrons have short loops of Henle and are far more numerous than the juxtamedullary ones, whose long loops of Henle descend deep into the medulla along the pyramids. These are responsible for the development of a high concentration gradient for water reabsorption.

Blood Flow

One-tenth of the 1200 ml/min of kidney blood flow is filtered through the glomerulus, producing a daily filtration volume of 170 l. The tubules are

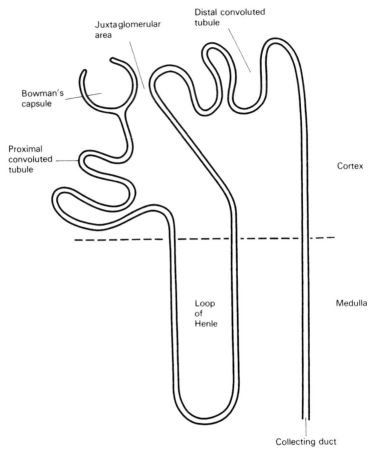

Figure 2.8 Structure of cortical renal tubule.

then responsible for selective reabsorption of almost all of this fluid. The filtration pressure within Bowman's capsule is equal to the arterial capillary blood pressure (70 mmHg), less both the osmotic pressure of the plasma proteins (25 mmHg) and the intratubular pressure (10 mmHg) – the net filtration pressure being of the order of 35 mmHg (Fig. 2.11c).

Renal Function

The main function of the tubular cells is to reabsorb both fluid and electrolyte selectively and to transfer them to the capillary network that surrounds the tubule and ultimately into the renal vein. Several processes exist within the tubule for the reabsorption of various constituents of the urine. The reabsorption of inorganic ions (e.g. sodium and potassium, and

Jo Coleman

Information Update Service

Butterworth-Heinemann

FREEPOST SCE 5435

Oxford

Oxon

OX2 8BR

UK

Keep up-to-date with the latest books in your field.

Visit our website and register now for our FREE e-mail update service, or join our mailing list and enter our monthly prize draw to win £100 worth of books. Just complete the form below and return it to us now! (FREEPOST if you are based in the UK)

www.bh.com

Please Complete In Block Capitals

Title of book you have purchased:...

....

Subject area of interest:...

Name:...

Job title:..

Business sector (if relevant):..

Street:..

Town:.. County:..................................

Country:... Postcode:...

Email:...

Telephone:...

How would you prefer to be contacted: Post ☐   e-mail ☐   Both ☐

Signature:.. Date:......................................

☐ Please arrange for me to be kept informed of other books and information services on this and related subjects (✔ box if not required). This information is being collected on behalf of Reed Elsevier plc group and may be used to supply information about products by companies within the group.

> FOR OFFICE USE ONLY

Butterworth-Heinemann,
a division of Reed Educational
& Professional Publishing Limited.
Registered office: 25 Victoria Street,
London SW1H 0EX.
Registered in England 3099304.
VAT number GB: 663 3472 30.

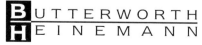

BUTTERWORTH HEINEMANN

A member of the Reed Elsevier plc group

also substances such as glucose) is an active process requiring energy; these substances are reabsorbed at a rate that depends on the body's requirement. Reabsorption of water, in contrast, is a passive process and depends on the concentration gradient established by the active reabsorption of other ions. In this way, the proximal convoluted tubule is responsible for the coarse control of the urine volume and composition and it is left to the loop of Henle and the collecting duct, in the case of water reabsorption, and the distal convoluted tubule, in the case of ions, to produce the fine control over urine composition.

In addition to active and passive reabsorption from the tubules some substances are secreted by the tubules themselves, including some naturally occurring steroids and other glucuronides (products of metabolism) produced by the liver, hippuric acid and some drugs – for example, penicillin.

Reabsorption of drugs from the tubule depends on their being in a fat-soluble form suitable for taking up by the cells. This occurs only when the drug is in the un-ionised state. Acidic drugs are highly ionised in an alkaline medium and vice versa. In the case of an acidic drug, like aspirin, maintaining the urine alkaline – and therefore the aspirin in an ionised form – will prevent its reabsorption by the tubules. This explains the use of forced alkaline diuresis in the treatment of aspirin overdose.

In normal circumstances the molecular weight of a substance determines whether or not it will diffuse across Bowman's capsule and into the tubule. The molecular threshold is about 70 000, which means that whereas substances like sodium, potassium, glucose, amino acids, urea, uric acid, creatinine and water are all small enough to pass into the tubular lumen, albumin, red cells, white cells and platelets are too large. Albumin with a molecular weight of 69 000 is just too large and this substance is the first to appear in the urine as an indication of kidney damage, however mild.

Loop of Henle

The loop of Henle and collecting duct systems are together responsible for the fine control of urine volume. This is achieved by the countercurrent mechanism, which depends on the fact that as the loop of Henle dips further into the medulla, more marked in the juxtamedullary than in the cortical nephrons, the surrounding tissue becomes progressively more concentrated. This increased concentration is effected by active reabsorption of sodium chloride from the ascending loop of Henle, possibly under the influence of antidiuretic hormone (ADH), and resecretion into the descending limb. As more sodium is reabsorbed, the further down into the medulla the nephron passes, the more concentrated the medullary tissue becomes. Unlike the descending limb, the ascending loop of Henle is normally impermeable to water, which is therefore reabsorbed only from the distal tubule and collecting ducts whose permeability to water reabsorption is under the control of ADH. As the collecting duct passes further down into the medulla, a greater volume of water is reabsorbed until ultimately the concentration of sodium in the urine equals that in the medullary tissue surrounding the tubule. This explains why the longer the juxtaglomerular loops of Henle are, the more water can be reabsorbed.

Distal Convoluted Tubule

Although the distal tubule is concerned only with the selective reabsorption of about one-eighth of the total ion content of the urine, it is this part of the nephron which produces fine control of urine volume and composition. As in the proximal tubule, active transport systems exist but, in addition, reabsorption is under the influence of two important hormones.

Aldosterone

This steroid hormone is secreted by the zona glomerulosa of the adrenal cortex and stimulates reabsorption of sodium ions from the distal tubule in response to a low sodium concentration. In exchange for sodium, potassium ions are excreted and, conversely, reduced concentrations of aldosterone will reduce the extracellular sodium concentration. Water is also lost passively along the concentration gradient created by the sodium loss. Aldosterone secretion is stimulated by surgery, anxiety, trauma and haemorrhage and probably also by adrenocorticotrophic hormone (ACTH). In addition, aldosterone is released as part of the renin–angiotensin system for maintaining blood pressure.

Antidiuretic Hormone (ADH, Vasopressin)

ADH is a peptide hormone produced by the posterior pituitary gland in response to two main stimuli:

1. A rise in the osmotic pressure of the plasma, which produces ADH release and therefore water retention. This is mediated via the osmoreceptors in the hypothalamus.
2. A fall in plasma volume detected by the volume receptors in the great thoracic veins and right atrium. In addition to these two primary stimuli, ADH release may be increased by stress, haemorrhage, shock, catecholamine release and also surgery and certain anaesthetic agents, particularly ether, halothane and morphine.

Renin–Angiotensin System

In addition to its excretory role, the kidney exerts control over arterial blood pressure. This results from the juxtaglomerular apparatus sensing changes in renal arterial blood pressure. A fall in pressure promotes secretion of renin which converts an α-globulin (angiotensinogen) into angiotensin I which is, in turn, converted into angiotensin II by a specific converting enzyme in the lung. Angiotensin II is a potent arteriolar vasoconstrictor that produces a widespread rise in systemic arterial blood pressure, thereby increasing renal perfusion pressure. It also stimulates the adrenal cortex to produce aldosterone which, in turn, increases extracellular fluid volume by sodium and water retention. Unilateral renal artery stenosis promotes renin secretion and is thought to be the cause of hypertension in this condition.

Autoregulation in the Renal Circulation

Quite apart from the renin–angiotensin system, the renal circulation also exhibits autoregulation. This is a property of the renal vasculature itself, and means that the kidney can maintain an adequate and constant blood flow despite changes in systemic arterial blood pressure within the range of 80–200 mmHg systolic and hence glomerular filtration. This is brought about by changes in renal vascular resistance in response to arterial pressure changes and is thought to be a local response of the vessels themselves and independent of hormonal influence. This phenomenon also exists in the cerebral and coronary circulations.

Atrial Natriuretic Peptide (ANP)

This hormone is released from the wall of the atria of the heart in response to over-stretching of the muscle fibres, i.e. over-filling. It produces a diuresis, secondary to salt loss and is also a vasodilator, which results in an increase in renal blood flow.

Erythropoietin

The rate of production of red blood cells by the bone marrow depends on the level of erythropoietin, a hormone which is formed by the action of a renal erythropoietic factor (REF) on a circulating globulin produced by the liver. The main stimulus to the release of this factor appears to be hypoxia and, although it has been suggested that it is released from the juxtaglomerular apparatus, this is unrelated to the renin–angiotensin system mentioned above. Hypoxia and haemorrhage stimulate erythropoietin production and, conversely, blood transfusion decreases the erythropoietic activity of the bone marrow.

● FLUID AND ACID–BASE BALANCE

Man comprises about 70% water, a 70 kg adult male having a fluid volume of about 45 l (Fig. 2.9). This is divided between the intracellular and the extracellular space in a ratio of about 2 : 1, the intracellular fluid volume being 30 l and the extracellular fluid volume 15 l. The extracellular fluid is subdivided further into 12 l of interstitial fluid and 3 l of plasma.

The normal fluid balance of a 70 kg man involves the exchange of about 3000 ml of fluid per day. This is taken in by drinking, in food and in the metabolic activity of the body, particularly in the production of carbon dioxide and water from carbohydrate metabolism. Fluid is normally lost in the form of urine (1500 ml), through the skin (900 ml), in expired air (400 ml) and in the faeces (200 ml).

Fluid distributed throughout the body is an aqueous solution containing various amounts of positively and negatively charged ions (cations and anions). Their distribution is illustrated in Figure 2.10.

In addition to these there are some un-ionised substances – for example, glucose and urea. It is essential that a balance exists between anions and cations so that in plasma, for example, the number of sodium and potassium ions approximately balance the number of chloride and bicarbonate ions. Figure 2.10 shows that whereas potassium is present in far greater amounts within the cells, the intracellular sodium concentration is small and indeed sodium ions are excluded from the cells by an active process known as the 'sodium pump'. Only when cells are functioning inadequately or dead is sodium able to leak in and potassium to leak out. Sodium–potassium exchange is a temporary but integral part of nerve-impulse transmission.

Knowing that sodium is distributed only throughout the extracellular space – in other words 15 l of body fluid – it is possible to estimate the

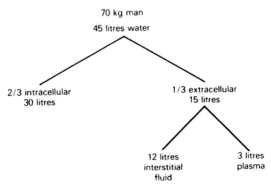

Figure 2.9 Normal fluid balance of a 70 kg man.

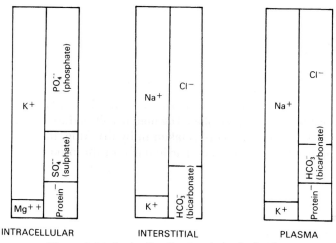

Figure 2.10 Ionic distribution in body fluids.

Table 2.4 Normal daily requirement of electrolytes

	mmol/day	g/day
Na^+	70–160	
K^+	50–80	
Ca^{2+}	5–10	0.9–1.0
Sulphate		0.3–3.0
Phosphate		0.88
Nitrogen (amino acids)		1.5

degree of a total body sodium deficit. If, for example, the serum sodium concentration is 120 mmol instead of 140 mmol/l, this implies that the body is deficient by 20 mmol per litre of body fluid, which contains sodium; in other words 20 times 15 mmol in all, i.e. 300 mmol sodium. A litre of normal saline contains 150 mmol, so in addition to their normal sodium requirement the patient requires 2 l of saline to restore their sodium depletion. Table 2.4 indicates the body's normal daily requirements for electrolytes.

Formation of Extracellular Fluid

The extracellular fluid compartment consists of both the plasma and the extravascular fluid in the ratio of about 3 : 12 l. The ionic content of these two fluid compartments is similar, with the exception of plasma proteins, which are retained entirely intravascularly, and are responsible for the maintenance of intravascular fluid (see Fig. 2.10). They exert an osmotic pressure of about 25 mmHg, tending to retain fluid within the intravascular space. At the capillary level, Figure 2.11a illustrates how at the arterial end of the capillary the hydrostatic pressure, being greater than the osmotic pressure of the plasma proteins, tends to force fluid out of the capillaries, while at the venous end, where the osmotic pressure is greater than the hydrostatic pressure, the fluid re-enters the capillary.

In addition to this formation and removal by the blood vessels themselves, the lymphatics are also present to reabsorb tissue fluid. A lack of plasma proteins, leading to a fall in the plasma osmotic pressure, therefore tends to produce an increase in extravascular fluid (oedema), which may either occur in dependent parts such as the ankles or sacrum or, more seriously, in the lungs as pulmonary oedema. Under normal circumstances, the osmotic pressure of the plasma proteins (25 mmHg) greatly exceeds the net hydrostatic pressure in the pulmonary vascular bed (8 mmHg), but hypoproteinaemia or pulmonary hypertension will produce pulmonary oedema (Fig. 2.11b). Hence the maintenance of the colloidal osmotic pressure of the plasma is vital and may be augmented not only by giving plasma protein but also by other osmotically active substances, for example, dextran, gelatin and starch solutions and plasma protein fraction (human plasma protein fraction (HPPF), human albumin solution (HAS)). The composition of plasma is illustrated in Figure 2.10. Apart from maintaining osmotic pressure, the main functions of the plasma proteins are to act as a temporary protein reserve, to contribute towards blood viscosity, and to act as buffers in maintaining acid–base balance.

Acid–Base Balance

Maintaining a constant ratio between acid and base (alkali) in the body is vital to the maintenance of normal pH within the physiological range of 7.38–7.42. This is mainly because many of the enzyme systems of the body function efficiently only at physiological pH; pH is an expression of the hydrogen ion (H^+) concentration or degree of acidity of the fluid, but because of the way in which it has derived a fall in pH (e.g. 7.4–7.2) represents a rise in hydrogen ion concentration and, since hydrogen ions are the active part of any acid, this produces an increase in acidosis. Conversely, a rise in pH represents a fall in hydrogen ion concentration and therefore an alkalosis. There are four, and only four, primary disorders of acid–base balance (Table 2.5) and these are either of respiratory or of metabolic origin. The respiratory acid concerned is carbon dioxide which when combined with water forms carbonic acid. Failure to excrete carbon dioxide leads to respiratory acidosis, while overexcretion (e.g. overbreathing) leads to respiratory alkalosis. The most important metabolic acid is lactic acid, produced primarily by anaerobic cellular respiration. Lactic acid

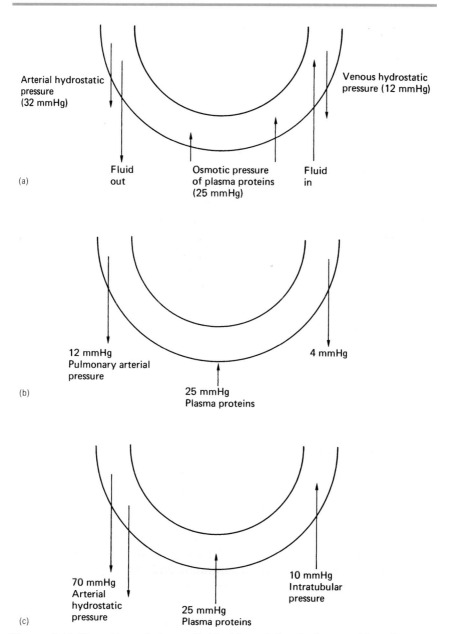

Figure 2.11 Formation of tissue fluid: (a) peripheral tissues, (b) pulmonary circulation, (c) glomerular filtration in the kidney.

Table 2.5 Primary disorders of acid–base balance

Primary problem	Secondary compensation
Respiratory acidosis	Metabolic alkalosis
Respiratory alkalosis	Metabolic acidosis
Metabolic acidosis	Respiratory alkalosis
Metabolic alkalosis	Respiratory acidosis

accumulation produces a metabolic acidosis. Metabolic alkalosis is relatively rare and unimportant and is usually produced by abnormal ingestion of some alkali – for example, aluminium hydroxide for peptic ulceration.

When faced with a primary problem of acid–base balance, the body's natural reaction is to try to compensate for this and the compensatory mechanisms represent the diametrically opposite acid–base state to that of the primary problem (Table 2.5). For example, a respiratory acidosis is compensated for by the body creating a metabolic alkalosis and a metabolic acidosis is compensated by the body producing a respiratory alkalosis. The following shows the fundamental biochemistry behind acid–base balance:

$$CO_2 + H_2O \ \rightleftarrows \ H_2CO_3 \text{ (carbonic acid)} \ \rightleftarrows \ H^+ + HCO_3^- \text{ (bicarbonate, base, alkali)}$$

Lungs — (fast compensation) Kidneys — (slow compensation)

Carbon dioxide and water combine to form carbonic acid, a weak acid which dissociates within the body into hydrogen ions and bicarbonate ions. This reaction may proceed in either direction and the body has only two ways of correcting acid–base balance. The lungs can excrete or conserve carbon dioxide, a relatively rapid process because the brain can alter the respiratory rate to excrete or conserve carbon dioxide at very short notice. The kidneys can excrete hydrogen ions (acid) or bicarbonate ions (HCO_3^-, alkali, base) selectively, but this is a relatively slow method of compensation requiring several hours to become established. The natural compensatory mechanism of the body is to use renal methods when the respiratory system is at fault, and the respiratory system when either the renal or other metabolic processes are at fault so that the kidneys eventually compensate for a respiratory acidosis by excreting abnormally large quantities of hydrogen ions.

Buffering Systems

Renal compensation takes several hours to become established, but it is vital that the pH of the body does not change. To prevent this there exists a system within the blood to buffer or minimise the pH change resulting from alterations in the concentrations of acid or base until the body is able to produce definitive compensation. It is remarkable and convenient that the principal buffering system which exists within the body again involves the carbon dioxide–bicarbonate system. The equation above shows that carbon dioxide when dissolved in water produces hydrogen and bicarbonate ions. The following equation indicates the relationship between pH and the ratio of carbonic acid to bicarbonate, i.e. acid to base:

$$pH = pK + \log(base/acid)$$

$$\therefore pH \propto (bicarbonate)/(carbonic\ acid)$$

$$pH \propto 20/1$$

In normal circumstances the ratio of base to acid is about 20 : 1, so there is considerable reserve of base over acid that can neutralise the addition of any acid and thus prevent a change in pH. Provided that the kidneys definitively excrete the excess acid within the space of a few hours, thus allowing the bicarbonate reserve to be regenerated, this buffering system works excellently. In addition, man constantly produces both hydrogen and bicarbonate ions as part of normal cellular respiration, and if the kidneys selectively excrete hydrogen ions and conserve bicarbonate as necessary, the buffering system of the blood is maintained. Both the plasma proteins and haemoglobin are also able to absorb hydrogen ions temporarily, thus providing extra buffering capacity to the blood. This system therefore is capable of resisting change in pH in the short term until the body is able to excrete or conserve the relative acid or base to compensate for the metabolic insult.

Interpretation of Acid–Base/Blood-gas Results

Most laboratories supply their results in the following form:

- pH
- P_{CO_2}
- base deficit
- standard bicarbonate
- P_{O_2}
- oxygen saturation.

In order to interpret acid–base balance it is vital to know whether the patient has been treated or is simply compensating for his/her own metabolic disorder. In an untreated patient the pH represents the primary problem, thus if the pH is acid the patient has a primary acidosis, though this may be either respiratory or metabolic in origin or a mixture of both. If the arterial P_{CO_2} is above normal in the case of a primary acidosis then the patient must have a respiratory acidosis, either on its own or as part of a mixed respiratory and metabolic acidosis. The P_{CO_2} therefore indicates the respiratory component of the acidosis.

The metabolic component is derived from the standard bicarbonate. By definition, the standard bicarbonate is the bicarbonate concentration of the blood when the P_{CO_2} of the blood has been corrected to normal, in other words so that there is no respiratory component to any acid–base imbalance. The standard bicarbonate is normally 25 mmol/l. The base refers to the amount of bicarbonate in excess of (base excess) or less than (base deficit) the standard figure of 25. If the base excess is -10, this represents a bicarbonate level of 15 mmol/l. Since the bicarbonate we are considering is free bicarbonate from the equations, a fall in free bicarbonate must imply that a proportion of the remainder has been used to combine with free hydrogen ions; a fall in bicarbonate represents compensation for an acidosis. Hence the combination of standard bicarbonate and base deficit or excess indicates the degree of the metabolic component of the acidosis or alkalosis.

In addition to the interpretation of acid–base data, and sometimes more importantly, an arterial blood-gas sample provides information as to the state of gas exchange within the lungs. This is done by measuring the P_{CO_2} and P_{O_2} levels. Measurement of both these values within the normal range obviously indicates satisfactory lung function. Since oxygen diffuses across the alveolar membrane less readily than carbon dioxide, when this function is partially impaired, hypoxia, resulting from inadequate saturation of the haemoglobin (indicated by a fall from the normally 95–100% oxygen saturation of haemoglobin), may well occur despite a normal level of P_{CO_2}.

Measurement of Arterial Blood Gases

In the past the only available electrode for acid–base and blood-gas measurement was a pH electrode and for this reason, although pH itself could be measured directly, P_{CO_2} had to be inferred from the actual pH of the blood. Nowadays, however, individual electrodes, sensitive to either pH, P_{CO_2} or P_{O_2}, are commonly used in automatic blood-gas analysers.

3

Haematology and Blood Transfusion

The circulating blood volume of a 70 kg adult is 5 l, 1 l of which is
contained in the heart, arterial and capillary circulations, 1 l within
the pulmonary circulation and 3 l in the venous circulation. Blood is a
suspension of cells in plasma, the overall volume of the cells being about
45% of the total blood volume.

● RED BLOOD CELLS

The normal red blood cell count is 5 million per cubic millimetre,
each cell having a life of about 120 days. A significant proportion of cells
within a 3–4 week-old unit of transfused blood will therefore have reached
the end of their useful lives. Red cells are formed from reticulo-endothelial
cells in the bone marrow, the immediate precursor being the reticulocyte.
In cases of high marrow activity after haemorrhage, a significant reticulocyte count may occur in the peripheral blood. The main function of the
red blood cells is to transport oxygen in combination with the haemoglobin inside the cell. This is a protein of molecular weight 67 000 which
combines with oxygen in the lungs and gives up oxygen in the peripheral
tissues. (Further details of oxygen carriage are discussed in Chapter 2.)
Cyanosis is the name given to the blue appearance of tissues resulting from
deoxygenated blood circulating through them. At least 5 g of reduced
haemoglobin is necessary for cyanosis to be present; this condition is therefore extremely rare in anaemia and not pathological in situations of high
red cell counts such as polycythaemia.

Red blood cells are removed from the circulation by the reticulo-endothelial system in the bone marrow, liver and spleen. The cellular protein and haemoglobin are broken down to amino acids, which are re-used in the body together with the iron which is stored as ferritin. The remainder of the haem molecule is converted to bilirubin and biliverdin, which combine with glucuronic acid in the liver and are excreted into the bowel. Interruption of bile pigment excretion leads to jaundice.

● WHITE BLOOD CELLS

The normal white blood cell count is 5000–10 000 cells/mm^3. Unlike the red cells, white cells exist in several different forms. The polymorphonuclear leucocytes (granulocytes) comprise about 70% of the white cell count. These are subdivided according to their staining characteristics into basophils (1%), eosinophils (3%) and neutrophils (66%). The neutrophils are phagocytes, able to engulf and remove foreign particles and bacteria from the blood, and are the main defence mechanism of the body against infection. Eosinophils are increased in allergic conditions such as asthma and hay fever and the basophils are thought to be circulating mast cells capable of releasing histamine.

The lymphocytes, comprising 25% of the total white cell count, are divided into large and small types and are involved in the production of antibodies, which combine with and neutralise foreign substances known as antigens. Lymphocytes therefore provide a memory system of protection for the body against unwanted substances or organisms. The excessive formation of antibodies in this way is responsible for several hypersensitivity reactions to drugs (Chapter 21). In normal circumstances antibodies combine with foreign antigens to neutralise them and therefore prevent their effects, but in some conditions excessive antigen and antibody combination may release histamine or similar substances resulting in a hypersensitivity reaction. These reactions sometimes occur in response to intravenous administration of certain anaesthetics, in particular induction agents and muscle relaxants.

The remaining white blood cells, 5–6% of the total, are monocytes, another group of phagocytic cells.

● PLATELETS

The normal platelet count is 250 000/mm^3, thrombocytopenia being the name given to a pathological reduction in the amount of platelets circulating in the peripheral blood. Their main function is to aggregate at the site of injury, causing a plug and preventing capillary bleeding.

Their subsequent breakdown may release vasoconstrictive amines such as 5-hydroxytryptamine, producing local vasoconstriction and again preventing bleeding. Platelet consumption during severe bleeding may reduce their circulating numbers. This is common in massive blood transfusion when the normal clotting factors and the platelet count are both exhausted. Transfusion of fresh frozen plasma containing clotting factors, and platelets themselves, may be necessary to arrest haemorrhage. In normal circumstances a platelet count of 60 000 is sufficient to prevent pathological haemorrhage. The clumping of platelets forming a platelet plug is enhanced by two factors in the coagulation cascade, and platelet breakdown yields a further platelet factor which is important in blood clotting.

● COAGULATION OF BLOOD

In normal circumstances a balance is maintained in the body between coagulation and clot breakdown (fibrinolysis). Blood clots are formed when the plasma protein fibrinogen changes into insoluble fibrin, which, in turn, traps red cells and platelets to form a blood clot. The clotting factors are present in plasma, which will produce a clot without the presence of blood cells. Fibrinogen changes into insoluble fibrin under the influence of thrombin which, in the presence of calcium ions, is produced by the action of thromboplastin on prothrombin (Fig. 3.1). Tissue damage (the extrinsic coagulation system) releases thromboplastin, which together with platelet breakdown (intrinsic system), both initiate the coagulation cascade, activating factor X via factor VII (extrinsic pathway) or via factors IX and VIII (intrinsic pathway). The presence of certain factors is also necessary for the system to work efficiently, and the absence of certain

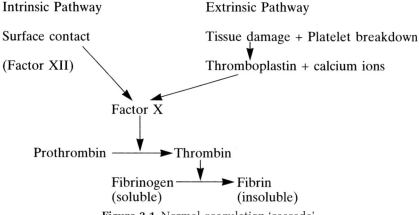

Figure 3.1 Normal coagulation 'cascade'.

other factors produces coagulation disorders – for example, factor VIII, the antihaemophilic factor, is absent in haemophilia. Prothrombin is made in the liver and vitamin K is necessary for its production. Absence of vitamin K (e.g. in cases of liver damage and jaundice) may affect coagulation. Heparin, as a prothrombin antagonist, is itself indirectly antagonised by vitamin K.

● FIBRINOLYSIS

The fibrinolytic system is the natural remover of unwanted blood clot and platelet aggregates, and acts by dissolving the fibrin network and producing fibrin degradation products. Activation of a circulating protein (plasminogen) is produced by tissue or blood activators, which in a similar cascade to the coagulation process enhance conversion of plasminogen to plasmin, the substance responsible for fibrin breakdown. Pathological fibrinolysis (Fig. 3.2) may occur in response to certain circulating fibrinolysins (e.g. urokinase released by the prostate) and may be prevented by antifibrinolytic agents such as aprotonin (trasylol) or tranexamic acid (cyclokapron).

Disseminated Intravascular Coagulation

This disease of intravascular coagulation may be associated with many conditions, for example, severe haemorrhage, pancreatitis, drug overdose, Mendelson's syndrome, or after major surgery and cardiopulmonary bypass. Abnormal coagulation occurs within the microcirculation using up the available clotting factors and reducing peripheral flow. This results in many of the presenting symptoms related to malfunction of organs such as lung, kidney, liver and brain. Subsequent proliferation of intravascular coagulation produces reduced efficiency of normal clotting and profuse bleeding due to excessive consumption of fibrinogen and platelets. The correct

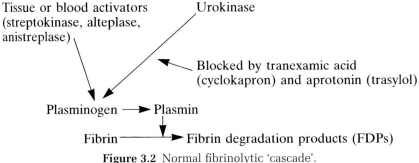

Figure 3.2 Normal fibrinolytic 'cascade'.

treatment is to remove the cause 'triggering' the disseminated intravascular coagulation (DIC) and possibly to prevent further coagulation by anti-coagulating the patient with heparin. This treatment may seem illogical, but it prevents further consumption of coagulation factors and allows restoration of normal clotting function. There is little point in replacing clotting factors or platelets until the 'trigger' is removed.

● ANTICOAGULANTS

These drugs are given to antagonise the normal clotting mechanisms in the blood, either to prevent pathological thrombosis after venous stasis and surgery or to prevent blood clot forming on, for example, artificial heart valves after operation. The two main anticoagulants are heparin and warfarin.

Heparin

Heparin is a naturally occurring anticoagulant – produced by mast cells – which forms a reversible combination with plasma proteins, the complex preventing the action of thrombin on fibrinogen. The action of heparin is antagonised by protamine but also naturally in the body by the enzyme heparinase. The duration of action of heparin is therefore only 4–6 h and repeat doses or intravenous infusion are necessary to maintain full anticoagulation. Heparin is used to prevent thrombosis and embolism and has an immediate anticoagulant effect. Its use allows stabilisation of anticoagulation before more prolonged treatment with warfarin.

Warfarin

This anticoagulant acts by combination with vitamin K in the liver, inhibiting prothrombin synthesis. The onset of action is 24–48 h before full anticoagulation is achieved. The action of warfarin is antagonised by vitamin K but, again, this is a slow process.

Protamine

This ionic antagonist of heparin is used when rapid reversal of anticoagulation is required. Normal physiological reversal of heparin takes between 4 and 6 h and protamine is useful, for example, after cardiopulmonary bypass or renal dialysis when local heparinisation is used to prevent coagulation. Rapid infusion of protamine sulphate may cause myocardial depression and hypotension, so this drug should be given slowly by intravenous infusion rather than as a bolus dose.

● PLASMA

Plasma comprises 55% of the blood volume and is essentially a solution of electrolytes, mainly sodium chloride and bicarbonate in water, which also contains plasma proteins. Plasma is involved in the carriage of blood cells and oxygen, the maintenance of acid–base balance and the transfer of gaseous and metabolic waste products to the lungs and kidneys. Apart from its electrolyte content the plasma proteins form an essential part of this solution. Two of these proteins, albumin and globulin, are present in large quantities, while two others, prothrombin and fibrinogen, are present in smaller amounts. The globulin fraction of the plasma is largely responsible for maintaining immunity and antibody production (immunoglobulins), while albumin is the protein most responsible for combination with both drugs and metabolic products.

Main Functions of Plasma Proteins

Maintenance of Osmotic Pressure

The presence of high molecular weight substances within the plasma produces an osmotic pressure intravascularly, tending to draw fluid into the blood vessels. This is essential for the prevention of oedema, hypo-proteinaemia being associated with peripheral oedema and fluid leak into the tissues (see Fig. 2.11a).

Protein Reserve

Although the body's need for protein cannot be met for more than a few hours by the metabolism of plasma proteins, these may provide a reserve during periods of excessive demands by the liver as a result of energetic exercise.

Buffering Activity

The plasma proteins act as a buffer by combining with both acids and alkalis. As discussed in Chapter 2, the maintenance of normal plasma pH is essential to body function, and the plasma proteins provide an additional buffering system to that of the bicarbonate/carbonic acid system.

Viscosity

Due to its viscous nature the resistance to blood flow is governed by the plasma proteins and the cellular elements of the blood. Optimum blood viscosity is essential for adequate peripheral blood flow through tissues.

Carriage of Drugs within the Plasma

When drugs are injected or absorbed into the bloodstream they are almost entirely carried in the plasma to their sites of action. The active part of any drug is that which is in free solution within the plasma, while that in combination with plasma proteins is inactive. The degree of protein binding of drugs therefore governs their activity and, more important still, if two protein-bound drugs are administered simultaneously one may displace the other from the plasma proteins, thereby potentiating its action. An example of this is when a diabetic patient, established on oral hypo-glycaemic drugs, is given aspirin, which is also protein bound. This may displace the hypoglycaemic drug from the plasma proteins and produce excessive hypoglycaemia by increasing the relative amount of free drug within the plasma. There are several other examples of drug interaction due to competition for plasma protein binding and simultaneous drug therapy is often difficult to control and predict.

● PREVENTION OF DEEP VENOUS THROMBOSIS

The methods available are divided into pharmacological and mechanical, the latter being further divided into active and passive. The simplest mechanical method utilises elasticated TED stockings to reduce the volume of blood within the leg, preventing venous pooling and therefore throm-bosis. Active intermittent calf compression using pneumatic leggings not only increases venous return and reduces pooling, but also activates fibrinolysis (Fig. 3.3).

Pharmacological methods of deep venous thrombosis (DVT) prevention include the infusion of dextran 70, 500 ml every 24 h until the patient is

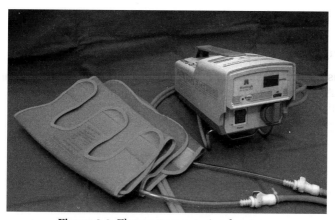

Figure 3.3 Flotron compression leggings.

fully mobile, or subcutaneous heparin (Minihep), 5000 units every 8 or 12 h over a similar period. Probably the most effective method, which should routinely be used for all high-risk patients and those on the oral contraceptive pill is to combine TED stockings with a Minihep regimen. Low molecular weight heparin (Clexane 20 mg), which is said to prevent pathological clotting but to preserve the normal prothrombin to thrombin reaction, has been shown to be particularly useful in orthopaedic joint replacement surgery. It has the additional advantage of needing only once-daily administration.

● TRANSFUSION OF BLOOD

The transfusion of blood and blood products is now widely used in anaesthetic practice, the availability of adequate supplies of whole blood being an essential part of major surgery. Although several other solutions are available for fluid and electrolyte replacement during surgery, none at present has the ability to carry oxygen in adequate amounts throughout the body. In some animals, transfusions may be administered from one to another without blood grouping or cross-matching, but in man, blood contains certain factors connected with the red cells which may make them incompatible with the cells from another individual; samples from both the donor and the recipient must therefore be checked for compatibility.

● BLOOD GROUPING AND CROSS-MATCHING

The four major blood groups identified in man are O, A, B and AB, present in 46%, 42%, 9% and 3% of the population, respectively. Patients belong to one or other group depending on the presence or absence of agglutinogens A and B on the surface of the red cells. Group A individuals have agglutinogen A on the surface of their red cells, while those with agglutinogen A and B belong to group AB and those with neither A nor B belong to group O.

Blood plasma contains agglutinins anti-A and anti-B which, when combined with the appropriate agglutinogen, will cause agglutination of the red cells. Agglutinin anti-A is present in the plasma of groups B and O, while anti-B is found in group A and group O. Group AB has neither anti-A nor anti-B agglutinins in the plasma and therefore does not possess any factor likely to cause blood group incompatibility by agglutination. Group AB patients are therefore known as universal recipients. Although group O blood contains both anti-A and anti-B, by the time these agglutinins are diluted after transfusion into a patient with normal blood volume, the amounts in the plasma will be insufficient to cause agglutination. Group O is therefore known as universal donor blood.

Routine cross-matching procedures include grouping the patient's blood, using sera containing anti-A or anti-B, and subsequently incubating samples of both donor and recipient blood together to look for signs of agglutination. Blood grouping also involves the detection and compatibility of various minor agglutinogens, C, D and E, the most important of which is D – the Rhesus factor. Patients with factor D (about 85% of the population) are said to be Rhesus positive. Unlike the ABC system, patients do not possess anti-D until they have been sensitised by exposure to blood containing factor D. If they are then Rhesus negative they will manufacture anti-D which will produce agglutination upon subsequent exposure to factor D. This means that it is always possible to transfuse patients who are Rhesus positive with Rhesus-negative blood, but if the patient has already been sensitised, the reverse is impossible. Universal donor blood is therefore not only group O, but also Rhesus negative.

Since the agglutinogens A and B are present only on the surface of red cells, blood grouping and cross-matching is necessary only when transfusions of blood are being given. Plasma and other blood products may be given without cross-matching procedures without risk of agglutination.

● PRACTICAL ASPECTS OF BLOOD TRANSFUSION

Storage

Whole blood should not be left at room temperature for longer than is necessary to complete the transfusion, this normally being within a maximum of 4–6 h. Blood required for transfusion should be either placed in a refrigerator specifically designed for the purpose and maintained at 4°C, or transferred in specially designed cool containers for immediate use in theatre.

Checking

A systematic check of each unit of blood is vital before administration. This should be preceded by a check that the patient's blood group has been established, by reference to the identification label attached to the patient and not to the notes. The blood transfusion form must contain adequate data for identification with the patient concerned and simultaneously with the blood to be transfused. The correct procedure is for two people to cross-check the form with the patient, and then each bag of blood against the form. Of particular importance are the blood groups of both the patient and the cross-matched blood, the date of expiry of the blood (normally 3 weeks after collection), the patient's identification attached to the bag of blood and, finally, the appropriate number of the bag. Scrupulous attention to these details will avoid mistakes which may be fatal.

Administration of Blood

Blood is normally administered through a peripheral drip at a rate of 500 ml over a maximum of 4–6 h. Considerable variation may occur, of course, when patients are being transfused in theatre or in response to major blood loss and in this event not only must the blood be carefully checked but certain other precautions should also be taken. Since the blood will be cool the use of a warming coil and water bath to allow the transfusion to be given at body temperature will prevent cooling of the patient.

The use of microfilters in addition to the normal filter within the intravenous administration set will prevent considerable quantities of broken red cells and aggregates of white cells and platelets from reaching the patient and being deposited within the small capillaries of the lung. These filters are relatively cheap and should be used wherever possible. Although opinions on the use of blood microfilters vary, their ability to reduce or prevent transfusion of microemboli is not in question. Two main types of filter exist. The screen filter, for example, Pall Ultipor (Fig. 3.4), is simply a mesh with a pore size of 20 μm, which tends to clog up with use, but is very efficient. Depth filters have an average pore size of 20 μm and rely on adsorption. They tend to become less efficient with use as their adsorptive capacity is reduced. It has been shown that pressurising blood through

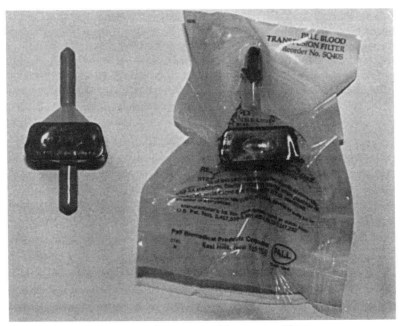

Figure 3.4 Screen-type blood microfilter.

filters, particularly the screen types, results in significant histamine release, and this practice is not now recommended.

● HAZARDS OF BLOOD TRANSFUSION

The scrupulous detail attached to every aspect of blood grouping and cross-matching by the National Blood Transfusion Service has minimised complications of blood transfusion caused by mismatching. Nevertheless, these do occur occasionally and may result in appreciable and serious degrees of intravascular coagulation if not detected early. Minor and relatively subclinical reactions to blood transfusion may occur more frequently, manifested usually as tachycardia, flushing, pyrexia or skin rashes. In this event, intravenous chlorpheniramine (Piriton), an antihistamine, may be used to alleviate symptoms. In all cases where a transfusion reaction is suspected, the transfusion should be stopped and a sample of the patient's blood should be returned with the transfused blood to the laboratory. Serious agglutination reactions leading to capillary obstruction may cause severe pain – usually in the abdomen or loin – and subsequent haemolysis of the cells will produce haemoglobinuria and renal failure.

Blood transfusions may also lead to cross-infection, particularly of conditions such as hepatitis B and C and syphilis, though these are prevented by modern screening methods within the National Blood Transfusion Service. All donated blood is also routinely screened for HIV antibody, although this may still be negative in a recently infected individual in whom insufficient time for antibody production has passed. Other infective complications may arise around the transfusion site, but these are rarely serious.

● MASSIVE BLOOD TRANSFUSION

With the exception of mismatching and infection, most complications of blood transfusion occur as a result of large quantities of blood being given too quickly. Massive blood transfusion is defined as the transfusion of half a patient's blood volume within an hour and may produce several complications. Stored blood inevitably contains not only intact red cells but broken cells, platelet aggregates, white cell aggregates and other debris. In addition, stored blood is depleted in 2,3-diphosphoglycerate (2,3-DPG) necessary for optimum oxygen carriage, and this takes several days to be restored. Blood is collected into bags which already contain an anticoagulant, either acid–citrate–dextrose (ACD) or citrate–phosphate–dextrose (CPD). In both cases the clotting factors in the blood will be depleted, as both platelets and fibrinogen are viable for only 24–48 h after collection.

Hypothermia

Blood stored at 4°C needs to be warmed to body temperature by using a warming coil attached to the intravenous infusion set to avoid progressive hypothermia with large transfusions and, in particular, acute cooling of the heart (Fig. 3.5).

Filtration

Microfilters prevent debris accumulating within the microcirculation of the lungs and are essential during massive transfusion (Fig. 3.4).

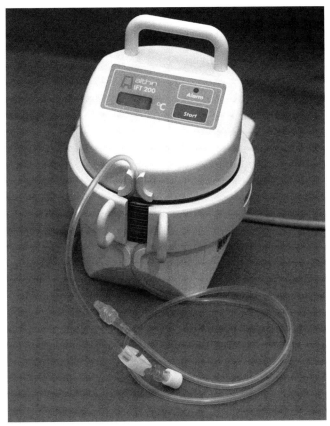

Figure 3.5 Electric (dry) blood warming coil.

Serum Potassium

Cellular breakdown within stored blood inevitably increases the serum potassium concentrations. Although these rarely produce pathological hyperkalaemia, electrocardiographic (ECG) monitoring is essential to detect early signs, particularly peaked T-waves.

Citrate Toxicity

The citrate used as an anticoagulant in stored blood combines with calcium within the patient and may produce serious reductions in the serum calcium concentration. This occurs only with rapid and large blood transfusions but requires intravenous calcium therapy to prevent the effects of hypocalcaemia, particularly on the myocardium. During a massive transfusion the administration of 10 ml 10% calcium gluconate should be considered with every fourth unit of blood.

Metabolic Acidosis

Anaerobic respiration in red cells in stored blood, together with the acid anticoagulants used, inevitably means that large transfusions will produce a metabolic acidosis. Patients may be able to compensate for this, but impaired cardiac function is an indication for correction with bicarbonate. This should not be done over-enthusiastically because one of the end products of citrate metabolism within the liver is bicarbonate, and massive transfusion may produce a metabolic alkalosis on the first or second postoperative day.

Coagulation Disorders

The lack of normal clotting factors and platelets within stored blood may result in severe depletion and bleeding during surgery, particularly when the available factors are being consumed at a rapid rate. Pathological consumption of clotting factors in the form of DIC may also occur as a side-effect of massive blood transfusion. Clotting factors may be replaced by the transfusion of fresh frozen plasma or platelets and this should always be contemplated towards the end of the operation or immediately afterwards when haemostasis has been achieved or when it is causing problems.

Circulatory Overload

Massive transfusion is best carried out in conjunction with central venous pressure monitoring to give some indication of the degree of transfusion required. Massive blood loss is often difficult to assess and, particularly in older people with poor cardiac reserve, acute heart failure and pulmonary oedema are easily precipitated after transfusion.

OTHER BLOOD PRODUCTS

Although the replacement of blood lost during surgery is best achieved with whole blood, many transfusion centres now issue either plasma-reduced blood or packed cells from which the plasma has been used to prepare other blood fractions such as platelets or clotting factors. The use of concentrated red cells is particularly advantageous when patients require preoperative transfusions. They have a normal blood volume but a reduced red cell level and therefore haemoglobin concentration, and do not require transfusion of plasma as well as blood.

Due to the risks of transmitting infection, transfusion of dried plasma is now almost obsolete in the UK, but human plasma protein fraction (HPPF) or human albumin solution (HAS) has been widely used until recently. Essentially, both are pasteurised plasma, heated to 60°C to destroy both potential infection and antigens but not to denature the plasma proteins. In this form it is particularly useful when the plasma volume requires expansion in place of an adequate or high red cell content. More recently, the use of albumin has been questioned and it has been suggested that albumin therapy has been associated with an increase in mortality in seriously ill patients.

SAGM BLOOD

It is now generally accepted that unless whole blood is specifically required, stored blood is supplied either in a plasma reduced form or as red cells resuspended in SAGM (saline–adenine–glucose–mannitol). This additive is not an anticoagulant but will prolong the life of stored red cells, making them suitable for use for 4 or even 5 weeks after donation. The blood is still collected into CPD as an anticoagulant and so the potential complications related to this will not be prevented. If surgical blood loss is to be replaced with SAGM blood, it may be necessary simultaneously to replace plasma losses with either HAS or a volume expander such as Haemaccel.

DEXTRAN

This polysaccharide (sugar) solution is used as a plasma volume expander. The numbers (40, 70, 110) after the name refer to the average molecular weight of the dextran molecules in thousands. Thus dextran 70 with a molecular weight of 70 000 resembles serum albumin. Normally, albumin is not excreted by the kidney (though in sickness albuminuria is an early feature), implying that the renal molecular threshold is about 65–70 000. The transfusion of dextran therefore not only results in expansion of the intravascular volume by 500 ml, but also, by increasing the osmotic pressure of the plasma, tends to draw additional fluid into the intravascular space. Dextran 70 will not be excreted through the kidneys until the molecules are broken down and become smaller. Dextran 40 will remain within the circulation for a shorter time, but because it is less viscous than plasma containing plasma proteins, will reduce blood viscosity, and is used to increase peripheral blood flow in vascular disease. Dextran 70 also has an antiplatelet action that prevents aggregation, and is therefore used in the prophylaxis of DVT. The dextrans, however, do not carry oxygen, can only be given up to a maximum of 1 l per day and interfere with blood cross-matching. They may produce hypersensitivity reactions, especially in patients with an allergic tendency, e.g. asthmatics. Their use should be confined to those who need blood-volume expansion without red cells or as an emergency when blood is not available.

● GELATIN SOLUTIONS (HAEMACCEL, GELUFUCIN)

Haemaccel and Gelufucin are gelatin solutions of average molecular weight 30 000, and are often used in place of dextran. Their molecular size means that they are not retained within the blood vessels for as long as dextran 70 but are useful as plasma volume expanders. They are also increasingly used in conjunction with SAGM suspended red blood cells for the replacement of whole blood loss during surgery. Haemaccel has a longer shelf life than dextran, so is more useful in major accident packs where prolonged storage may be required. Hypersensitivity reactions of similar frequency to dextran have been reported, but newer methods of preparation and purification have reduced the incidence considerably.

● HETASTARCH SOLUTIONS (HESPAN, PENTASPAN)

The large molecular weight (450 000) of the hydroxyethyl starch solution Hespan makes it considerably longer acting than either the dextran or gelatin solutions. It may have considerable advantages in the treatment of massive haemorrhage in a patient with multiple injuries but, by remaining in the circulation for a long time, may delay the subsequent administration of blood, if circulatory overload is to be avoided.

Medium molecular weight starch (250 000, Pentaspan) is also available and has similar effects to the higher molecular weight dextran solutions. It is more appropriate for perioperative and intensive care use than in resuscitation from major trauma.

4

Intravenous Induction Agents

Intravenous induction of anaesthesia is invariably used in adults, although gas induction is almost always possible except where this is unacceptable to the patient. The aim of an intravenous anaesthetic induction agent is to take the patient from a conscious state into surgical anaesthesia within a few seconds and to maintain them there for several minutes until the maintenance anaesthetic has taken over. The action of intravenous induction agents depends largely on a bolus dose being injected fairly rapidly and reaching the brain, the brain level being proportional to the plasma level of the drug. Diffusion of the drug from plasma into brain occurs mainly because of the concentration gradient. The plasma level rises rapidly due to fast injection; if the injection rate is too slow anaesthesia may not be induced. Thiopentone (the 'truth drug'), for example, is effective in sub-anaesthetic doses by simply allowing the patients to talk in an uninhibited fashion. The plasma level of an intravenous agent then falls due to dilution, redistribution, protein binding and metabolism. As the brain level falls, the effect of the drug wears off and the patient wakes up.

● THIOPENTONE

Thiopentone (Pentothal, Intraval) is an ultra-short-acting barbiturate that produces a smooth induction of anaesthesia within one arm–brain circulation time. Its action, which lasts between 5 and 10 min, is terminated by rapid dilution and redistribution. The metabolism and subsequent excretion of thiopentone, however, is prolonged due to its redistribution into body fat and may take up to 48 h. Thiopentone may produce severe hypotension primarily as a result of peripheral vasodilatation which may be complicated by myocardial depression, particularly in sick, hypovolaemic patients. Thiopentone also causes respiratory depression and apnoea by decreasing the respiratory centre's sensitivity to carbon dioxide and may also cause laryngeal spasm and bronchospasm, particularly in asthmatics. Although usually given intravenously, rectal thiopentone may be given to children to induce anaesthesia, and intravenous thiopentone as an infusion has been used to control convulsions in epilepsy. Thiopentone should not be given to patients who are sensitive to barbiturates or to those suffering from porphyria (Chapter 15).

● METHOHEXITONE

Methohexitone (Brietal) is another ultra-short-acting barbiturate with a shorter duration of action than thiopentone. Although still available, its use has declined recently, largely due to the introduction of propofol. In common with many of the shorter-acting induction agents, methohexitone administration may be associated with several excitatory phenomena such as coughing, hiccoughing, salivation, extraneous movement, hypertonus and apnoea. Nevertheless, when brief anaesthesia is important, methohexitone is extremely useful. Its actions are similar to thiopentone, but its cardiovascular depression is less pronounced. The actions of methohexitone are likewise terminated by redistribution and metabolism, excretion occurring over 24 h. Methohexitone should not be given to epileptics because it may precipitate convulsions.

● PROPOFOL

Propofol (Diprivan) is a non-barbiturate induction agent which provides a smooth induction, largely free from many of the side-effects seen with methohexitone. It is cardiovascularly stable, producing a modest reduction in blood pressure, but may produce significant respiratory depression if used by continuous infusion in a spontaneously breathing patient. Significant hypersensitivity reactions are very rare, but since Diprivan is suspended in soya-bean emulsion (see Intralipid), the large volumes necessary for total intravenous anaesthesia (TIVA) or prolonged sedation in intensive care in some patients may produce problems with hyperlipidaemia.

Unlike thiopentone, whose clinical effects are terminated by redistribution, the effects of propofol are controlled by rapid hepatic metabolism. A significant proportion of the drug is metabolised as soon as it passes through the liver, the so-called 'first-pass effect'. The patients wake rapidly due to this metabolism and the absence of active metabolites, and therefore recovery is free from side-effects or 'hang-over' effects. These metabolic characteristics make propofol extremely suitable for TIVA.

● ETOMIDATE

Etomidate (Hypnomidate) is another non-barbiturate intravenous induction agent, widely used in Europe, mainly because of its lack of severe depressant effects on the cardiovascular system. Excitatory side-effects are common and it seems to have no distinct advantages over other agents. Pain on injection is common, and thrombophlebitis may sometimes occur, particularly when injected into a small vein. Etomidate has been shown to produce adrenal suppression and low levels of serum cortisol when used as a continuous infusion in intensive care. For this reason its use has now been restricted to single doses for induction of anaesthesia.

● KETAMINE

Ketamine (Ketalar) is a dissociative anaesthetic agent, given either intravenously or intramuscularly. It is said to preserve the pharyngeal and laryngeal reflexes, thus protecting the airway during anaesthesia. Ketamine is particularly useful for patients with airway problems requiring sedation for repeated operations (e.g. burns and radiotherapy), its considerable analgesic effect being of great benefit. Ketamine is a cardiovascular stimulant producing noradrenaline release, resulting in hypertension and tachycardia, and should not be used in hypertensive patients. It may produce hallucinations and nightmares while waking in some patients, particularly those who have not been premedicated; patients recovering from ketamine anaesthesia should therefore be left undisturbed to reduce the incidence of side-effects.

● TOTAL (CONTINUOUS) INTRAVENOUS ANAESTHESIA

Although the intravenous anaesthetic agents above were developed as induction agents, there is no reason why continuous administration of such an agent, for example, propofol in the form of an intravenous infusion, could not be used to maintain anaesthesia. Considerable research has been undertaken into intravenous anaesthesia, particularly its advantages in the lack of pollution and duration of post-anaesthetic sedation. Intermittent bolus injections of propofol, rather than continuous infusion are already used, particularly in minor gynaecological surgical anaesthesia and bronchoscopy. It is probably better to use a rapidly metabolised agent such as propofol, to avoid the cumulative effect of a drug like thiopentone, although excessively large infusion volumes may be required.

Figure 4.1 illustrates the principles behind TIVA. It relates the plasma concentration of the drug to time and if one assumes that the line 'X' represents the plasma level which produces anaesthesia in 100% of patients,

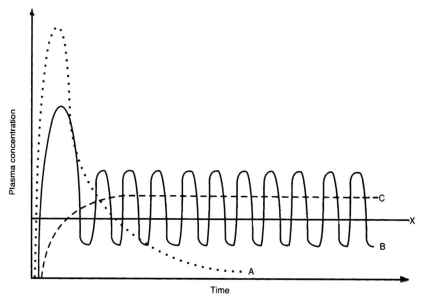

Figure 4.1 Pharmacokinetic principles of TIVA.

there are several ways in which this can be achieved, the so-called loading and maintenance infusion rates of the drug. 'A' illustrates the administration of a bolus dose which rapidly achieves an excessively high plasma concentration of the drug, which is short-lived due to rapid metabolism. 'B' indicates the effect of intermittent bolus doses of the drug, with the inevitable fluctuations in plasma concentration and adequacy of anaesthesia above and below line 'X'. 'C' represents a continuous infusion regimen, with the plasma concentration gradually rising to an adequate anaesthetic level. The achieving of the final anaesthetic concentration in 'C' can be speeded up by using a rapid infusion rate of say ten times the maintenance infusion rate to 'load' the patient for 10 min, followed by 10 min at five times this maintenance rate, and then a normal steady infusion rate.

Advantages of TIVA

Because of the rapid hepatic metabolism of propofol, accumulation does not occur and so the waking time should be the same irrespective of the duration of the normal maintenance infusion. Recovery is pleasant with no hangover. Nausea and vomiting are rare unless due to surgical reasons or opiates.

Disadvantages of TIVA

As has been discussed above, the depth of anaesthesia can be a problem, particularly since at present we do not have 'depth-of-anaesthesia' monitors.

The incidence of awareness can be significant in the paralysed patient and special care is needed to avoid this.

● HAZARDS OF INTRAVENOUS INDUCTION AGENTS

The most severe hazards associated with intravenous induction of anaesthesia are probably cardiovascular collapse either associated with hypovolaemic shock, or in patients with cardiovascular disease. Relative overdose of these agents is a common problem in sick and elderly patients, and also in young patients, particularly those who are shocked as a result of blood or fluid loss. Hypotension is posturally sensitive, particularly with thiopentone when the effects are largely due to peripheral vasodilatation and therefore usually respond to rapid fluid administration. Intravenous induction agents may produce apnoea and should not be used in patients with obstructed or difficult airways in whom ventilation may be impossible.

Hypersensitivity reactions have been reported to nearly all the intravenous induction agents, particularly thiopentone, although the mechanism is uncertain (Chapter 21). Propofol and etomidate, however, appear to be free from true hypersensitivity effects, which is a great advantage. By contrast, Althesin and propanidid (Epontol) both caused considerable hypersensitivity reactions, probably due to the solubilising agent, Cremophor EL, in which they were dissolved. It is largely as a result of this that they were withdrawn. Specific hazards are associated with individual sensitivity to barbiturates and diseases like porphyria (Chapter 15).

Extravascular Injection

Extravascular injection of intravenous induction agents may produce severe irritation, particularly with thiopentone, which is an extremely alkaline agent and may produce localised tissue necrosis. Accidental extravascular injection should be followed by injection of hyaluronidase into the area to encourage diffusion and absorption.

Intra-arterial Injection

Accidental intra-arterial injection of thiopentone, particularly in the antecubital fossa, may produce severe symptoms of arterial obstruction within the microcirculation of the hand, and indeed permanent ischaemia has been reported. This appears to be related to the alkaline nature of the solution forming crystals within the small vessels and obstructing blood flow within the hand. Accidental intra-arterial injection should be followed by injection of a vasodilator and, if necessary, a sympathetic block of the affected limb with the intention of producing a maximum degree of vasodilatation.

5

Uptake and Distribution of Volatile and Intravenous Anaesthetic Agents

•Volatile anaesthetic agents •Intravenous anaesthetic agents

● VOLATILE ANAESTHETIC AGENTS

Physical Properties

There are several physical properties that influence the efficiency of a particular compound as an anaesthetic agent. It is particularly important to be able to produce a high concentration of the agent at atmospheric pressure since it has been shown that one needs to be able to achieve 10 times the normal anaesthetic maintenance concentration of a volatile agent to make it useful for both induction and maintenance of anaesthesia. The saturated vapour pressure (SVP) provides such an index since it indicates the maximum proportion of atmospheric pressure (760 mmHg) which can be occupied by a saturated vapour of the substance. Thus halothane with an SVP of 247 mmHg theoretically allows a maximum concentration of 33% (247/760 × 100) to be achieved, thus fulfilling the requirements of a useful anaesthetic agent, the normal maintenance halothane concentration being 0.7–1%. Similarly, the SVPs of enflurane and isoflurane are 175 and 238, respectively.

Trichloroethylene, in contrast, with an SVP of only 60 mmHg did not fulfil these requirements: induction with trichloroethylene was both difficult and prolonged. Other physical properties of the agent, such as its solubility in rubber or metal, may also influence the uptake.

The most important factor in the uptake of a volatile anaesthetic agent is its alveolar concentration which, in turn, depends on minute volume ventilation. The lungs are not normally resistant to the free diffusion of anaesthetic agents and lung disease is therefore relatively unimportant.

The inspired agent is diluted by and must equilibrate with the air that remains in the lungs as functional residual capacity (FRC).

Minimum Alveolar Concentration

Minimum alveolar concentration (MAC) indicates the minimum alveolar concentration of an agent required to produce lack of reflex response to skin incision in man. Some common values are: halothane 0.765%; ether 1.92%; trichloroethylene 0.17%; enflurane 1.68%, isoflurane 1.15%; sevoflurane 1.70%; desflurane 6.0%. Once the volatile anaesthetic agent is present in adequate quantity within the alveolus, further uptake depends on its passing into the circulation.

Uptake into Circulation

The rate of uptake from the alveolus into the blood depends upon the following.

Concentration Gradient Across Alveolar Membrane

This gradient is between the inspired concentration and the mixed venous (pulmonary arterial) concentration of the agent, the latter being dependent on tissue uptake.

Solubility of Agent in Blood

This is governed by the blood-gas solubility coefficient. Some typical values are: nitrous oxide 0.47; isoflurane 1.4; enflurane 1.9; halothane 2.36; ether 12.1; sevoflurane 0.40; desflurane 0.70. The higher the blood-gas solubility coefficient the more soluble is the agent in blood. If the solubility is low, only small quantities of the agent will leave the alveolus and dissolve in the blood and therefore the alveolar concentration will rise rapidly. Since this is the concentration which determines the tension of the agent in arterial blood, the latter will rise rapidly and determine the concentration gradients to other tissues and particularly the brain. Agents that are relatively insoluble in blood (e.g. nitrous oxide) rapidly produce high blood tensions and therefore a high concentration gradient from blood to brain and high brain levels. This is synonymous with rapid induction and, since recovery is a direct reversal of this process, with rapid recovery also. Conversely, agents with a high blood solubility (e.g. ether) take a long time to achieve adequate blood tension and subsequently brain tension. To a certain extent this may be compensated for by a high inspired concentration, but recovery is inevitably prolonged.

Pulmonary Blood Flow

As the pulmonary blood flow rises, more of the agent is removed from the alveolus and therefore the arterial blood tension takes longer to rise, and induction takes longer. Conversely, with a decrease in pulmonary blood flow, induction is rapid since alveolar and therefore arterial tensions rise quickly. Pulmonary blood flow in this situation is synonymous with cardiac output.

Changes in Ventilation

These have little effect in the case of insoluble agents since the alveolar concentration is always high. Soluble agents, however, are influenced by increased ventilation because, as a result of this, alveolar concentration may suddenly rise.

Tissue Uptake

This is dependent on the following.

Concentration Gradient

This gradient is between the blood and tissues, and therefore on the alveolar concentration. Once equilibrium is reached, no further uptake occurs.

Tissue Blood Solubility

Most anaesthetic agents are equally soluble in tissue and blood, with the exception of halothane, which is three times more soluble in brain and muscle than in blood and extremely soluble in fat. This last property is common among certain anaesthetic agents (e.g. halothane, enflurane and isoflurane), and fats are known to store inhalational anaesthetics.

Tissue Blood Flow

It is convenient to divide the tissues into four groups:

- *Vessel-rich group*: Brain, liver, heart and kidney, receiving a total of 70–75% of the cardiac output. The concentration of anaesthetic agent will rise rapidly in all these organs, equilibrium being reached within about 10 min.
- *Intermediate group*: Skeletal muscle and skin: 20% of the cardiac output.
- *Fat group*: This is 5% of the cardiac output.

• *Vessel-poor group*: Bones, etc. less than 1% of the cardiac output. Equilibration in the fat and vessel-poor groups takes place extremely slowly.

Concentration Effect

If two anaesthetics are given simultaneously, say nitrous oxide and halothane, one (N_2O) being present in high concentration, then as this is removed into the blood the other gases in the alveolus rapidly assume greater proportions. The rate of this effect obviously depends on the uptake of the high concentration gas into the blood and is therefore most pronounced with a very soluble anaesthetic agent (e.g. ether) and the factors are lessened if the halothane itself is already present in a high concentration.

Diffusion Hypoxia (Fink Phenomenon)

At the end of an anaesthetic, nitrous oxide is exhaled and if at this point the patient is allowed to breathe air, the lungs will, for a while, contain a mixture of nitrous oxide, nitrogen, oxygen, carbon dioxide and water, thus lowering the overall concentration of oxygen and producing relative hypoxia. In addition, as the nitrous oxide is breathed out, the total exhaled volume is greater than the inspired volume and therefore the alveolar carbon dioxide concentration falls. This leads to a fall in arterial carbon dioxide concentration, which depresses ventilation and accentuates the hypoxia already produced.

Metabolism and Distribution

As will be discussed in Chapter 10, the vast majority of volatile anaesthetic agents are excreted unchanged in the expired air. Nevertheless, a small proportion of almost every agent is metabolised within the liver and these

Table 5.1 Common metabolites and their potential toxicity

Agent	Metabolites	Potential toxicity
Halothane	Trifluracetic acid	Hepatotoxic
	Trifluracetaldehyde	
	Bromide and chloride ions	
Enflurane	Free fluoride ions	Nephrotoxic
Isoflurane	Minimal metabolism	
Trichloroethylene	Dichloracetylene	Ototoxic
(with hot soda-lime)		
Sevoflurane	Compounds A & B	?Nephrotoxic

metabolites are subsequently excreted in the bile and urine. The common metabolites and their potential toxicity are indicated in Table 5.1.

● INTRAVENOUS ANAESTHETIC AGENTS

Uptake

Uptake depends on a number of important factors.

1. The rate of injection.
2. Concentration of the agent.
3. The volume injected.
4. The site of injection, e.g. artery, vein (central or peripheral).
5. The circulation time.

The circulation time is dependent on the cardiac output, which itself is influenced by premedication, other drugs and the age and general fitness of the patient. The lower the cardiac output the longer the arm to brain circulation time.

Distribution

The redistribution of intravenous anaesthetic agents is the main factor influencing the waking time after a single intravenous dose. The action of intravenous agents depends on rapid administration of a large dose producing a high blood-to-brain concentration gradient. This level is then rapidly reduced by dilution within the bloodstream over a few minutes and then decays more slowly as the agent is redistributed to other body tissues in a similar way to the volatile anaesthetic agents. Redistribution to fat is a slow process since the fat blood flow is too small to account for this being the major route by which the action of intravenous agents is terminated. The ultra-short-acting barbiturates (e.g. thiopentone and methohexitone) are metabolised relatively slowly at the rate of about 10–15% of the total dose per hour.

A high proportion of the total dose of intravenous induction agents is protein bound and therefore inactive, the degree of binding depending upon the pH of the plasma. A fall in pH leads to a fall in the unbound plasma concentration of thiopentone and, conversely, a given dose of thiopentone will last longer if a patient is hyperventilated. This effect is similar with methohexitone.

In contrast to the barbiturate intravenous agents, which are only relatively slowly metabolised over many hours, other agents such as propofol (Diprivan) are metabolised in the liver so rapidly that it is this metabolism that terminates their action. The inactive metabolites are conjugated and then excreted in the bile and subsequently the faeces and urine.

Ketamine is rapidly metabolised within the liver to alcohols, which are subsequently excreted in the urine. Although the commonly used intravenous induction agents do not produce active metabolites, diazepam, which is sometimes used for induction, although broken down relatively rapidly in the liver, may still produce a prolonged effect. This is due to its active metabolites, particularly desmethyldiazepam and temazepam, although the effect is more prominent if the drug is given in repeated doses (Chapter 44). Accumulation of the intravenous induction agents after repeated administration is not a problem in those agents such as propofol, which are rapidly metabolised, but may produce pronounced effects in barbiturates, thiopentone and methohexitone, which accumulate in the body and are only slowly metabolised (Chapter 4).

6

Gases Used in Anaesthesia

•Oxygen •Carbon dioxide •Nitrous oxide •Entonox •Cyclopropane •Helium
•Compressed medical air

● OXYGEN

History

In 1674 John Mayow of Oxford demonstrated the existence of oxygen (O_2) when he showed that both fire and respiration could continue until one-fifth part of the air in an enclosed chamber had been used up. However, Mayow's work was little known and credit for the realisation of the importance of this gas as a normal constituent of air is usually given to Joseph Priestley, a Unitarian minister, as a result of work he carried out in about 1775. He called oxygen 'dephlogisticated air' and the name 'oxygène' was given by Frenchmen Antoine Lavoisier and Pierre Laplace.

Commercial Preparation and Storage

Oxygen is usually produced commercially by a method known as fractional distillation of liquid air. This method uses the fact that as the temperature of liquid air gradually rises its component gases are given off individually because of the difference in their boiling points. The boiling point of oxygen is $-182.5°C$.

Oxygen is supplied to hospitals by tankers in liquid form and stored in tanks at $-165°C$ at 10.5 bar pressure. The tank is vacuum insulated and liquid oxygen is evaporated into gas and then supplied by pipelines to the various sites for use.

Properties

Oxygen makes up 20.9% of normal air. It has a molecular weight of 32 and a specific gravity of 1.105 compared with air, which is 1.0. It does not itself ignite, but in its presence combustible material (e.g. wood or cloth) burns much more vigorously. Thus dust, oil or grease may ignite in the heat caused by the compression wave produced when an oxygen cylinder is suddenly turned on. Precautions against this eventuality include (a) cautiously and slightly opening the cylinder valve before attaching it to the anaesthetic machine to blow out any dust, (b) opening the rotameter needle valves beforehand to 'leak' the sudden pressure rise off downstream, and (c) banning all oil and grease from areas when oxygen is likely to be released under pressure.

● CARBON DIOXIDE

History

Carbon dioxide (CO_2) was isolated by Joseph Black in 1757. Henry Hill Hickman, in 1824, published the results of his production of anaesthesia in animals by using this gas. He failed in his attempts to introduce it as an anaesthetic in man. Its significance in human physiology was not realised until the work of Haldane in England in 1926. This led to a widespread realisation of the dangers of carbon dioxide accumulation under anaesthesia and a fashion developed for producing hypocarbia, i.e. a reduction of the blood P_{CO_2} below its normal level, under anaesthesia. In recent years it has become apparent that this too has its disadvantages and usually attempts are now made to maintain approximate normocarbia.

Commercial Preparation

Carbon dioxide is usually produced commercially by the action of heat on calcium or magnesium carbonates:

$$CaCO_3 \rightarrow CaO + CO_2$$

(calcium carbonate)   (calcium oxide)   (carbon dioxide)

Properties

Carbon dioxide is a colourless gas which in high concentration has a pungent smell. Its molecular weight is 44 and its specific gravity 1.5. It occurs as a natural constituent of air but only in a concentration of 0.03%. It is non-inflammable and does not support combustion, hence its use as the insufflating gas in laparoscopy.

Anaesthetic Uses of Carbon Dioxide

Carbon dioxide is no longer routinely stored on anaesthetic machines. Where a rotameter is available, it remains the responsibility of the anaesthetist to connect this gas, thus avoiding the problem of leaving the gas supply accidentally on.

Traditional uses of carbon dioxide, for example, to facilitate gaseous induction and to restart breathing at the end of surgery have been made obsolete by modern drugs and monitoring. The main use of carbon dioxide now is for insufflation of the peritoneum for laparoscopic procedures.

NITROUS OXIDE

History

In 1772 Joseph Priestley first prepared nitrous oxide (N_2O), and in 1800 Sir Humphrey Davy first demonstrated its anaesthetic properties. In 1844 in the USA an itinerant chemist, Gardner Quincy Colton, demonstrated its anaesthetic properties to an audience which included a dentist named Horace Wells. The latter realised its potential use in dental practice, but after some success his attempt to show its use as a surgical anaesthetic at the Massachusetts General Hospital was something of a debacle. It was rapidly superseded by ether and did not regain popularity for nearly 20 years.

Joseph Clover first used nitrous oxide to provide a relatively pleasant induction to ether anaesthesia and Boyle's machine was introduced in 1917. This permitted the vaporisation of ether in a stream of nitrous oxide and oxygen. Today, nitrous oxide with oxygen provides the basis for the vast majority of inhalational anaesthetics in countries where advanced anaesthetic equipment is available.

Commercial Preparation

Nitrous oxide is prepared by heating ammonium nitrate in large iron retorts at 240°C:

$$NH_4NO_3 \quad \rightarrow \quad 2H_2O \quad + \quad N_2O$$

(ammonium nitrate)   (water)   (nitrous oxide)

Properties

Nitrous oxide is a sweet-smelling, non-irritant, colourless gas, with a molecular weight of 44 and a specific gravity of 1.5. It is neither inflammable nor explosive, but like oxygen supports combustion of other oxidisable materials if an initial temperature high enough to decompose nitrous oxide into nitrogen and oxygen is supplied (450°C).

Nitrous oxide is an excellent analgesic (hence its use to relieve pain in labour), but is a weak anaesthetic agent. Consequently it may be impossible to produce full anaesthesia in a robust adult with nitrous oxide and oxygen alone without using a hypoxic mixture, i.e. a nitrous oxide of over 80%. Similarly, when using muscle-relaxant anaesthesia, nitrous oxide should almost always be supplemented with an inhalational or intravenous agent. Otherwise there is the real possibility that the patient may develop some awareness or recall under the anaesthetic (Chapter 21).

Nitrous oxide is generally regarded as non-toxic, but there have been occasional reports of reversible agranulocytosis after prolonged administration of the gas in intensive care. The association of teratogenesis and abortions in female staff exposed to nitrous oxide remains unproved. Environmental effects on the ozone layer are also minimal. Another possible adverse effect of nitrous oxide occurs due to its rapid diffusion compared with nitrogen in air. For every molecule of nitrogen removed from an air-containing space, 35 molecules of nitrous oxide will enter. There is thus an increase in the gas space when it is compliant, for example, in a pneumothorax or air embolus, and an increase in pressure when the space cannot expand, for example, in middle ear cavity surgery. Nitrous oxide should not therefore be used in these circumstances. 'Diffusion' hypoxia can occur immediately after nitrous oxide is discontinued because it diffuses into the lung alveoli from the blood much faster than nitrogen can diffuse in from the room air. This can be avoided by administering 100% oxygen at the end of the anaesthetic. Nitrous oxide is also thought to increase the incidence of nausea and vomiting and many anaesthetists prefer to use air as the carrier gas instead of nitrous oxide routinely.

● ENTONOX

'Entonox' is the British Oxygen Company (BOC) name for premixed gases in one cylinder containing 50% nitrous oxide and 50% oxygen. It is curious that this mixture is gaseous at its normal cylinder pressure of 137 bar (2000 psi). The pressure at which nitrous oxide alone liquefies varies with the temperature, but around room temperature of 20°C it liquefies at 50 bar. Oxygen, at its usual cylinder pressure of 137 bar, is in the gaseous form. However, when oxygen is bubbled through liquid nitrous oxide in a cylinder, the latter vaporises and a gaseous mixture of nitrous oxide and oxygen is formed. By continuing to introduce oxygen into the cylinder, various proportions of nitrous oxide and oxygen can be made and the mixture of nitrous oxide and oxygen in equal proportions known as Entonox is supplied in cylinders at a pressure of 137 bar.

Entonox cylinders vary from a portable 500 l size to large 5000 l cylinders intended for pipeline use. At normal environmental temperatures the nitrous oxide and oxygen remain in the gaseous phase, but if the temperature falls below −7°C some nitrous oxide liquefies and separates from the oxygen. In these circumstances, if the cylinder is used vertically with the valve at the top it is possible when the cylinder is nearing exhaustion to obtain a hypoxic mixture of almost pure nitrous oxide. Fortunately, the nitrous oxide can be restored to the gaseous phase by inverting the cylinder three times after it has been rewarmed.

The Entonox cylinder has a two-stage valve. The first one is a reducing valve which reduces the pressure of the gas to about 4 bar. The second valve is a one-way valve and opens only with the negative pressure of inspiration from the patient but closes when the positive pressure of expiration pushes down a sensing diaphragm. This safety feature allows Entonox to be delivered only when the patient inspires.

Entonox is most popular as a convenient and effective method of pain relief in obstetrics, but may also be useful in other circumstances, for example, for trauma and changing burns dressings.

● CYCLOPROPANE

The anaesthetic properties of cyclopropane were first discovered by Lucas and Henderson of Toronto in 1929, but its use as a clinical anaesthetic agent was developed by Waters and his colleagues at Madison, Wisconsin, in the years just after 1930.

The gas is colourless, sweet-smelling and non-irritant except in high concentrations. Its molecular weight is 42 and the specific gravity 1.42. It is easily liquefied and was available in orange cylinders at a pressure of 5 bar. It is probably the most explosive agent and because of this, its costs and many side-effects it is no longer used in clinical practice.

● HELIUM

Isolated by Sir William Ramsey in 1895, helium is an inert odourless gas with a molecular weight of 4 and specific gravity of 0.178 compared to 1.0 of air. Helium is prepared from natural gas and stored in brown cylinders on its own or in brown cylinders with brown and white shoulders when mixed with oxygen.

The main anaesthetic use of helium is for the inhalation induction of anaesthesia in patients with partial respiratory obstruction. A 20:80 mixture of oxygen and helium has a density one-third that of air. The patient therefore requires less effort to breathe this mixture when it is used as a carrier gas for the inhalation agent, thereby facilitating inhalation induction of anaesthesia.

● COMPRESSED MEDICAL AIR

Since the introduction of powerful volatile agents and total intravenous anaesthesia, the use of nitrous oxide as the carrier gas has declined and the use of medical air has increased. Medical air is now supplied in cylinders coloured grey with a white and black shoulder and also via pipelines. Most modern anaesthetic machines also have rotameters for delivering air.

For hospital use, air from the atmosphere is compressed, cooled and then stored, from where it is cleaned by means of separators and dried before finally passing through filters to make it bacteria free. It is supplied at a pipeline pressure of 4.0 bar for anaesthetic use and at 6.9 bar for driving machinery such as surgical drills.

7

Anaesthetic Gas Supply: The Anaesthetic Machine

•British Standards Institution •Units of pressure •Gas cylinders •Identification colours of cylinders •Cylinder testing •Cylinder valves •Pin-index valve •Information carried on gas cylinders and valves •Gas pipelines •Flexible pipelines •Pressure regulators or pressure-reducing valves •Pressure gauges •Flow restrictors and high-pressure relief valves •Flowmeters •Oxygen failure warning devices •Oxygen bypass •Checking the anaesthetic machine •Suction systems

This chapter discusses the transport and supply of anaesthetic gases from their source in cylinders or a pipeline through to the anaesthetic machine and its outlet. Chapter 8 describes the various anaesthetic breathing systems, by which the anaesthetic gases are carried from the outlet of the machine to the patient. Chapter 18 describes the airway devices used for delivery of the gases from the distal end of the anaesthetic breathing system to the patient's lungs.

The most popular anaesthetic machine in common use is often referred to as Boyle's machine, although it is much changed from the original model introduced in 1917 by Edmund Boyle, a London anaesthetist. Basically, the anaesthetic machine remains a trolley with a working surface, special positions (yokes) for attaching anaesthetic gas cylinders or pipelines, pressure regulators for reducing the high pressure from most gas cylinders, means of metering the anaesthetic gases (rotameters) and vaporisers (which are essentially sophisticated vaporising bottles). Modern anaesthetic machines are like 'work stations' and also include ventilators and monitoring devices built into the machine (Fig. 7.1). Unlike previous machines, modern machines are driven by electrical and electronic hardware and are quite sophisticated.

● BRITISH STANDARDS INSTITUTION

This institution produces pamphlets called British Standards (or BS) which cover hundreds of engineering and industrial products and techniques;

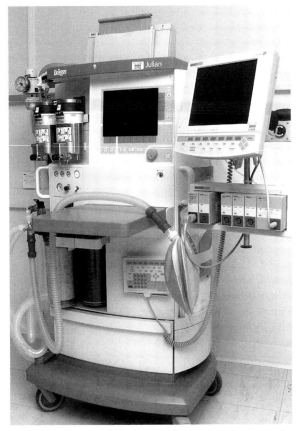

Figure 7.1 The Dräger 'Julian' – a modern anaesthetic workstation.

several have been produced in the UK covering all aspects of medical gas pipelines, cylinders and cylinder valves.

● UNITS OF PRESSURE

Unfortunately, despite attempts at standardisation, a profusion of units of pressure still exists. In this book the units cited will usually be those most commonly found in a particular situation, for example, in this chapter, bar and pounds to the square inch (psi) are those found on most gas cylinders and cylinder valves. Other units are millimetres of mercury (mmHg), kilopascals (kPa), kilograms/square centimetre (kg/cm^2) and centimetres of water (cmH_2O). A simple conversion is as follows:

One atmosphere, also called one bar, is approximately equal to 101 kPa, 15 psi, 760 mmHg or 1035 cmH_2O.

● GAS CYLINDERS

These are usually made of steel, the types of steel being referred to as high carbon, low carbon and manganese for hospital use, or chrome–molybdenum for lightweight, portable cylinders. These terms refer to some of the constituents added to the iron in the manufacture of the steel, the percentage of the components being laid down in a BS. Cylinders are supplied in different sizes from A to J, size A being the smallest and size J being the larger variety for hospital storage bank (Fig. 7.2). Size E cylinders are commonly found on anaesthetic machines.

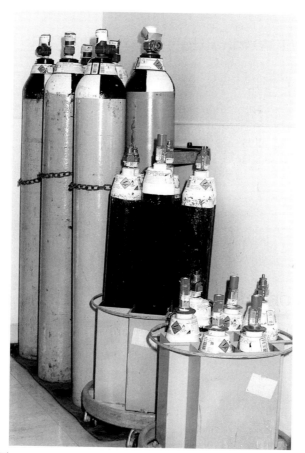

Figure 7.2 Different gas cylinders in theatre storage area.

Table 7.1 BS cylinder colour code

Name of gas	Symbol	Valve end colour	Body colour
Oxygen	O_2	White	Black
Nitrous oxide	N_2O	Blue	Blue
Cyclopropane	C_3H_6	Orange	Orange
Carbon dioxide	CO_2	Grey	Grey
Helium	He	Brown	Brown
Nitrogen	N_2	Black	Grey
Oxygen and carbon dioxide	$O_2 + CO_2$	White and grey	Black
Oxygen and helium mixtures	$O_2 + He$	White and brown	Black
Air (medical)	AIR	White and black	Grey
Oxygen and nitrous oxide mixture (Entonox)	$O_2 + N_2O$	White and blue	Blue

● IDENTIFICATION COLOURS OF CYLINDERS

The colour coding of the cylinder contents is also laid down in a BS, but unfortunately as yet there is no international agreement on this coding. The BS cylinder colour code is shown in Table 7.1. In some cases the valve end (shoulder) of the cylinder has special identification colours. In the case of gas mixtures, these colours are applied in four segments, two of each colour (e.g. Entonox).

● CYLINDER TESTING

During the manufacture of the cylinders, sample strips are taken from one of each batch of 100 cylinders and subjected to tensile (or stretching), impact and bend tests. Each completed cylinder also undergoes hydraulic pressure testing by a high 'proof' pressure of 200 bar applied internally. The details of all these tests are described in BS.

In addition to these tests on new cylinders, hydraulic pressure testing is repeated every 5 years. The date of testing is indicated either by symbols stamped on the shoulder of the cylinder or on the valve (see below) or by a colour-coded disc fixed round the neck of the cylinder.

● CYLINDER VALVES

The cylinder valve is screwed into the neck of the cylinder. It is usually made of chromium-plated brass or bronze. There are two types in common use, the bull-nosed and the pin-index. Pin-index valves are the most common types used. Full cylinders are supplied with a red plastic seal which prevents dust or grit from entering the valve outlet. It is nevertheless recommended that after removing the seal, but before attaching the cylinder to the machine, the valve be momentarily opened and closed to blow away any foreign matter which would otherwise be blown into the regulator. It is important to ensure that the handler's face is averted. Once the cylinder is securely attached to the anaesthetic or other apparatus, the cylinder valve is opened by slowly turning the valve spindle two complete turns anti-clockwise with the valve key or handwheel provided.

● PIN-INDEX VALVE

Pin-index valves are designed in such a way that it is possible to connect only the correct gas cylinder to the appropriate yoke on the anaesthetic machine (Fig. 7.3a). The upper of the three holes in the pin-index valve is the gas outlet. The lower two holes are placed on the circumference of a circle whose centre is the centre of the gas outlet hole and whose radius is 14.3 mm (9/16 in.). The positions of these holes are precisely laid down for each of the common medical gases by a BS, for example, 2 and 5 for oxygen (Fig. 7.3b) The only gas without two lower hole positions is Entonox which has one central hole at position 7 (between 3 and 4). These pin-index holes are blind, having no internal connection within the cylinder valve. They correspond with pins in the appropriate position for the same gas in the yoke of the anaesthetic machine. A sealing washer (Bodok seal) is essential between the pin-index valve and the valve yoke.

● INFORMATION CARRIED ON GAS CYLINDERS AND VALVES

Some interesting and useful symbols and figures are carried on gas cylinders and valves. Some of these tend to be obscured by successive layers of paint and by batch number labels applied by the manufacturer, but among other information it should be possible to find the following.

Identification of Gas

The name or chemical symbol of the gas or gas mixture is indelibly stamped on the cylinder valve and painted on the cylinder, which also bears a label with the same information, and, for gas mixtures, the proportion of the constituents. This is, of course, in addition to the identification of the cylinder contents by colour coding.

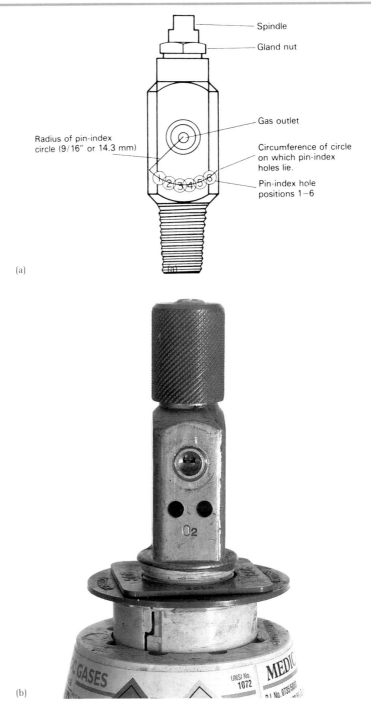

(a)

(b)

Figure 7.3 (a) Pin-index valve and (b) pin-index valve on oxygen cylinder.

Cylinder Size

The cylinder size is identified by a capital letter code (e.g. A, B, C) stencilled on the cylinder or shown on a label. The capacity of the cylinder is also marked on the valve end of the cylinder.

Tare Weight

The tare or empty weight of the cylinder plus valve is stamped on all cylinders containing liquefiable gases, i.e. nitrous oxide, carbon dioxide and cyclopropane. The cylinder contents for these gases can be measured accurately by weighing the cylinder and deducting the tare weight. The weight of 100 l of the gas is given on a label on the cylinder, for example, 100 l N_2O weighs 0.182 kg.

Maximum Permissible Working Pressure

This is stamped on the cylinder valve. The pressure might easily be exceeded if the cylinder were stored in the sun or beside a radiator.

Hydraulic Test Date

This has already been mentioned under 'Cylinder testing'. When the date is stamped on the cylinder valve or cylinder shoulder it is represented by the last two figures of the date and the quarter of the year indicated by one of the figures 1–4 with a circle round it. Thus 81 3 BR means that the cylinder was tested in the third quarter of 1981. Beside the date mark is stamped a test mark in the form of initials or a hieroglyphic to indicate the British Oxygen Company (BOC) testing centre where the test was carried out, for example, BR = Brentford.

● GAS PIPELINES

The central store of the gases is in the form of a liquid tank or a bank of big cylinders or both. From the central stores, the gas is carried by pipelines of special high-quality copper to the wall outlet. When the pressure in these pipelines falls, valves in the central stores open to release evaporated gas into the pipelines. The wall outlets are fixed points at places where gases are frequently used, for example, the operating theatre (Fig. 7.4). From these fixed outlets gases can be delivered to the anaesthetic machine by means of flexible pipelines.

Safety devices to prevent leak of gases in the high-pressure pipelines include the provision of stop valves at strategic points so gas can be

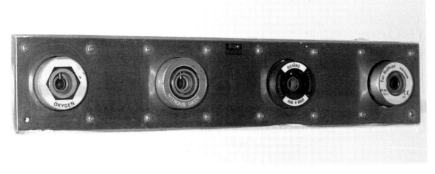

Figure 7.4 Fixed wall outlets for anaesthetic gases and vacuum.

diverted. Also there are low-pressure alarms installed in places where there are wall outlets to detect any fall in the pressure of the gas. The fixed wall outlets are identified by gas names and by colour as specified in the BS, for example, white for oxygen, blue for nitrous oxide and white and black for air. Further safety precautions include the 'Permit to Work' system. This means that whenever repairs are needed or new pipelines are installed, all the personnel are informed and then work is carried out only by qualified engineers.

● FLEXIBLE PIPELINES

The anaesthetic machine is connected to the gas outlets by means of flexible pipelines to facilitate movement. These pipelines have a 'fixed' end to the anaesthetic machine and a 'detachable' end which can be inserted into the outlet wall socket of the pipeline. The fixed connection is made possible by a nut and linear union in which the thread is gas specific and non-interchangeable (non-interchangeable screw thread, NIST). The detachable end is made non-interchangeable by an indexing collar of diameter specific for each gas which is also colour coded.

Two useful tests can be performed for pipelines. The tug test is a sharp tug on the pipeline to ensure that the connections are properly engaged. The single hose test is useful in detecting cross-connection, for example, only oxygen should flow in the rotameter when the oxygen pipeline is connected.

The usual hospital medical gas pipeline pressure is 4 bar (400 kPa or 60 psi). For hospitals using large amounts of oxygen, it is usual for the oxygen to be supplied and stored in liquid form in tanks from where it is vaporised.

● PRESSURE REGULATORS OR PRESSURE-REDUCING VALVES

The most important function of pressure regulators is to provide gases to the flowmeters at a constant pressure. Otherwise, as the pressure in the cylinder gradually falls, constant readjustment of the needle valve leading to the flowmeter would be required to maintain a constant flow rate. On modern anaesthetic machines the pressure regulators usually reduce the pressure to 4 bar (400 kPa or 60 psi) and, instead of being sited on top of the cylinder, are usually tucked under the working surface of the machine. Pressure regulators are not required for pipeline gases because they are supplied at a pressure of 4 bar.

● PRESSURE GAUGES

These indicate the pressure in the gas cylinder to which they are attached or the gas pipeline pressure. The commonest type of pressure gauge is the Bourdon gauge (Fig. 7.5a) which acts in the same way as the popular children's party toy of a curled tube of paper which straightens when blown into (Fig. 7.5b).

In the Bourdon pressure gauge the curled tube is made of metal and requires great pressure to produce a slight straightening movement. The closed end of the tube is linked to a pointer which indicates the pressure.

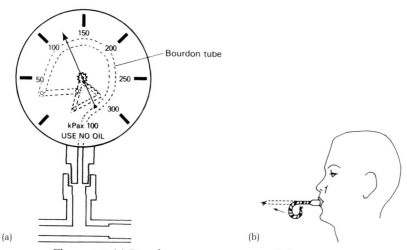

(a) (b)

Figure 7.5 (a) Bourdon pressure gauge and (b) its principle.

● FLOW RESTRICTORS AND HIGH-PRESSURE RELIEF VALVES

As the gas supplied from the pipelines to the anaesthetic machine is at 4 bar and does not require a pressure regulator, any obstruction to the machine outlet will result in a rapid rise in pressure in the pipelines and in the vaporisers, resulting in damage. To assist in restricting these surges, flow restrictors are placed in the pipelines upstream of the flowmeters and pressure relief valves are fitted at the backbar blowing off at approximately 74 kPa (555 mg) to protect the pipeline and vaporisers.

● FLOWMETERS

Flowmeters may be divided into two groups: (a) constant pressure/variable orifice flowmeters and (b) variable pressure/constant orifice flowmeters. Only the former are in common use in modern anaesthetic machines.

Constant Pressure/Variable Orifice

The commonest example of this group is the rotameter (Fig. 7.6), the most popular flowmeter in use in anaesthetics. This consists of a glass tube mounted vertically within which a rotating bobbin is free to move. Although invisible to the naked eye, the tube tapers very gradually so that it is wider at the top than at the bottom. This means that there is an annular orifice between the bobbin and the walls of the glass tube, and this orifice increases in size as the bobbin moves up the tube.

The anaesthetic gas enters the lower part of the tube through a simple needle valve. This causes the bobbin to rise up within the tube, the gas escaping through the annular orifice. The bobbin settles at a level where its weight is balanced by the pressure drop across the orifice. As the needle valve is opened, admitting more gas into the lower part of the tube, the bobbin is forced higher in the tube as the higher gas flow requires a larger orifice to maintain the pressure drop at a constant level, i.e. that required to support the bobbin. The needle valve is operated by control knobs which are labelled and colour coded. The oxygen control knob is of a larger diameter and also mounted on a larger stem, hence it protrudes further than other knobs.

The rotation of the bobbin is caused by the gas blowing through oblique cuts made in the rim of the bobbin. Provided that the glass tube is mounted vertically, and provided that there is no dirt in it, the bobbin spins freely in the centre of the tube without touching the side. This eliminates any error which might be caused by friction and makes the rotameter more accurate.

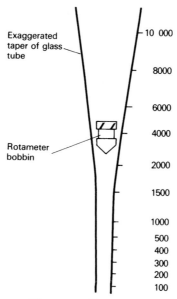

Figure 7.6 Rotameter.

The glass tube is calibrated to show the gas flow, the measurement being taken from the top of the bobbin. Not only are the tubes non-interchangeable for different gases but each is also calibrated with its own bobbin and must not be used for any other. In modern machines it is becoming common for oxygen and nitrous oxide control valves to be mechanically linked by a chain belt mechanism so that <25% oxygen cannot be set by the needle valves.

On the Boyle's machine the flowmeters are grouped in a bank on the top left of the machine. After passing through them the gases mix in the hollow tube on the top rear of the machine. There they may be used to vaporise volatile anaesthetic agents (Chapter 9) before passing to the outlet from the anaesthetic machine.

● OXYGEN FAILURE WARNING DEVICES

It has been recommended that the ideal warning device should have the following features:

1. Be operated only by the oxygen supply.
2. Not be operated by mains or battery power.
3. There should be a warning of impending failure, and a further warning that failure has occurred.

4. The signals are audible and of sufficient length, volume and character.
5. When the device is triggered:
   (a) Other gases and vapours should cease to flow.
   (b) The breathing circuit is opened to the atmosphere.
   (c) The inspired oxygen concentration should be at least equal to that of air, and build-up of carbon dioxide should not occur whether respiration is spontaneous or controlled.

Devices are now available which cut out the nitrous oxide and other gas supply if the oxygen pressure falls below 50% and also have an audible warning device which is powered through a small reservoir of oxygen, situated underneath the machine and maintained at 4 bar.

● OXYGEN BYPASS

The maximum flow rate of oxygen through the rotameter is usually 10 l/min. An additional oxygen bypass at 35 l/min is available for emergencies. Except in older machines, the oxygen bypass button is spring loaded to prevent accidental prolonged dilution of the inhaled anaesthetic mixture.

● CHECKING THE ANAESTHETIC MACHINE

Because of the variety of oxygen failure warning devices, pressure relief valves, ventilators and breathing systems which may be used, it is not possible to give one description of a method of testing the entire anaesthetic apparatus which is to be used for a particular anaesthetic. In the UK, guidelines are published by the Association of Anaesthetists of Great Britain and Ireland (AAGBI) and manufacturers usually provide their own recommendations.

The following is a description of the basic testing of the anaesthetic machine which the anaesthetist should carry out at the beginning of each list. It is assumed that the machine has both a pipeline and single cylinder supplies of nitrous oxide and oxygen.

Oxygen Analyser

The analyser is checked, calibrated and placed to monitor gases leaving the common gas outlet.

Medical Gas Supplies

The pipeline hoses for nitrous oxide and oxygen are disconnected from their outlets, the cylinders turned off and all the flowmeter controls turned on. If appropriate, the electrical supply to the machine is turned on.

The oxygen cylinder is turned on and it is established that flow occurs only through the oxygen flowmeter. The cylinder is checked for adequate contents and the flow is set to 5 l/min, and the oxygen analyser should approach 100%.

The nitrous oxide cylinder is turned on and a check done to confirm that flow starts in the nitrous oxide flowmeter. The flow is adjusted to 5 l/min.

The oxygen cylinder is turned off, the flow of oxygen through the flowmeter stops and the primary audible alarm should operate.

The oxygen pipeline supply is turned on and this should restore the flow of oxygen and cancel the oxygen alarm. A 'tug test' is performed and it is confirmed that the pipeline pressure is 400 kPa (4 bar).

The nitrous oxide cylinder is turned off and the pipeline connected to restore flow of nitrous oxide. A 'tug test' and pressure gauge check are performed which should read 400 kPa. The nitrous oxide flowmeter is turned off.

If other gases are to be used, these should be checked in a similar manner.

All flowmeter valves are turned off.

The emergency flush valve is turned on to ensure that there is no decrease in pipeline pressure and to confirm that the analyser approaches 100%.

Vaporisers

These should be checked to make sure that they are fitted correctly to the machine, that any backbar locking mechanism is fully engaged and that the control knobs rotate through their full range.

Breathing Systems

The configuration of the breathing and scavanging systems to be used should be checked and tests performed for leaks and obstructions.

Ventilator

The normal operation of the ventilator and its controls is checked and the function of the pressure relief valve confirmed by occluding the patient port. The disconnect alarm is tested and a check is made to ensure that an alternative means to ventilate the patient is available should the ventilator malfunction.

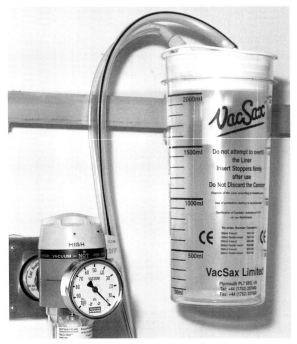

Figure 7.7 Suction control unit.

● SUCTION SYSTEMS

Suction apparatus is one of the most important pieces of equipment that the anaesthetist uses. The suction used in the theatre area is delivered by pipeline but portable systems are also available. The fixed suction systems used in operating theatres form part of the piped medical gases and vacuum systems and have to comply with the same BS in terms of installation and maintanence. A central pump generates the subatmospheric pressure required for the suction apparatus and is connected by fixed pipelines to a terminal wall outlet which is colour coded yellow. The fixed wall outlet will only accept a colour-coded flexible hose with a specific probe connector from the vacuum control unit. The vacuum control unit allows adjustment of the degree of vacuum applied to the distal suction tubing. The force of suction is indicated on a gauge on the vacuum control unit. Within this system there is a filter and float valve to provide protection from particulate matter. The control unit connects the distal tubing to a reservoir (Fig. 7.7). It is important not only that suction should reach adequate subatmospheric pressures, but that these pressures can be reached quickly if required. At times it is also necessary to be able to control the pressures to lower levels, as in applying suction to a neonate's respiratory tract. In most instances it is essential that a large enough volume can be moved by the apparatus. For example, suction that can achieve a high pressure but only shift a few millilitres per minute would be useless at removing a large volume of vomit. The degree of pressure attainable by pipeline suction should be of the order of 500 mmHg subatmospheric (two-thirds of an atmosphere).

8

Anaesthetic Breathing Systems

This chapter on the transport of anaesthetic gases to the patient and elimination of carbon dioxide from the patient describes the apparatus from the gas outlet on the anaesthetic machine to the point of delivery to the patient. This apparatus is usually referred to as an 'anaesthetic breathing system'. The airway devices used to transport gases from the distal end of the breathing system to the patient's lungs are described in Chapter 18.

Confusion in the classification of anaesthetic breathing systems arises partly from inconsistencies in nomenclature (especially of the terms 'semi-open' and 'semi-closed', which are used in different classifications for the same system) and partly from the number of variations in some of the types of systems. For example, over 60 variations of the circle system may be produced by changing the position in the circle of some of its component parts, such as fresh gas flow entry point, soda-lime canister, expiratory valve and non-return valves. Before classifying anaesthetic breathing systems, some of their important principles will be enumerated.

● PRINCIPLES OF ANAESTHETIC BREATHING SYSTEMS

1. There must be an adequate inspired oxygen concentration. With some anaesthetic breathing systems this may be supplied simply by room air.
2. There must be efficient elimination of carbon dioxide.
3. The system must not greatly increase the dead space.
4. The apparatus should not greatly increase the resistance to inspiration or expiration, the exception being the occasional application of a positive end-expiratory pressure.
5. The system should allow spontaneous and intermittent positive pressure ventilation (IPPV).
6. The system should protect the patient from barotrauma.

7. The system should be simple, safe, reliable, lightweight and cheap.
8. The system should be easy to scavenge.

The ideal system has not yet been developed but essentially all the systems have a length of corrugated tubing, reservoir bag and adjustable pressure-limiting (APL) valve as basic components to satisfy some of the principles mentioned.

Corrugated Tubing

The heavy, black antistatic tubing previously used for anaesthetic breathing systems has now been generally replaced by lightweight plastic tubing. It is still corrugated to prevent kinking but the inside bore is usually made smooth to reduce the resistance to breathing. Earlier systems had different connections, quite often non-interchangable to connect tubing, often resulting in kinks and misconnections. The modern connections are available as standards laid down by the International Standards Organisation and British Standard Institute. Three types of connections are generally used: a 30 mm tapered connector for linking scavenging systems to the breathing system, a 22 mm connector for connections within the breathing system and a 15 mm connector for linking the breathing system to airway devices such as tracheal tubes and laryngeal mask airway (LMA). The 15 mm connector, which is too cumbersome for paediatric tracheal tubes, is replaced by an 8.5 mm connector, which has adaptors for connecting it to a 15 mm connector.

The breathing systems are marketed as disposable single-use items but generally not used as such. The routine is usually to change a bacterial filter between cases and only dispose of the breathing system once a day or even once a week.

Reservoir Bag

The function of this bag is to store the gases exhaled during expiration and to provide these to the patient during inspiration. The movement of the bag during spontaneous respiration gives an idea of the pattern of breathing but is not an accurate indicator of tidal volumes. The reservoir bag is available in sizes usually of 0.5, 1 and 2 l and made of very compliant rubber such that any increase in its size when a pressure of 40 cmH$_2$O has been reached will result in no further increase in pressure. This protects the patients' lungs from barotrauma even when the APL valve is accidently left in the closed position.

Adjustable Pressure-limiting Valve (Fig. 8.1)

This is a one-way, spring-loaded valve with a disc that prevents the movement of air in the breathing system when the patient inspires but opens

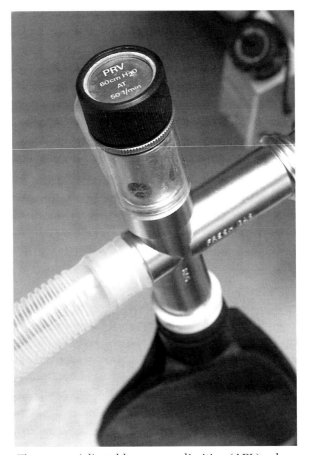

Figure 8.1 Adjustable pressure-limiting (APL) valve.

at a pressure of about $1\,cmH_2O$ to allow exhaled and surplus gases to be vented during expiration. The disc is made of hydrophobic material so that it does not stick due to water condensation. When the valve is fully screwed down, the disc will open at $60\,cmH_2O$ positive pressure, acting as a safety feature. Once the expired gases leave the APL they can be conveniently scavenged. The APL valve should be fully open during spontaneous respiration, partially closed during manual ventilation and fully closed during ventilator IPPV.

● CLASSIFICATION OF ANAESTHETIC BREATHING SYSTEMS

There is no general agreement about the classification of anaesthetic breathing systems, but the following classification divides the systems into three main groups:

1. open 'systems'
2. systems with an 'adequate' fresh gas flow, i.e. sufficient for carbon dioxide elimination, and
3. systems with an 'inadequate' fresh gas flow which rely on soda-lime for elimination of carbon dioxide.

Groups 2 and 3 contain various subgroups. Instead of trying to master the characteristics of all these subgroups, examples of the most popular systems used in the UK are emphasised below.

The efficiency of individual systems in fulfilling the principles given above, especially as regards providing adequate oxygen and eliminating carbon dioxide, may vary considerably depending on whether the system is being used for spontaneous or controlled respiration.

Open Systems

The classical example of this technique is the application of a volatile anaesthetic agent, such as diethyl ether, by a drop technique onto a gauze mask (e.g. a Schimmelbusch mask) or simply onto a handkerchief (the original 'rag and bottle' technique). Provided that the mask is held clear of the face, the oxygen supply is derived from the room air and there is no rebreathing as the expired gases escape freely into the atmosphere. Provided that the mask is held off the patient's face, this system has no resistance and no dead space.

Breathing Systems with Adequate Fresh Gas Flow

Systems Using Non-rebreathing Valves

The first example of this group of circuits incorporates a non-rebreathing valve, such as the Ambu-E valve (Fig. 8.2). The inspiratory side of this system incorporates a reservoir bag to deal with the peaks of the patient's inspiratory flow rate. The bag should not be referred to as a 'rebreathing' bag as this is not its function. The purpose of the bag is to continue filling with fresh gases during the patient's expiratory and expiratory pause phases so that it can deal with the patient's inspiratory peak flow which can easily reach 25–30 l/min in the case of an adult. On inspiration, the valve cycles into the inspiratory position so that the patient is supplied with pure fresh gases. The expiratory port then opens and the patient breathes out into the atmosphere. These valves facilitate the precise adjustment of the anaesthetic mixture as there is no contamination of the fresh gas flow by expired gases. Indeed, the patient's minute volume may be calculated by adjusting the fresh gas flow so that the reservoir bag neither

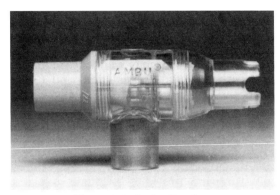

Figure 8.2 Ambu-E valve.

fills nor empties. A disadvantage of these valves is that they tend to stick if there is a build-up of moisture, or if the fresh gas flow appreciably exceeds the minute volume. This last problem may be avoided by incorporating an overflow valve, for example, a Heidbrink valve on the inspiratory side. This system is also relatively expensive in its use of gases and vapours.

Semi-closed Systems

This group of systems is commonly described by the useful but non-descriptive classification of Mapleson systems A–F, as shown in Figure 8.3. This group contains many of the most popular anaesthetic breathing systems used in the UK. Instead of describing each of the Mapleson systems in detail, it is proposed to describe some of the more frequently used ones and indicate to which of the Mapleson systems they belong.

Magill system (Fig. 8.4). This is an example of a Mapleson A system. The valve is a Heidbrink valve and there is a reservoir bag. Its popularity has declined because of the relatively cumbersome nature of the valve when it is modified to take a scavenging attachment. At the beginning of expiration the corrugated tubing fills first with the dead space gas and then with alveolar gas. As this expired gas flow meets the fresh gases, the pressure under the expiratory valve increases. When the pressure reaches $2\,cmH_2O$, the valve flap lifts and alveolar gas is vented into the atmosphere. Towards the end of expiration the pressure in the tubing begins to fall and the fresh gases begin to flow towards the patient again, flushing any remaining alveolar gas out through the valve. With a high fresh gas flow, dead space gas from the tubing and even fresh gas may be vented through the valve before it closes, but even if they are breathed in by the patient neither contains carbon dioxide. Hence this system preferentially eliminates alveolar gas, and rebreathing does not occur until the fresh gas flow falls below the alveolar ventilation, i.e. about 70% of the minute volume.

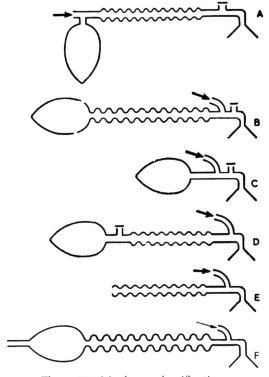

Figure 8.3 Mapleson classification.

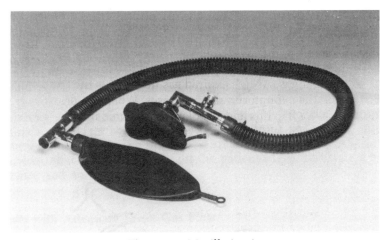

Figure 8.4 Magill circuit.

To use this system for controlled ventilation, the Heidbrink valve has to be partially screwed down. Venting of gases through the valve occurs only when the reservoir bag is squeezed, i.e. during the inspiratory phase, so that it is mainly fresh gas which is eliminated. For this reason the Magill system is inefficient for controlled ventilation.

Ayre's T-piece. This corresponds to the Mapleson E system and variations on this system are used widely in paediatrics (Chapter 37). When this system is being used for spontaneous respiration, during expiration fresh gas and expired gases from the patient pass down the expiratory limb. During the expiratory pause these mixed gases are flushed further down the limb by fresh gas. Whether any of the expired gases are reinspired depends on the rate of fresh gas flow and duration of the expiratory pause. The adverse effect of any rebreathing is reduced by the fact that as it will occur only at the end of inspiration, rebreathed gases tend to reach only as far as the patient's dead space, so they do not contaminate the alveolar gas. A fresh gas flow of about twice the minute volume is adequate to prevent significant rebreathing. If the fresh gas flow exceeds the peak inspiratory flow rate, no rebreathing will occur. This requires a fresh gas flow of about three times the minute volume. If the volume of the expiratory limb exceeds the tidal volume, the patient will not inspire any room air. Whether this happens with shorter expiratory limbs depends on the adequacy of the fresh gas flow. Controlled ventilation with the T-piece system is performed most simply by intermittent occlusion of the expiratory limb. This may expose the lungs to high inspiratory pressures and IPPV is more commonly and safely performed by the Jackson Rees modification of the T-piece (Fig. 8.5), which is the Mapleson F system. Controlled respiration is achieved by squeezing an open-ended bag inserted in the expiratory limb, the desired amount of lung inflation being achieved by adjusting the size of the orifice in the end of the bag, usually with the anaesthetist's little finger. The characteristics of the system are the same as during spontaneous

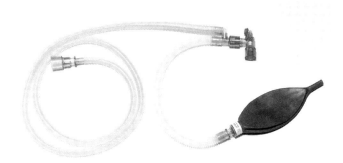

Figure 8.5 Jackson Rees modification of T-piece.

respiration, contamination of inspired gases with the mixed gases from the bag not occurring provided that the expiratory limb has a volume at least equal to the tidal volume and provided that the fresh gas flow is adequate. Ventilation of the expiratory limb with air is the principle used by several paediatric ventilators, the air not reaching as far as the patient, provided that the expiratory limb is of sufficient length. This is also the principle underlying controlled respiration with the Bain system (see below).

Coaxial systems (Bain; Lack). Although first used by Macintosh and Pask in the early 1940s, interest in these systems was rearoused in the 1980s. The most popular of these is the Bain system (Figs 8.6 and 8.7a). In this system, fresh gases are led along the narrow inner tube to the region of the face mask or tracheal tube. The expired gases pass along the outer tube before being vented through the expiratory valve. It may be seen that this corresponds to the Mapleson D system which, for spontaneous respiration, has characteristics similar to the Mapleson E or T-piece systems already described. Thus a fresh gas flow of about twice the minute volume is required to prevent rebreathing. However, the Bain system is more useful as a means of controlled respiration. It has been shown that a fresh gas flow of 70 ml/kg body weight is sufficient to maintain normocarbia, while a fresh gas flow of 100 ml/kg body weight will produce relatively mild hypocarbia. This occurs over a wide range of minute volumes, provided that this exceeds the fresh gas flow. Controlled respiration with the Bain system is achieved by manual compression of the reservoir bag after partially closing the expiratory valve, or by totally closing the expiratory valve and ventilating the expiratory limb with air after removing the reservoir bag (as described above for T-piece systems). It is important to insert an additional metre of corrugated tubing between the ventilator tubing and the end of the expiratory limb of the Bain system to prevent the anaesthetic gases being diluted with air.

The normocarbia produced by IPPV using the Bain circuit has advantages over the hypocarbia produced by many other systems of controlled respiration in that it causes less reduction of cardiac output and spontaneous respiration is resumed more rapidly at the end of the operation. Other advantages are that the tubing is light, long (1.8 m) and flexible and the change from spontaneous to controlled ventilation is easily made because the valve is remote from the patient. Bain systems as supplied by manufacturers are intended to be disposable. Pollution control is easy with a modified APL valve and, as mentioned above, controlled ventilation may be carried out by the simplest of ventilators applied to the expiratory limb. The only type of ventilator that is unsuitable is one driven by the fresh gas supply from the anaesthetic machine (e.g. Manley).

Apart from its relative inefficiency as a method of spontaneous respiration, the main disadvantages of the Bain's system lie in the fragility of the

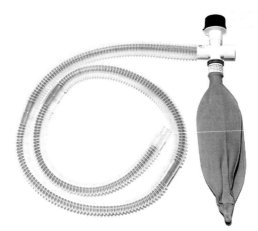

Figure 8.6 Bain coaxial system.

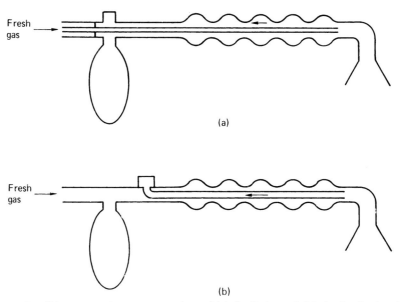

Figure 8.7 Diagrammatic representation of (a) the Bain and (b) the Lack circuits.

plastic tubing and the difficulty of detecting leaks in, or separation of, the small-bore fresh gas tube. The latter has become less of a problem with the introduction of semi-transparent outer tubing. However, before use a simple test should be made to confirm that both inner and outer tubes are intact. The outer tube is tested by closing the APL valve, occluding the patient end of the Bain system with the thumb and turning on a fresh gas flow of about 6 l/min. If the outer tube is intact the reservoir bag will inflate and gentle manual compression will confirm that there are no leaks from the outer tube. The little finger is then inserted inside the end of the expiratory tube to occlude the patient end of the inner (fresh gas) tube. If the inner tube is intact, this occlusion of the fresh gas flow will cause the rotameters to dip below their previous reading or the pressure relief valve to blow off.

The Lack system (Fig. 8.7b) is a coaxial system in which the fresh gases are carried to the patient through the outer tube (the reservoir bag is also on the inspiratory side), expiration occurring down the inner tube to the expiratory valve which is remote from the patient. It is a Mapleson A system, like the Magill circuit, and like the latter requires relatively modest fresh gas flows (approximately equal to minute volume) during spontaneous respiration to prevent rebreathing. It is thus more efficient than the Bain system for spontaneous respiration, while retaining the Bain's advantages of easy scavenging and a valve remote from the patient.

Circle Systems Without CO_2 Absorption

This type of system is of relatively recent origin. The aim of these systems (used mainly with controlled respiration) is to avoid the hypocarbia that almost inevitably occurs during IPPV with circle systems incorporating CO_2 absorption. It has been found that with relatively large tidal volumes (10–15 ml/kg body weight) only mild hypocarbia occurs with fresh gas flows of the order of those for the Bain circuit. It is important to keep the expiratory valve and the point of addition of fresh gases to the circuit well separated to prevent the expulsion of too high a proportion of the fresh gases unused from the system.

Entrainment in T-piece systems (injectors). In this T-piece modification, the inspiratory limb is not at right angles to the patient and expiratory limbs, but is angled towards the patient's limb, or even parallel to it. Intermittent injection of oxygen at high pressure through a needle-sized fresh gas flow orifice pointing in this direction entrains a larger volume of air through the expiratory limb. Stopping the oxygen flow allows the patient to breathe out. This has proved to be a convenient method of maintaining oxygenation of patients during microlaryngoscopy and bronchoscopy.

Insufflation. This form of anaesthesia has been usually confined to ear, nose and throat (ENT) departments. Formerly a hollow hook placed in the corner of the mouth, or the side tube of a Boyle–Davis gag was used to insufflate anaesthetic mixtures, usually during tonsillectomy. This technique may be regarded as a variety of T-piece, the expiratory limb being represented by the patient's mouth and pharynx. Though popular, this was a relatively crude and uncontrolled method of anaesthesia, and nowadays the atmospheric pollution produced would be unacceptable.

A slightly more refined technique is sometimes used for microlaryngo-scopy and laser surgery (Chapter 25). The anaesthetic mixture or more commonly oxygen and air are delivered through a small tube (e.g. a suction catheter) whose tip lies somewhere within the trachea. Anaesthesia is then usually maintained with a total intravenous technique in the spontaneously breathing patient.

Systems with an Inadequate Fresh Gas Flow

These systems derive from the theory that if sufficient oxygen is added to the system to provide the patient's basal requirements, and if some method of carbon dioxide absorption is used, the same anaesthetic mixture can be breathed over and over again.

The main justification for these systems is economy in the use of anaes-thetic gases and vapours. Other advantages are the conservation of expired heat and moisture, and less pollution of the theatre atmosphere. Both spon-taneous breathing and controlled ventilation techniques are satisfactory. In a truly 'closed' system there is less risk of an explosion with explosive anaesthetic mixtures.

Some disadvantages include higher resistance in the systems, bulky equipment, the slow uptake of volatile agents with low flows and the need for accurate monitoring of gases (see below).

Soda-lime

Soda-lime is the substance most commonly used to absorb CO_2. The composition of soda-lime, which varies slightly from manufacturer to manufacturer, is roughly calcium hydroxide, 94%; sodium hydroxide, 5%; potassium hydroxide, 1%.

Inert silicates are added to prevent powdering of the granules, which are of the size referred to as 4–8 mesh. The size of the granules is important to allow a large enough surface area for absorption and to prevent high resistance to gas flow. To the granules are added about 14% of moisture content, which is essential for the reaction with CO_2 to take place. A mixture of barium and calcium hydroxides (Baralyme) is the only commonly used alternative to soda-lime.

The reaction of CO_2 with soda-lime is shown in the formulae below. The calcium hydroxide is responsible for the major part of the CO_2 absorption, but combination occurs first with the more active sodium and potassium hydroxide to form sodium or potassium carbonate which then react with the calcium hydroxide, the sodium and potassium hydroxides being recon-stituted in the process.

$$CO_2 + H_2O \rightarrow H_2CO_3$$

$$H_2CO_3 + 2NaOH \text{ (or 2KOH)} \quad \rightarrow \quad Na_2CO_3 \text{ (or } K_2CO_3) + 2H_2O$$

(sodium	(potassium	(sodium	(potassium
hydroxide)	hydroxide)	carbonate)	carbonate)

$$Na_2CO_3 \text{ (or } K_2CO_3) + Ca(OH)_2 \quad \rightarrow \quad CaCO_3 \qquad 2NaOH \text{ (or 2KOH)}$$

(calcium	(calcium	(regenerated to
hydroxide)	carbonate)	react again)

Chemical indicators are added to some brands of soda-lime so that a colour change occurs when the soda-lime becomes exhausted. Examples are Clayton yellow which changes from pink to yellow and ethyl violet which changes from colourless to violet when the soda-lime loses its efficiency. Too much reliance should not, however, be put on these chemical indicators; it is better to note the period during which the soda-lime has been in use. As a rough guide for this purpose, 1 kg soda-lime should last an anaesthetised adult of average weight for about 8 h.

When soda-lime canisters lie on their sides there is a tendency for the granules to fall away from the upper part of the canister so that the gases may be preferentially channelled through this area without giving up their CO_2. For this reason, soda-lime canisters should be mounted vertically whenever possible.

Soda-lime and Trichloroethylene

Soda-lime should never be used in the presence of trichloroethylene as the combination of heat and alkali may result in the breakdown of trichloroethylene into two toxic gases – dichloracetylene and phosgene. These produce cranial nerve palsies or even death. Trichloroethylene is no longer available in the UK for anaesthetic use.

Circle Systems

It has been stated above that there are many combinations for the relative positioning of the main components of the circle system. These components are two unidirectional valves, two T-piece connections to be placed next to the patient and at the fresh gas inflow point, a soda-lime canister, a reservoir bag and an overflow valve.

One possible arrangement of the components is shown in Figure 8.8. Without discussing the other possibilities in detail, it would, for instance, be pointless to have the overflow valve between the fresh gas inflow and the patient so that fresh gases were vented from the system without ever passing to the patient.

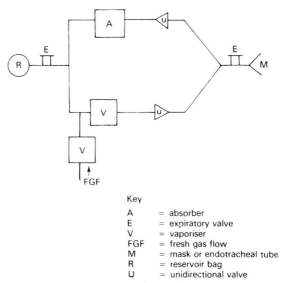

Key

A	=	absorber
E	=	expiratory valve
V	=	vaporiser
FGF	=	fresh gas flow
M	=	mask or endotracheal tube
R	=	reservoir bag
U	=	unidirectional valve

Figure 8.8 Example of a circle arrangement.

As indicated above, the circle systems may be used without soda-lime for spontaneous or controlled respiration, with fresh gas flows down to as low as the patient's alveolar ventilation without any build-up of CO_2. For the average adult this means a fresh gas flow of about 4 l/min. When the fresh gas flow is reduced below the alveolar ventilation it is essential to have a soda-lime canister in the circuit to prevent build-up of CO_2.

Theoretically it is possible to use a circle system as a totally closed system. Once anaesthesia is established, only the patient's basal requirement of 200–250 ml oxygen need be added to the system, the carbon dioxide being absorbed by the soda-lime and the patient losing no volatile anaesthetic to the atmosphere because of the closed system. In practice, this perfect balance is never attained for various reasons, such as the continued uptake of anaesthetic from the system by the patient, and imperfect absorption of CO_2. Concentrations of oxygen and anaesthetic in the system may vary considerably. In practice an oxygen flow rate of at least 0.5 l and total gas flow of at least 1 l is recommended. These systems are gaining popularity again because of the availability and use of accurate oxygen analysers, anaesthetic agent and end-tidal CO_2 monitors.

Position of the vaporiser in the circuit. In circle systems the vaporiser may be outside the circuit (VOC) or inside the circle (VIC). In the case of VOC, the fresh gas passes through the vaporiser before joining the circuit where the concentration of anaesthetic will always be lower than the vaporiser setting as long as uptake by the patient is taking place. Eventually, as equilibrium is reached and the patient ceases to take anaesthetic from the circle, the concentration in the circle will rise towards the vaporiser setting.

The exception to this rule occurs when controlled respiration is used. This applies to any of the systems where compression of the reservoir bag may cause a backflow into the vaporising chamber of gases which have already picked up the volatile anaesthetic. This 'pumping' action may produce concentrations of volatile anaesthetic higher than the vaporiser setting; to prevent this phenomenon vaporisers or anaesthetic machines are now provided with a non-return valve to eliminate the backflow in the system.

In the case of VIC, the gases may pass through the vaporiser many times. In spontaneous respiration the resulting deep anaesthesia and respiratory depression slow the uptake of anaesthetic by the patient so that there is a certain built-in safety factor with this arrangement. However, if controlled respiration is used, this inherent safety is lost and high and potentially lethal concentrations of anaesthetic may be inspired.

9

Vaporisers and Inhalers

● VAPORISATION

Molecules in a liquid are constantly moving, the liquid not disintegrating because of the strong, mutual attraction of the closely packed molecules. Some of the molecules near the surface of the liquid move vertically with sufficient speed to overcome the attraction of the other molecules of the liquid. They become free in the atmosphere above the liquid where they are referred to as the vapour of the liquid. The rate of escape of the molecules is determined by the velocity of their movement, which depends on the temperature of the liquid. As the temperature rises the number of molecules that escape from the surface of the liquid increases, so that the concentration of vapour above the liquid increases. Conversely, as the temperature of the liquid falls, the speed of movement of the molecules is reduced and the concentration of the vapour also falls.

Latent Heat of Vaporisation

This is a most important physical principle when discussing the vaporisation of volatile anaesthetic agents. Vaporisation requires the use of energy, as the natural tendency for the molecules of the liquid to adhere together has to be overcome. The energy is provided as heat, and this is called the latent heat of vaporisation of the liquid.

The latent heat varies from liquid to liquid, but is surprisingly high. For instance, while only 1 calorie of heat is required to raise the temperature of 1 ml water by 1°C, it requires 580 calories to convert 1 ml water into water vapour (steam) without change of temperature (i.e. the latent heat of vaporisation of water is 580).

The heat required for vaporisation may be supplied from an external source, or may be taken from the liquid itself. In the latter case the temperature of the liquid falls, and this is what happens when a volatile anaesthetic liquid is vaporised. As we have seen above, a fall in temperature results in the volatile liquid vaporising less readily, so that the amount of liquid converted into vapour falls. This means that as a stream of gases passes over a volatile anaesthetic liquid in a vaporiser, the concentration of vapour picked up will steadily fall due to the liquid cooling unless it is heated or some form of temperature-compensating mechanism is introduced.

The concept of latent heat also explains other phenomena seen in anaesthesia, for example, the ice that tends to form on the lower part of nitrous oxide cylinders as the gas is run off. The explanation here is that the lower part of the cylinder contains liquid nitrous oxide which has to be vaporised to replace the gaseous nitrous oxide being run off through the valve in the upper part of the cylinder. This vaporisation needs heat, which is taken first from the liquid nitrous oxide itself so that its temperature falls. Heat is taken next from the steel walls of the cylinder which become so cold that the water vapour in the atmosphere condenses on the outer surface of the cylinder and immediately freezes.

● VAPORISERS AND INHALERS

Vaporisers and inhalers are pieces of equipment designed for vaporising volatile anaesthetic liquids. Vaporisers are usually described as having either plenum or draw-over characteristics. A plenum vaporiser is designed for use in a plenum anaesthetic system, i.e. a system where the vaporising gases arise from a high-pressure source such as a pipeline or cylinders. In this type of system no effort is required on the patient's part to draw the gases through the vaporiser, so it is not necessary that the resistance to flow of gases through the vaporiser be particularly low. Examples of this type of vaporiser are the Fluotec and Abingdon vaporisers.

In draw-over vaporisers (the inhalers all belong to this group) the vaporising vehicle (usually air) is drawn through the vaporiser by the patient's own respiratory effort. This means that the resistance of the vaporiser must be low so that the patient does not have to make too great an effort. Examples of this type of vaporiser are the EMO (Epstein–Macintosh–Oxford) inhaler and the OMV (Oxford Miniature Vaporiser). While plenum vaporisers cannot be used in draw-over systems, there is no reason why draw-over vaporisers cannot be used in plenum systems.

The basic arrangement of most modern vaporisers is similar to that of the bottles formerly supplied with the Boyle's anaesthetic apparatus. The construction is shown in Figure 9.1a–c. These vaporisers are essentially bottles with an on–off control lever. In Figure 9.1a the lever is in the 'off' position so that the entire flow of gases bypasses the vaporising bottle. In Figure 9.1b the lever is in the 'on' position so that the entire flow of gases passes into the vaporising bottle. The control lever may be placed in any intermediate position, thus varying the proportion of gas flow diverted over the volatile liquid. Some Boyle's bottles had a further method of

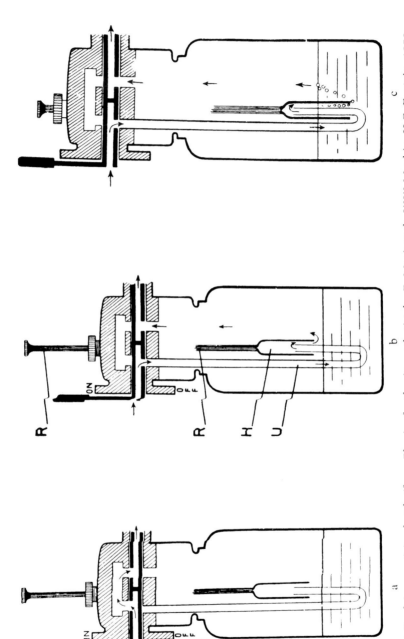

Figure 9.1 Boyle's vaporising bottle (from *Physics for the Anaesthetist*, by R. Macintosh, W.W. Mushin, H.G. Epstein, 1958, courtesy of Blackwell Scientific).

controlling the vapour concentration. This consisted of the rod R which could be used to lower the hood down over the open end of the tube U. As the hood was lowered, the flow of gases escaping from the open end of the tube U was diverted closer and closer to the surface of the volatile liquid. Finally, as shown in Figure 9.1c, the hood could be lowered so that the gases were bubbled through the volatile agent, thus producing the maximum concentration of vapour achievable with this apparatus. Unfortunately the concentration of vapour steadily fell as vaporisation produced cooling of the liquid. With a volatile agent like ether the temperature, and therefore the concentration of ether vapour produced, fell so low that it might be inadequate for anaesthesia. For this reason it was not uncommon to put two Boyle's bottles in series or to surround the Boyle's bottle with a vessel containing warm water in an effort to maintain the ether temperature and therefore the concentration.

Temperature-compensating Devices

Many modern vaporisers conform to this basic configuration of a bottle with a main control knob or lever which divides the gas stream into two parts, one bypassing the vaporising chamber and the other passing through it. In addition, many vaporisers now contain some temperature-compensating device, so that for any setting of the main control lever, the concentration of vapour leaving the vaporiser is constant. These temperature-compensating mechanisms are usually in the form of a bimetallic strip or a thermosensitive capsule.

Bimetallic Strip

The bimetallic strip mechanism depends on the fact that different metals expand to different amounts when heated. A bimetallic strip consists of two bars of different metals riveted together, so that when the whole strip is warmed it bends as the metal with the greater coefficient of expansion lengthens relative to the other bar. The bimetallic strip is made to operate a valve regulating the proportion of the gas stream which bypasses the vaporising chamber. This can be seen in Figure 9.2, which shows a Fluotec mark 2 vaporiser. As the halothane in the vaporising chamber cools, the bimetallic bar tends to open the valve so that a higher proportion of the gas stream is diverted over the surface of the halothane. Conversely, if the halothane warms up, the bimetallic strip-operated valve tends to close and a higher proportion of the gas stream bypasses the vaporising chamber. In this way, the concentration of halothane emitting from the vaporiser remains constant despite alterations in temperature of the liquid halothane produced either by vaporisation or by changes in the ambient temperature.

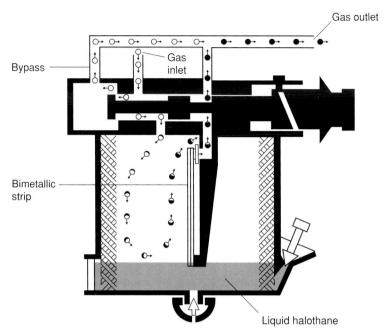

Figure 9.2 Fluotec mark 2 vaporiser in 'on' position (courtesy of Cyprane Ltd, Keighley, Yorkshire).

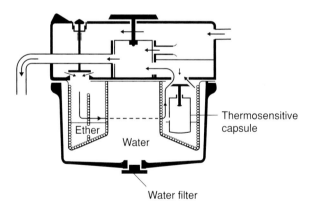

Figure 9.3 Cross-section of EMO vaporiser.

Thermosensitive Capsule

An example of a thermosensitive capsule is shown in the diagram of the EMO vaporiser (Fig. 9.3). In this case the capsule consists of a metal bellows which operates a plunger which opens and closes a valve. The bellows is surrounded by ether vapour in a closed container. In this case

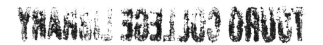

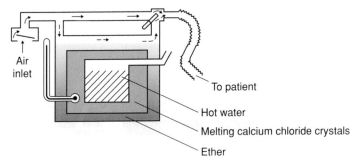

Air
inlet

To patient

Hot water

Melting calcium chloride crystals

Ether

Figure 9.4 Oxford vaporiser mark 1.

the valve alters the proportion of the gas stream which passes through the vaporising chamber. The capsule sits within the vaporising chamber so that a fall in the temperature of the ether in that chamber is accompanied by a fall in temperature of the ether vapour within the closed container. This causes an opening of the valve so that a higher proportion of the gas stream passes through the vaporising chamber. The converse applies if the temperature of the ether in the vaporising chamber rises. A similar method of temperature compensation is found in the Abingdon vaporiser.

Some vaporisers, for example the EMO and OMV, have a water-jacket or container surrounding the vaporising chamber. This is not a temperature-compensating device, but acts as a heat reservoir so that the temperature of the volatile agent does not tend to fall as quickly as if the vaporising chamber was surrounded simply by air.

Two other methods of dealing with the problem presented by the changes in vapour concentration associated with changes of temperature will be mentioned.

The first was the ingenious principle of the mark 1 Oxford vaporiser for ether (Fig. 9.4). In this apparatus the vaporising chamber was surrounded by a vessel containing melting calcium chloride crystals. These have a constant temperature while in the melting state, and maintain the ether at a constant temperature. The other method is the 'copper kettle' apparatus which gained considerable popularity in the USA. This vaporiser consisted of a vaporising chamber made of copper, which has a high thermal conductivity, and was attached to an anaesthetic tabletop of the same material. This arrangement ensured that the contents of the vaporising chamber remained at room temperature. The vaporiser was supplied with its own relatively low flow of oxygen which was divided into fine bubbles as it passed through the volatile agent. In this way, the oxygen flowing through the vaporiser was always completely saturated with anaesthetic vapour; this stream then joined the main stream of anaesthetic gases. Provided that the flow rates of the two streams and the temperature of the liquid (which stayed constant) were known, the final concentration of the vapour in the emerging gas stream could be read off from tables. This relatively com-plicated system never gained popularity in the UK.

Flow Compensation

In the Fluotec mark 2, the output of the vaporiser depended on the flow rate of the gas passing through it and charts had to be followed to ensure stable concentration. Later models of the Fluotec vaporisers do not have this problem as the liquid is fully saturated over a wide range of flow rates.

Pressure Effects

Back-pressure from the ventilator or obstruction to the outlet of gas can result in fluctuations in vapour output or damage to the vaporiser. This is prevented by inserting safety valves downstream of the vaporiser and by increasing the resistance to flow through the vaporiser (Chapter 8).

Improvements in the design of vaporisers include the incorporation of wicks in the vaporiser chamber to ensure full exposure of the gas to the volatile agent and thus compensation for any fall in the level of the liquid.

Safety features in the modern vaporisers include colour coding for vapor-isers and colour-coded fillers for specific volatile agents, for example, red for halothane, orange for enflurane and purple for isoflurane. Selective switches ensure that only one vaporiser can be left open at one time, thus avoiding accidents.

● THE EMO INHALER

The EMO ether inhaler (Fig. 9.5) is a temperature-compensated, draw-over ether vaporiser which was introduced in 1956. It is used with the OIB (Oxford Inflating Bellows) which consists of two unidirectional flap valves and a spring-loaded bellows. There is also a stopcock for adding oxygen directly to the bellows.

Ether concentrations of up to 20% can be obtained by moving the lever on top of the vaporiser, these concentrations being kept accurate over a wide range of temperatures by the temperature-compensating device already mentioned, which is located inside the casing of the vaporiser. The apparatus also has a water-jacket with a capacity of about 1200 ml.

This apparatus may be used simply with air as the vaporising vehicle with either spontaneous or controlled respiration. For the former, a Heidbrink or non-return valve may be used. Controlled respiration may be performed with the OIB and a closed Heidbrink valve by intermittently raising the face mask, or a thumb placed over the suction port of a Portex connection if the patient is intubated. More conveniently, an inflating valve such as

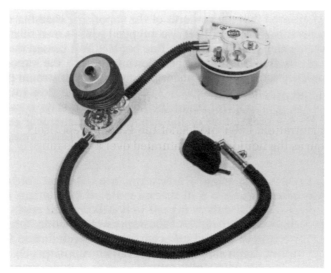

Figure 9.5 EMO inhaler.

the Ambu-E may be used, but in this case the magnet supplied with the OIB must be placed over the flap valve on the patient side of the OIB. If this is not done, the valve will not cycle into the expiratory (open from patient to atmosphere) position and the patient will become progressively overinflated with each breath.

The one situation in which the magnet must not be left in place over the flap valve is when the patient is breathing spontaneously with a Heidbrink valve. This will result in the patient rebreathing back into the bellows instead of out through the Heidbrink valve, which is very dangerous.

Oxygen may be added to the EMO system either by a T-piece system plugged into the inlet port of the EMO or via the stopcock on the OIB. The former is preferable (except when the OIB is being used simply for resuscitation) as oxygen added at the OIB will dilute the concentration of ether emitting from the EMO. It is important to remember that while ether and air are for practical purposes non-detonable, the addition of oxygen produces a most explosive mixture.

Further refinements of the EMO system are the addition of OMVs for halothane (which should be placed between the EMO and OIB) or its conversion into a plenum system for use with nitrous oxide and oxygen. The prior administration of about 2% halothane for 2–3 min has a powerful depressant effect on the coughing evoked by ether, so that induction with the latter may be greatly facilitated.

Another important modification of the EMO system is the so-called Tri-Service (Army, Air Force and Navy) system. This involves the substitution of OMVs for the EMO inhaler. This can be used for spontaneous or controlled respiration anaesthesia and its portability and efficiency was proved in the Falklands campaign.

Almost any operation can be carried out with the EMO system using air and ether alone. This fact, plus the robustness, reliability and portability of the EMO, makes it a most important piece of anaesthetic equipment worldwide, especially in underdeveloped countries where compressed gases may be either unobtainable or prohibitively expensive.

10

Volatile Anaesthetic Agents

*•Ether •Halothane •Trichloroethylene •Enflurane •Isoflurane •Desflurane
•Sevoflurane*

Volatile anaesthetic agents depend on uptake by the lungs and subsequent diffusion across the alveolar capillary membrane into the bloodstream. Apart from using this method of administration, however, the volatile anaesthetic agents exert their effects like any other drug dissolved in blood, and therefore in terms of anaesthesia, possess the important properties of hypnosis, analgesia and relaxation in varying degrees.

Uptake by the lungs (Chapter 5) depends on the physical properties of the agent concerned as well as on variations in minute volume and alveolar ventilation. The importance of saturated vapour pressure in terms of the maximum vapour concentration of any particular agent, together with blood/gas solubility coefficients, have both already been emphasised. The values of these, for the volatile agents considered in this chapter, are listed in Table 10.1.

Although volatile agents are generally used for maintaining anaesthesia it is perfectly feasible to use them for induction, particularly in children; for this purpose some agents are much better than others; for example, sevoflurane is much more pleasant to inhale than either halothane or isoflurane. In general, however, we must consider the agents in terms of their contribution towards a balanced anaesthetic technique and therefore their relative properties in terms of hypnosis, analgesia and relaxation. These are summarised in Table 10.2 and it can be seen that the only agent to possess all three properties is ether, which at the same time is explosive when used with N_2O or O_2 and therefore little used today. The volatile agents are broadly divided into ethers and hydrocarbons. The addition of halogen radicals (fluoride, chloride, bromide) to molecules of increasing size tends to increase their potency.

In addition to their pharmacological contribution to general anaesthesia, the volatile anaesthetic agents must be considered in terms of their effects on blood pressure, cardiac output, respiration, peripheral vascular resistance (PVR) and intracranial pressure (ICP), via an increase in cerebral blood

Table 10.1 Physical properties of volatile anaesthetics

	Boiling point (°C)	Saturated vapour pressure at 20°C	Solubility coefficient		MAC (%)	% Metabolised
			Blood/gas	Oil/H_2O		
Halothane	50	243	2.36	330	0.77	18–20
Ether	35	442	12.1	3.2	1.92	6
Trichloroethylene	87.5	60	9.5	400	0.17	Small
Enflurane	56.5	174.5	1.9	120	1.68	3
Isoflurane	49	250	1.4	174	1.15	0.3
Desflurane	23.5	664	0.4	18.7	6	Minimal
Sevoflurane	58.5	160	0.7	47	1.7	2.5

Table 10.2 Pharmacological properties of volatile anaesthetics

	Hypnosis	Analgesia	Relaxation
Halothane	++		++
Ether	+	+	+
Trichloroethylene	+	++	(+)
Enflurane	++	?(+)	++
Isoflurane	++	?(+)	++
Desflurane	++	?	++
Sevoflurane	++	?	++

Table 10.3 Clinical pharmacology of volatile anaesthetic agents

	Halothane	Enflurane	Isoflurane	Desflurane	Sevoflurane
Heart rate	↓↓	→	→	↓	→
Blood pressure	↓↓	↓↓	↓↓	↘	↘
Myocardial contractility	↓↓	↓	→	→	→
PVR	↓	↓	↓↓	↓	↘
Cardiac output	↓	↓	→	→	→
CBF	↑	↑	→	→	→
Respiratory depression	↓	↓	↓	↓	↓
Bronchial irritation	−	(+)	++	−	−

flow (CBF); in many instances their routes of metabolism and excretion are also important (Table 10.3).

● ETHER

Although not used in modern anaesthetic practice, ether is a very safe agent in relatively untrained hands (e.g. in developing countries), and uniquely it possesses hypnotic, analgesic and relaxant properties. However, it is a relatively soluble anaesthetic agent and therefore takes a long time to induce anaesthesia if used for an inhalational induction (Chapter 5), but ether is relatively cheap and is widely used in underdeveloped countries. It tends to produce raised levels of adrenaline and therefore an increased pulse rate and a relatively steady blood pressure. Hyperglycaemia, bronchial and coronary artery dilatation, an increase in respiratory rate and dilatation of the pupils are also results of catecholamine release. The relatively high blood solubility of ether means that recovery from this agent may be prolonged although it is excreted entirely unchanged.

● HALOTHANE

Halothane is widely used in a great many different anaesthetic techniques. It is an excellent hypnotic and, being relatively insoluble in blood, produces rapid induction of anaesthesia. It is also a good relaxant though not sufficient alone to allow abdominal surgery except in infants. Even so, halothane possesses no analgesic properties and therefore requires supplementary analgesia, either in the form of premedication or intraoperatively. It produces significant effects on blood pressure by depressing both the myocardium and the conducting tissue of the heart. Halothane also causes an overall reduction in peripheral resistance by producing vasodilatation in skin which is partially balanced by vasoconstriction in skeletal muscle.

Vagal stimulation results in a decreased pulse rate and aggravates the hypotension produced. Like other agents it produces dose-related respiratory depression. About 18% of the inhaled halothane is metabolised by the liver, the remainder being excreted unchanged, but halothane has been shown to cause alterations in hepatic function, particularly after repeated exposure to the drug. Hepatitis following repeat halothane anaesthesia has been demonstrated unequivocally, but in only very few cases. Several possible causes have been suggested, from hepatic hypoxia to direct hepatotoxicity. Another likely cause is a hypersensitivity reaction to a metabolite of halothane (Chapter 21), but as the histological picture is identical to viral hepatitis it is possible that an exacerbation of such a disease may be the cause of the hepatitis. Other agents such as methoxyflurane have also been shown to produce hepatitis. Halothane relaxes the pregnant uterus and should not be used, except in very low concentrations, in pregnant patients. As part of its vasodilator action, it increases CBF and therefore ICP.

● TRICHLOROETHYLENE

Although little used now, trichloroethylene (Trilene) is an excellent analgesic and weak hypnotic, though its high blood solubility produces prolonged induction and recovery. It has relatively little effect on either blood pressure or pulse rate, though it may produce cardiac dysrhythmias of all kinds, leading to hypotension. It has also been used in obstetrics for inhalation analgesia and is extremely cheap. Trichloroethylene should not be used with soda-lime in a closed circuit because toxic metabolites (Chapter 8) may be produced which cause cranial nerve damage. Trichloroethylene is excreted by the lungs almost entirely unchanged.

● ENFLURANE

Enflurane possesses many similar properties to halothane and is a good hypnotic and relaxant, though its analgesic properties are in some doubt. Its effects on the cardiovascular and respiratory system are similar to halothane, producing an overall reduction in blood pressure and heart rate. The main advantage of enflurane seems to be that it is metabolised to a far lesser extent than halothane and has not yet been implicated in postoperative hepatitis (enflurane metabolism is less than 3%; halothane 18%). Enflurane does not cause catecholamine release or associated problems and appears to be acceptable for inhalational induction of anaesthesia. It is more irritant to inhale than halothane, but would appear to be a better drug for use in patients with cardiovascular disease in whom myocardial perfusion is borderline. Like halothane, enflurane increases ICP and also should not be used in epileptic patients in whom it may precipitate convulsions.

● ISOFLURANE

Isoflurane is a halogenated ether and an optical isomer of enflurane. Unlike both halothane and enflurane, however, it does not depress myocardial contractility or conduction. Isoflurane produces hypotension by peripheral vasodilatation and increasing doses of the agent will lower blood pressure and simultaneously increase the depth of anaesthesia. This tends to prevent the reflex tachycardia which results from other techniques of induced hypotension. Isoflurane is metabolised <0.3% making it a suitable agent for use in patients with liver disease. For this reason, it is highly unlikely to be associated with the production of hepatitis. Isoflurane is irritant to inhale and therefore relatively unsuitable for inhalational induction. It increases CBF and ICP, though it is probably the best anaesthetic agent for use in neurosurgical anaesthesia.

● DESFLURANE

Desflurane is a very rapidly acting inhalational agent, though its minimum alveolar concentration (MAC) of 6% indicates a relatively low potency. It is minimally metabolised and tends to produce a modest fall in blood pressure by vasodilatation, without affecting myocardial contractility. It is irritant to inhale and therefore not very suitable for inhalational induction. In many ways, it is similar to isoflurane with even more rapid recovery times, making it very suitable for day-case anaesthesia.

● SEVOFLURANE

This is another relatively potent inhalational agent which produces only moderate hypotension without myocardial depression. It is not irritant to inhale and so is suitable for paediatric inhalational induction, producing only relatively low levels of respiratory depression. Sevoflurane is metabolised to a similar extent to enflurane (2.5%) and it may be that toxic metabolites (Compounds A and B) limit its use, particularly in a closed circuit in combination with soda-lime. This is a potential problem since these newer agents tend to be very expensive and therefore should be used at low flow rates in a circle system to minimise costs. Neither desflurane nor sevoflurane has a major effect on CBF.

11

Neuromuscular Transmission and Muscle-relaxant Drugs

•History •Neuromuscular transmission •Types of neuromuscular block
•Individual drugs •Antibiotics and muscle-relaxant drugs
•Nerve stimulators •Postoperative apnoea

● HISTORY

The early explorers of South America brought back reports of a mysterious arrow poison used by the South American Indians. Small quantities of this poison – curare – probably reached Europe, but it was not until 1851 that Sir Benjamin Brodie published a book describing some experiments with the substance. These included a description of how an ass treated with curare was kept alive by artificial respiration (happily not by mouth-to-mouth respiration, but by a bellows inserted in a tracheostomy!).

In 1850 Claude Bernard, the great physiologist, showed how the site of action of curare is neither on the nerve nor on the muscle, but on the neuromuscular junction.

Crude curare was made from various sources, but in 1935 King isolated one of the active constituents – the alkaloid d-tubocurarine which came from the roots of a small plant, *Chondrodendron tomentosum*.

In 1940 Bennet described the use of d-tubocurarine to soften the convulsions produced by electroconvulsive therapy. In 1942 Griffith and Johnson of Montreal described the first use of d-tubocurarine to provide muscle relaxation for surgery; this paper marked one of the milestones of modern anaesthesia.

Suxamethonium was introduced into clinical practice in 1951 at the Karolinska Institute in Stockholm.

● NEUROMUSCULAR TRANSMISSION

The passage of an impulse down a nerve fibre is believed to be an electrical phenomenon. Similarly, the spread of an impulse across a muscle fibre causing it to contract is also thought to be electrical. However, the transmission of the impulse from the nerve fibre to the muscle fibre is carried out by the chemical substance acetylcholine, and this occurs at special junctional areas between the nerve fibre and muscle fibre, usually referred to as the neuromuscular or myoneural junction (Fig. 11.1).

The nerve-ending part of the neuromuscular junction is called the presynaptic or prejunctional area. Acetylcholine is manufactured, stored and, when a nerve impulse arrives, released from this area of the nerve ending.

Acetylcholine then crosses the extremely narrow gap to arrive at the muscle side of the neuromuscular junction. This is called the postsynaptic area or motor end-plate. The motor end-plate contains special acetylcholine receptor sites. On the arrival of sufficient acetylcholine the muscle membrane of the postsynaptic area becomes permeable to sodium ions, which pass into the muscle cell and produce sudden electrical depolarisation. If this current of depolarisation (also called the motor end-plate potential) reaches a certain magnitude the depolarisation spreads to the adjacent part of the muscle fibre (when it is called the muscle action potential) and is propagated across the surface of the muscle fibre, causing the contraction of the fibre in its wake.

In the meantime the acetylcholine is broken down in a fraction of a second by an enzyme called acetylcholinesterase, which is present at the motor end-plate. The neuromuscular junction is then ready to receive and transmit the next nerve impulse.

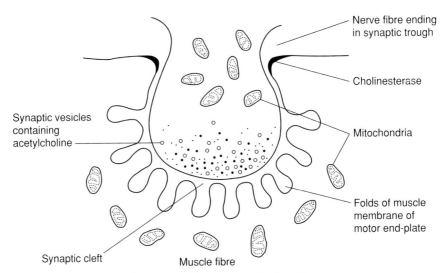

Figure 11.1 Neuromuscular junction.

● TYPES OF NEUROMUSCULAR BLOCK

Depolarising Block

Neuromuscular blocking agents of this group produce depolarisation at the postsynaptic membrane in the same way as acetylcholine. However, once depolarisation has occurred it is maintained, so that when acetylcholine is released by the nerve stimulus it can produce no further depolarisation and paralysis occurs. The relaxation produced by depolarising block is preceded by a short period of muscle fasciculation as the agent produces depolarisation.

Non-depolarising Block

The non-depolarising blocking agents (also formerly called competitive inhibitory blocking agents) are believed to attach themselves to the receptor sites on the postsynaptic membrane to which the acetylcholine molecules normally become attached. The acetylcholine is prevented from reaching the end-plate receptor site in sufficient quantity to produce depolarisation, thus explaining the name given to this type of block.

If acetylcholine is present in sufficient concentration it is capable of displacing the non-depolarising blocker from the receptor sites so that the neuromuscular junction can function again. This is achieved clinically by administering an anticholinesterase drug which inhibits the enzyme cholinesterase, whose normal function is to break down the acetylcholine at the neuromuscular junction. Thus the concentration of acetylcholine builds up and the block is overcome.

The anticholinesterase most frequently used in anaesthesia is neostigmine. Besides its action in reversing a non-depolarising block, however, neostigmine also has unwanted muscarinic effects (Chapter 13), the most important of which are bradycardia (or even cardiac arrest) and stimulation of bronchial and salivary secretion. These muscarinic actions of neostigmine are antagonised by atropine and glycopyrrolate, so it is customary to give these drugs with (or immediately before) the neostigmine in the usual adult dose of atropine 1.2–1.8 mg or glycopyrrolate 0.5 mg with neostigmine 2.5–5.0 mg. Nevertheless, the neostigmine usually just 'wins' in these proportions and it is unusual for patients in the recovery room after this combination of drugs to have a faster pulse than normal. This is not necessarily an indication of the patient's well-being, of course, but merely an indication that they have recently been given neostigmine.

As anticholinesterase drugs increase the concentration of acetylcholine at the neuromuscular junction, and as acetylcholine causes depolarisation, these drugs tend to have a depolarising blocking action of their own and to potentiate the effect of any depolarising agents that may be circulating.

It is therefore unwise to give a short-acting depolarising agent in an attempt to reintroduce neuromuscular blockade after a non-depolarising block has been reversed by neostigmine. If neuromuscular block does occur it is likely to be prolonged.

Phase II Block (Dual Block)

If depolarising blocking agents are given repeatedly to produce a prolonged period of relaxation, the depolarising block eventually changes its nature. The block increasingly shows the properties of a non-depolarising block, in particular it being possible at least partially to reverse the block by an anticholinesterase. The readiness with which this type of block becomes of clinical significance with intermittent suxamethonium varies from patient to patient but is seldom important with a total dose of under 500 mg in a fit adult. A marked degree of dual block is best avoided – if intermittent suxamethonium or a suxamethonium infusion is being used – by ensuring every now and again that the patient is adequately 'coming out' of the incremental doses of the drug.

● INDIVIDUAL DRUGS

Depolarising Agents

Suxamethonium

Suxamethonium (Scoline), the only depolarising agent still in common clinical use, was introduced in 1951. Usually 75–100 mg is given to intubate a male adult, the effect coming on in a circulation time and lasting for 3–5 min. The muscle fasciculations which it causes before paralysis may be violent. 'Suxamethonium pains' are skeletal muscle pains that occur in some patients after receiving suxamethonium. They are thought to be related in some way to the fasciculations, although their severity is not directly related to the degree of visible fasciculation. They occur most commonly and most severely in patients who are quickly ambulant after their anaesthetic and their incidence has been reported as being as high as 80%. In contrast, an incidence as low as 2% has been reported after major thoracic surgery. They are also uncommon in children and in the elderly. Their frequency and severity can be reduced by giving a small dose of a non-depolarising agent, for example, 1 mg vecuronium at least 2 min before the suxamethonium. Unfortunately this technique slightly reduces the efficacy of the suxamethonium, which may be a disadvantage if intubation is urgent or difficult.

Other side-effects of suxamethonium associated with the muscle fasciculations are increased intraocular pressure due to contraction of the intraocular muscles and an increase in serum potassium due to muscle fibre rupture. The former complication may be dangerous in certain eye procedures (e.g. where there is a perforating injury to the eye or in cataract operations). The rise in serum potassium due to muscle damage is not usually serious unless the potassium concentration is already raised. In both these events it is probably better to avoid depolarising muscle relaxants or, if they are considered essential, to precede them with a small dose of a non-depolarising agent as described above.

The only other significant side-effect of suxamethonium is its tendency to produce bradycardia, especially after the injection of a second dose. This effect is blocked by atropine and many anaesthetists recommend that this drug be given intravenously if not before the first, at least before the second dose of suxamethonium.

While the commonest use of suxamethonium is to provide good intubating conditions, it may be used to provide relaxation for longer operations by giving incremental doses (of about 25 mg in an adult) or by using a suxamethonium infusion, for example, suxamethonium 500 mg in normal saline 500 ml. Two problems make this less universally popular for prolonged muscle relaxation than the non-depolarising agents. The first of these is the possibility of dual block developing; the second is the relative difficulty of providing as smooth a level of muscular relaxation as with the longer-acting agents.

Suxamethonium (Scoline) Apnoea

Suxamethonium is usually rapidly broken down in the plasma by a naturally occurring enzyme called plasma (or pseudo) cholinesterase. This usually gives suxamethonium an action of only 3–5 min. However, a few people possess an atypical pseudocholinesterase enzyme which has very little ability to break down suxamethonium. This abnormal enzyme is inherited by transmission of an abnormal gene, affecting about one in 3000 people. In these patients suxamethonium has a more prolonged action, often in the 2–4 h range, the suxamethonium being broken down by alkaline hydrolysis, a process which does not play an important role in normal patients. Essentially the treatment consists of ventilating the patient, preferably with a mixture of nitrous oxide and oxygen until adequate respiration returns. Confirmation that the apnoea is due to this cause may be obtained by testing the patient's serum for atypical pseudocholinesterase. If the test is positive it is important to test close relatives in the same way to anticipate their extreme sensitivity to suxamethonium. Every effort should be made to avoid giving suxamethonium to those affected.

Non-depolarising Agents

The remaining agents discussed in this chapter all belong to this group. They are all slower in onset than suxamethonium, adequate conditions for intubation not usually occurring in under 2–3 min. As they do not produce depolarisation these agents do not produce muscle fasciculations or any of the complications associated with them. They are relatively long-acting, but their action is reversed by neostigmine. Probably the 'ideal' muscle relaxant would be a non-depolarising agent with an onset as rapid as that of suxamethonium and a very short action. Claims that various new agents almost fulfil these criteria have not been substantiated.

d-Tubocurarine Chloride (Tubarine)

This purified alkaloid is the only naturally occurring substance still available as a neuromuscular blocking agent, although it is now rarely used in the UK. It is relatively slow in onset (about 3 min) and lasts for 30–45 min, although none of the non-depolarising agents has an abrupt end-point. For endotracheal intubation a dose of 40–45 mg is required in a 70 kg man, this being reduced by one-third for abdominal muscle relaxation if intubation has previously been carried out under suxamethonium. As with other non-depolarising agents, incremental doses are about one-fifth of the intubation dose. In the presence of halothane and ether the dosage requirements for d-tubocurarine are reduced, but it is unlikely that these agents act in precisely the same way as d-tubocurarine.

One of the main side-effects of d-tubocurarine is its tendency to produce hypotension. It probably does this mainly by myocardial depression, but animal experiments suggest that it may have some blocking effect on the sympathetic ganglia and also some histamine-releasing action. As histamine may cause bronchospasm, theoretically this is not the relaxant of choice for asthmatics. The tendency to reduce blood pressure is made use of, especially in conjunction with halothane, as a method of producing controlled hypotension to reduce surgical bleeding. The local release of histamine after injection of d-tubocurarine is sometimes seen as erythema and weals along the line of the vein. These reactions are not serious and usually fade in a few minutes.

d-Tubocurarine is excreted unchanged by the kidneys, the biliary system providing an alternative route which may be particularly valuable when renal function is impaired.

In ill patients the effect of d-tubocurarine may be difficult to reverse completely with neostigmine, the respiration in particular remaining inadequate with 'see-sawing' movements of the abdomen and chest, and a 'tracheal tug', the larynx jerking downwards towards the chest with each inspiration. The mechanism of this resistance to neostigmine is unknown, but it seems to be commoner in the presence of a metabolic acidosis. This problem may arise with any of the non-depolarising drugs, as well as with d-tubocurarine.

Pancuronium Bromide (Pavulon)

This is a synthetic non-depolarising drug, and is unusual in that it has a steroid ring configuration. Its rapid onset makes it a popular choice where a non-depolariser is to be used for endotracheal intubation, and its duration of action probably lies between that of vecuronium and alcuronium. A 70 kg man would require 8–10 mg for good intubating conditions and a woman 8 mg. Incremental doses of about one-fifth these amounts are required.

The effects of pancuronium on the cardiovascular system are to produce a tachycardia (usually mild or moderate) and sometimes a slight increase in blood pressure. It is not believed to release histamine or cross the placenta in significant amounts.

Pancuronium is excreted largely unchanged by the kidneys, but metabolism in the liver and excretion in the bile is a valuable alternative excretory mechanism.

Vecuronium Bromide (Norcuron)

This has a speed of onset similar to pancuronium and a medium duration of action (20–30 min). The dose is the same as or slightly larger than that for pancuronium. It has the least effect on the cardiovascular system of any of the relaxants, causing neither tachycardia nor hypotension, and it does not release histamine. It is excreted mostly in the bile and only to a small extent through the kidneys, making it a useful drug in cases of renal failure. Its shorter duration of action makes it suitable for continuous infusion.

Rocuronium Bromide (Esmeron)

This is another medium-acting, non-depolarising agent similar to vecuronium, although its onset of action is faster. It is available in liquid form and, in contrast to vecuronium, does not induce bradycardia by vagal stimulation. In all other aspects, it is similar to vecuronium and is suitable for total intravenous anaesthesia (TIVA). Like vecuronium, its action is potentiated by volatile anaesthetic agents.

Atracurium Besylate (Tracrium)

Another non-depolarising drug, atracurium has a speed of onset and duration of action similar to that of vecuronium. About 40 mg is recommended to intubate a 70 kg patient. Atracurium is unique in that it is broken down in the plasma mainly by a process known as 'Hofmann elimination' which occurs at plasma pH and body temperature. The termination of action of this drug is not dependent on metabolism or excretion by either the liver or the kidneys, so it is useful in hepatic or renal failure (Chapter 32). Under normal circumstances its action is reversed using atropine/neostigmine.

Atracurium has minimal effects on the heart and blood pressure, and has a weak histamine-releasing action.

It should be noted that anaesthetic agents (e.g. halothane) or surgical manoeuvres (e.g. peritoneal traction) which cause vagal stimulation are more likely to produce a bradycardia when cardiovascularly inactive drugs like vecuronium or atracurium are being used rather than tachycardia-inducing agents like pancuronium.

Cisatracurium (Nimbex)

This drug is similar to atracurium, though longer acting. It is said to release less histamine and is more likely to require reversal with neostigmine, than atracurium. Its action is potentiated by volatile anaesthetic agents.

Mivacurium (Mivacron)

This drug is even shorter acting than vecuronium. Unfortunately, its onset of action is still significantly slower than succinylcholine. It is also metabolised in an unusual way for a non-depolarising drug in that it is broken down by plasma (pseudo-) cholinesterase, like succinylcholine. Like vecuronium and atracurium, one of its major advantages is its potential administration by continuous infusion as part of TIVA.

● ANTIBIOTICS AND MUSCLE-RELAXANT DRUGS

Several antibiotics, particularly the aminoglycosides, for example, gentamycin, neomycin and vancomycin, have neuromuscular blocking properties. They tend to potentiate non-depolarising block and deaths have been reported when large doses of some of these antibiotics have been given to patients under anaesthesia. Particularly high doses may be given intraperitoneally during colonic surgery. The block produced is partly reversed by neostigmine but calcium appears to be more effective.

● NERVE STIMULATORS

Portable, battery-powered nerve stimulators are becoming increasingly popular (Fig. 11.2). By means of two electrodes placed over a peripheral nerve (commonly the ulnar nerve at the wrist) they can apply a variety of different types of stimulation the effect of which is seen by contraction

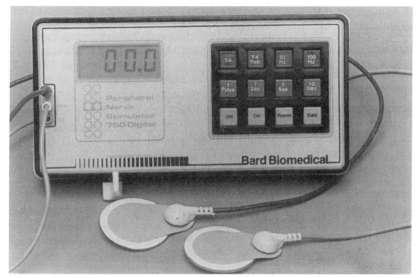

Figure 11.2 A typical battery-powered nerve stimulator.

of a muscle supplied by that nerve (usually the adductor muscle of the thumb). These types of stimulation are usually either single stimuli eliciting a twitch response, tetanic bursts at rates of 50 or 100 cycles/s or as groups of four stimuli at a rate of 2/s – the so-called 'train of four' stimulation.

By studying the effects of these different stimuli on the response of the adductor pollicis it is possible to estimate the degree of neuromuscular blockade. This is useful not only in adjusting increments or infusions of muscle relaxants, but also in deciding whether residual neuromuscular blockade is responsible for postoperative apnoea. The nerve stimulator is less useful in deciding between depolarising and non-depolarising blocks as nearly all prolonged blocks are non-depolarising in nature.

● POSTOPERATIVE APNOEA

There are many reasons why a patient may not breathe (or may breathe inadequately) at the end of an anaesthetic. In some cases remedial treatment may be possible; in others, given time, normal spontaneous respiration will return of its own accord. Whatever the cause, it is fundamental that the patient be ventilated until normal respiration is re-established.

Some of the many causes of prolonged apnoea are given below. In any one case, more than one of these factors is frequently involved.

Depression of the Respiratory Centre

Depression of the respiratory centre in the brain occurs by residual effect of a narcotic premedication or residual traces of induction or maintenance agents, for example, thiopentone or halothane.

Hypocapnia

This commonly plays at least a part in the apnoea often seen at the end of a controlled respiration anaesthetic. There is no stimulus to the medullary respiratory centre to recommence breathing until the arterial P_{CO_2} returns to its normal preoperative level.

Hypercapnia

This is a less common cause of apnoea, being due usually to a fault in the anaesthetic circuit, resulting in excessive sedation.

General State of the Patient

The gravely ill patient, for example, one with severe hypotension, is less likely to breathe at the end of the operation. In addition, some new illness, such as a myocardial infarction or cerebrovascular accident, may have occurred during the anaesthetic.

Atypical Plasma (Pseudo) Cholinesterase

The apnoea which occurs in patients with this abnormal enzyme when they are given suxamethonium is described on p. 113.

Low Normal Plasma (Pseudo) Cholinesterase

This most commonly occurs in the presence of liver disease, in patients who have been contaminated with certain organophosphorus insecticides and in patients given ecothiopate iodide eye drops.

Phase II Block

This type of block is mentioned on p. 112 and usually follows the administration of an excessive amount of suxamethonium.

Acid–Base and Electrolyte Disturbances

The difficulty in reversing the effects of d-tubocurarine in the presence of a metabolic acidosis has also been mentioned. A similar position may arise in the presence of a low serum potassium.

12

Analgesics and Anti-emetics

*•Opiate analgesics •Neuroleptanaesthesia •Opiate antagonists
•Opiate-like analgesics •Anti-emetics*

● OPIATE ANALGESICS

Analgesia is one of the fundamental requirements of a balanced anaesthetic and, apart from certain volatile or gaseous anaesthetic agents which possess analgesic properties, modern anaesthetists employ many opiate or related substances to produce intra-operative analgesia. As such, these drugs may be given either as premedicants or, equally commonly nowadays, during anaesthesia. More recently there has been a tendency for increasingly large doses of, in particular, the synthetic opiate fentanyl to be used intra-operatively to abolish many of the potentially harmful effects of anaesthetic and surgical 'stress'.

There are several pharmacological effects common to all the opiate analgesics and their derivatives:

Analgesia
Sedation
Respiratory depression
Depression of the cough reflex
Nausea and vomiting
Gastrointestinal sphincteric spasm
Histamine release
Addiction
Cardiovascular depression
Constipation and bowel atony

Although it has been possible with some of the newer synthetic opiate analgesics to produce drugs with fewer side-effects than morphine or pethidine, it has so far been impossible to obtain a drug free from either addiction or respiratory depression, while at the same time maintaining satisfactory analgesia. However, the wider therapeutic ratio (i.e. the ratio between the effective dose and the toxic dose of the drug) of fentanyl and phenoperidine has made it possible to give far larger doses of these drugs for intra-operative analgesia and stress. In addition to the side-effects of opiate analgesics given above, it is important to consider the various available drugs in terms of their duration of action because this is one of the factors governing the wide range available.

Morphine

As one of the oldest and most effective of the analgesic agents, morphine is used as the standard with which the newer analgesics are compared. Morphine is a potent analgesic and also possesses a distinct euphoric action. The important side-effects are as follows:

- *Respiratory depression*: This tends to limit the intramuscular dose that may be safely given to a spontaneously breathing patient up to 10–15 mg but the therapeutic ratio is sufficient to allow up to 100 mg to be given in 1 h without toxic effects if the patient is ventilated. Morphine may also be used as a respiratory depressant in intensive care to control patients on artificial ventilation.
- *Depression of the cough reflex.*
- *Nausea and vomiting*: This is a significant problem and it is a good idea to give an anti-emetic, for example, prochlorperazine, with morphine.
- *Smooth muscle constriction*: Constriction of the smooth muscle of the large bowel produces constipation and may also predispose to break-down of bowel anastomoses. Morphine may produce bronchospasm which, together with histamine release, makes its use undesirable in asthmatics.
- *Addiction*: Although addiction may be a problem with long-term administration of morphine, this is uncommon if the drug is used only to treat acute pain; it is cruel to withhold morphine from a patient in pain for fear that they may become addicted.
- *Hypotension*: Moderate cardiovascular depression and hypotension occur with normal doses of morphine. When given intramuscularly morphine lasts for 3 h and intravenously for 1–3 h.

Pethidine

Pethidine is a synthetic analgesic similar to morphine, producing analgesia together with respiratory depression, suppression of the cough reflex, nausea and vomiting, and hypotension, and is a drug of addiction. Pethidine does not produce as much euphoria and sedation as morphine nor does it release significant amounts of histamine. Some patients are sensitive to pethidine and sweat, vomit, suffer vertigo and may become confused. Pethidine relaxes smooth muscle and it may be useful for renal and biliary colic after large-bowel surgery. Given intramuscularly, 50–100 mg lasts for about 180 min and intravenously 20–30 mg lasts for 60–120 min.

Diamorphine (Heroin)

A powerful analgesic, sedative and respiratory depressant, diamorphine is about twice as potent as morphine and useful in patients undergoing postoperative ventilation and in left ventricular failure, where it helps by decreasing anxiety and by producing mild respiratory depression and sedation. The main problem of diamorphine is addiction and for this reason it is not available in the USA. The normal dose is 5–7.5 mg intramuscularly. It is also frequently added to bupivacaine in continuous epidural anaesthesia.

Papaveretum

This drug is a mixture of purified opium alkaloids containing 50% morphine and 50% other opium alkaloids, for example, codeine, thebaine and papaverine. Clinically 20 mg of papaveretum is equal to about 10 mg morphine. The actions and side-effects of papaveretum are similar to morphine. Following evidence of potential teratogenicity of noscapine, one of the alkaloids in papaveretum, the drug was withdrawn several years ago. A new preparation of noscapine-free papaveretum is now available.

Fentanyl (Sublimaze)

This synthetic analgesic drug is derived from pethidine and is similar to phenoperidine. Like phenoperidine it has virtually no effect on the cardiovascular system. Fentanyl has an extremely wide therapeutic ratio and is now used in varying doses from 2 to 20 µg/kg for intra-operative analgesia. To a certain extent the size of the dose influences its duration of action. With the smaller doses, analgesia and respiratory depression last for about 30 min after an intravenous injection, while with larger doses this may be prolonged for up to 2–3 h. Fentanyl is a powerful respiratory depressant but has relatively few other side-effects, and its use is restricted to intra-operative analgesia. In some countries a combination of fentanyl and droperidol (Thalamonal) is used both intramuscularly and intravenously, usually as premedication.

Fentanyl is also used in very large doses (20–50 µg/kg) during cardiac surgery to produce profound analgesia and obtund all reflex responses. This is particularly advantageous in patients with a compromised coronary circulation in whom any increase in cardiac work due to tachycardia or hypertension might precipitate relative myocardial ischaemia and angina.

Alfentanil (Rapifen)

Alfentanil is a short-acting version of fentanyl, particularly suitable for use in day-case anaesthesia or for administration by intravenous infusion as part of a total intravenous anaesthetic (TIVA) technique. Like fentanyl, it is a powerful analgesic, but the respiratory depressant effect is relatively short-lived and less profound, making it suitable for administration in limited doses to spontaneously breathing patients (6–8 µg/kg). It is cardiovascularly stable and provides good reversible analgesia and sedation when administered as an infusion to ventilated patients in intensive care.

Sufentanil

This is a very potent version of fentanyl (10 × fentanyl), used mainly during cardiac surgery since it produces profound analgesia and stress-free anaesthesia, leading to great cardiovascular stability. It is of course also a profound respiratory depressant.

Remifentanil (Ultiva)

This has been specifically designed for continuous administration as part of a TIVA technique. It is an ultra short-acting opioid and is non-cumulative, wearing off within minutes of discontinuation of the infusion. The side-effects of respiratory depression, etc., are similar to the acute effects of fentanyl.

Phenoperidine

Like fentanyl, phenoperidine is a synthetic pethidine derivative causing respiratory depression but with relatively little effect on the cardiovascular system. Its longer duration of action, about 2 h after intramuscular injection and 1 h after intravenous injection, makes it more useful than fentanyl for intensive care when both analgesia and respiratory depression are required in patients on artificial ventilation. In some patients phenoperidine also has an emetic action.

Methadone (Physeptone)

A synthetic analgesic, this is similar to morphine with similar side-effects. The chief difference between the two drugs is that the duration of methadone, 2 h, is half that for the analgesia following intramuscular morphine. Methadone also produces less euphoria and is used to treat opiate addiction and drug withdrawal.

● NEUROLEPTANAESTHESIA

Neuroleptanaesthesia is a dissociative anaesthetic state, similar to ketamine anaesthesia, produced by administering fentanyl and droperidol. Since only small doses of fentanyl are used the patients breathe spontaneously and, although sedated and analgesic, are able to move to command. Although this technique is advantageous in some conditions – for example, neuro- and vascular radiological procedures – where complete analgesia is not needed, supplementary agents are required to produce surgical anaesthesia. Neuroleptanaesthetic induction of anaesthesia is also used, particularly in poor-risk patients for vascular surgery, because this technique results in minimal disturbance of cardiovascular haemodynamics.

● OPIATE ANTAGONISTS

Until relatively recently all the available opiate antagonists such as nalorphine and levallorphan were opiate drugs producing analgesia in their own right and only producing antagonism of the opiate side-effects such as respiratory depression when given in conjunction with another drug such as morphine.

Nalorphine (Lethidrone)

This acts as a competitive inhibitor of morphine to antagonise the respiratory depressant effects, but it is not possible to antagonise these without also removing the benefit of analgesia. Mixtures of opiates and nalorphine have been unsuccessful in producing selective analgesia without respiratory depression. Repeated doses of nalorphine may cause hypertension and may exacerbate symptoms in drug addiction. Nalorphine has also been used to reverse opiate-induced neonatal respiratory depression.

Naloxone (Narcan)

Naloxone is a synthetic opiate antagonist derived from oxymorphone and does not possess any opiate activity of its own. In a dose of 0.1–0.4 mg it will antagonise any of the opiate analgesics, although analgesia and respiratory depression are antagonised equally. Its duration of action is between 45 and 90 min; naloxone may therefore need to be given in repeated doses when morphine or another long-acting drug has just been administered.

● OPIATE-LIKE ANALGESICS

The search for an analgesic as powerful as morphine but without the sedative or respiratory depressant side-effects has been intensive and several drugs have been produced. However, all of these have proved to be addictive to a certain degree and also tend to produce nausea and vomiting and in some patients – particularly the elderly – confusion or disorientation. They also possess properties of opiate antagonism for which some, for example, pentazocine, were initially developed. This is the concept of partial agonist/antagonist and thus they may be used to reverse respiratory depression caused by other opiates.

Pentazocine (Fortral)

This analgesic is derived from nalorphine, with mild respiratory depression. It has now been shown to be addictive and may cause disorientation and hallucinations. It raises pulmonary artery blood pressure so should not be used in patients with myocardial infarction, and it also produces moderate falls in systemic blood pressure; 30 mg pentazocine is equivalent to 10 mg morphine given intramuscularly.

Phenazocine (Narphen)

A more potent synthetic analgesic than pentazocine, 3 mg being equivalent to 10 mg morphine, phenazocine may be given by mouth or sublingually but in other ways is similar to pentazocine.

Buprenorphine (Temgesic)

This long-acting member of the group produces good cardiovascular stability and moderate respiratory depression. It may also produce nausea and vomiting in some patients. So far, reports of its use in premedication or intra-operatively are somewhat disappointing although its long duration of action may make it useful in the treatment of postoperative pain.

Meptazinol (Meptid), Nalbuphine (Nubain)

These partial opiate agonist drugs, like pentazocine, will reverse opiate-induced respiratory depression. They are potent analgesics with a similar effect to morphine, but they do not possess the euphoric properties of the opiates and have fewer side-effects. They may cause nausea, vomiting and confusion, particularly in elderly patients, but respiratory depression is less likely to occur.

Tramadol (Zydol)

This produces analgesia both as an opioid and by serotoninergic and adrenergic pathways. It has fewer side-effects than morphine, in particular less respiratory depression.

● ANTI-EMETICS

Several drugs used in anaesthesia, particularly the opiate analgesics, produce nausea and vomiting. This is usually produced by stimulation of the vomiting centre which lies close to the respiratory centre in the medulla of the brain. The chemoreceptor trigger zone, another area stimulated by emetic drugs, lies superficial to the true vomiting centre. Vomiting may be initiated not only centrally but also by peripheral effects such as food or other irritants in the stomach. The drugs used to prevent vomiting are commonly phenothiazines. This group of drugs, the chief of which is chlorpromazine, has many actions (e.g. sedative, hypotensive, anti-emetic, antihistaminic, atropine-like and vasodilatory). Various members of the group each have one predominant effect (e.g. anti-emetic) and possess many of the other actions (e.g. sedation) as secondary effects.

Cyclizine (Valoid)

Cyclizine is an antihistamine with a marked anti-emetic action. It also has sedative properties and the other common side-effects such as blurred vision, urinary retention and tachycardia relate to its anticholinergic effects. Its action lasts for 6 h. Cyclizine is also combined with potent emetic analgesics such as morphine (Cyclimorph) and dipipanone (Diconal).

Prochlorperazine (Stemetil)

This phenothiazine drug is used as an anti-emetic and in the treatment of nausea and vomiting due to motion sickness, migraine and Ménière's disease. Unlike some phenothiazines, prochlorperazine does not cause noticeable sedation and has fewer other side-effects. Some patients, however, may develop extrapyramidal signs such as tremor and rolling of the eyes together with confusion. Patients look frightened and alarmed but this oculogyric crisis may be treated with intravenous atropine, promethazine or benztropine (Cogentin).

Metoclopramide (Maxolon)

This drug is not a phenothiazine but acts as an anti-emetic, both centrally by depressing the vomiting centre and peripherally by stimulating gastrointestinal emptying and therefore removing the peripheral stimulus to vomiting. Metoclopramide has few side-effects and is a useful anti-emetic drug but, like perphenazine, may cause extrapyramidal reactions.

Anticholinergic Agents

Both atropine and more particularly hyoscine (scopolamine, Kwells) possess an anti-emetic action but also tend to cause central nervous system depression. This is why it is recommended not to drive a car after taking anti-emetics for sea sickness.

Droperidol, Haloperidol

These butyrephenone drugs also possess significant anti-emetic action by depressing the chemoreceptor trigger zone. They are probably the most powerful anti-emetics available but cause sedation and, in some patients, confusion and hallucinations. They are really suitable only for prolonged anti-emesis in patients who require appreciable sedation, or, for example, in faciomaxillary surgery when the jaw is being wired together and when postoperative nausea and vomiting may produce serious problems.

Domperidone (Motilium)

This long-acting anti-emetic acts as a dopamine antagonist on the vomiting centre in the brain. Its prolonged effect makes it particularly suitable for oncology patients receiving cytotoxic drugs and it does not appear to produce excessive sedation.

Ondansetron (Zofran)

This is a 5-hydroxytryptamine-3 receptor antagonist and therefore an inhibitor of the chemoreceptor trigger zone in the brain. It was developed for cancer chemotherapy and is very effective. It can be given as either 4 or 8 mg intravenously pre- or intra-operatively and has few side-effects, although constipation and headaches may occur.

13

Autonomic and Cardiovascular Pharmacology

•Cholinergic agents •Anticholinergic drugs •Anticholinesterases
•Sympathomimetic amines •Adrenoceptor-blocking drugs
• α-Adrenoceptor-blocking drugs •β-Adrenoceptor-blocking drugs
•Combined α- and β-adrenoceptor-blocking drugs •Angiotensin-converting
enzyme inhibitors •Calcium-channel blockers

This chapter deals with the more detailed pharmacology of the individual drugs already mentioned in Chapter 2.

● CHOLINERGIC AGENTS

These are drugs with an acetylcholine-like action.

Carbachol

This drug mimics the actions of acetylcholine and is more resistant to destruction by cholinesterase. It possesses both muscarinic (parasympathetic) and nicotinic actions, although unless atropine is given concurrently to block the muscarinic actions these will tend to predominate. Carbachol therefore mainly stimulates the parasympathetic system dilating peripheral blood vessels, reducing heart rate and lowering the blood pressure. It is used to increase bladder tone in postoperative retention and to promote gut movement in intestinal atony. It may cause increased salivation, nausea, vomiting, sweating and blurred vision.

Bethanechol

This cholinergic agent also possesses predominantly muscarinic effects and is used in a similar way to carbachol, as a parasympathetic stimulant (parasympathomimetic). The side-effects are similar to carbachol.

● ANTICHOLINERGIC DRUGS

Atropine

Atropine blocks the action of acetylcholine on the parasympathetic nervous system and by producing parasympathetic blockade causes (a) tachycardia, (b) drying of the secretions of the mouth, gut and tracheo-bronchial tree, (c) relaxation of the smooth muscle of the gut, and (d) dilatation of the pupil (in large doses only).

Main Uses of Atropine

1. To abolish bradycardia induced by vagal stimulation. It is not effective in bradycardia due to heart block or digoxin overdose.
2. As premedication to reduce secretions in the tracheobronchial tree and to reduce the effects of vagal stimulation during intubation and surgery.
3. To counteract the parasympathetic effects of neostigmine, when it is used to reverse muscle relaxants.
4. As eyedrops in the form of homatropine to dilate the pupil for long periods.

Hyoscine (Scopolamine)

Hyoscine resembles atropine and produces similar effects as a result of parasympathetic blockade. Hyoscine also possesses a central effect which is different from atropine. While atropine stimulates the central nervous system, hyoscine tends to depress the cortex and produce sedation. Hyoscine also affects other parts of the brain causing amnesia and reducing motion sickness. For this reason, hyoscine is used to treat travel sickness (Kwells). The cardiac effects of hyoscine are less marked than those of atropine when the drugs are given in comparable dose.

Glycopyrrolate (Robinul)

Glycopyrrolate is also an anticholinergic drug, blocking the action of acetyl-choline on the parasympathetic nervous system. Its main use is in combination with anticholinesterase drugs such as neostigmine for the reversal of neuromuscular blockade and a combined preparation of the two drugs is available (neostigmine 2.5 mg and glycopyrrolate 0.5 mg in 1 ml). Glycopyrrolate produces less cardiovascular stimulation than atropine and since it does not cross the blood–brain barrier, excitatory side-effects do not occur.

● ANTICHOLINESTERASES

Neostigmine (Prostigmine)

Acetylcholine is normally broken down by cholinesterase into choline and acetic acid. Neostigmine is an anticholinesterase which increases the concentration of acetylcholine by preventing its breakdown. The acetylcholine produced possesses both muscarinic and nicotinic effects, the muscarinic stimulating the parasympathetic nervous system causing increased salivation, gut activity and bradycardia. These effects are antagonised by atropine. The nicotinic effects of acetylcholine are exerted at the skeletal neuromuscular junction and therefore antagonise the effect of non-depolarising neuromuscular-blocking drugs, for example, pancuronium, vecuronium. Intravenous neostigmine, therefore, is used to antagonise the effects of these relaxants and is given in combination with atropine to prevent the muscarinic side-effects which would otherwise occur. Neostigmine will also reverse the muscle weakness of myasthenia gravis, although pyridostigmine is more commonly used, unless the patient cannot take oral medication. Too much neostigmine may produce depolarisation of the muscle end-plate, also causing muscle paralysis – the cholinergic crisis of myasthenia gravis. This is in contrast to the normal weakness which occurs in this condition due to a relative lack of acetylcholine.

Pyridostigmine (Mestinon)

This is another anticholinesterase drug which possesses less activity than neostigmine. However, as its muscarinic actions are weaker and its duration of action is longer it is more useful than neostigmine in treating myasthenia gravis. It is also given by mouth which is a major advantage in this condition.

Physostigmine

This agent is a more potent anticholinesterase than neostigmine, with a greater effect on the cardiovascular system, the eye and the salivary secretions. Unlike both neostigmine and pyridostigmine, physostigmine crosses the blood–brain barrier, increasing the central nervous concentration of acetylcholine as well as the peripheral levels. This has been used to great effect in counteracting excessive central depression resulting from some drugs, for example, phenothiazine, hyoscine and the tricyclic antidepressants, which are thought to act by reducing the central nervous concentrations of acetylcholine.

Edrophonium (Tensilon)

This short-acting anticholinesterase is mainly used as a diagnostic test in cases of muscle weakness, thought to be due to myasthenia-like acetylcholine deficiency.

● SYMPATHOMIMETIC AMINES

Adrenaline (Epinephrine)

The actions of adrenaline may be divided into alpha (α) and beta (β) (Table 13.1). The α-effects are further subdivided into α_1 (cardiac) and α_2 (peripheral circulation), while the β-effects of adrenaline are also subdivided into β_1 (cardiac effect) and β_2 (bronchial effects). Adrenaline stimulates the α_2-receptors of the sympathetic nervous system, producing peripheral vasoconstriction, and the β_1-receptors, producing an increase in pulse rate and myocardial contractility. It is used to treat cardiac arrest, stimulating the heart without causing peripheral vasodilatation which might otherwise cause a fall in blood pressure and decreased coronary perfusion. Adrenaline also relaxes the smooth muscle of the bronchi by its β_2-effect and hence is useful in treating bronchospasm. It is also used with local analgesics for its vasoconstrictor properties to decrease the rate of absorption of the local analgesic. Adrenaline is used in the first-line treatment of angioneurotic oedema and other hypersensitivity reactions, both for its cardio-respiratory effects and also because it reduces capillary fluid leakage and oedema formation.

Noradrenaline (Norepinephrine, Levophed) (Table 13.2)

Noradrenaline is a naturally occurring catecholamine which causes a pronounced increase in blood pressure by peripheral vasoconstriction and, to a lesser extent, by stimulating myocardial contractility. Noradrenaline, therefore, is predominantly an α_2-adrenoceptor stimulant, and because

Table 13.1 The α- and β-actions of adrenaline

α-Actions	β_1-Actions	β_2-Actions
Dilatation of pupil	Increased heart rate	Bronchodilatation
Peripheral vasoconstriction	Increased myocardial	
Coronary vasoconstriction	contractility	
Intestinal sphincter	Coronary vasodilatation	
contraction		
Piloerection in skin		
Sweat production		

Table 13.2 The α- and β-agonists and blockers

Adrenergic effect	Stimulated by	Blocked by
α	Adrenaline Noradrenaline (Ephedrine) (Amphetamine)	Phentolamine Phenoxybenzamine
β (Non-specific)	Isoprenaline (Dopamine) Ephedrine Amphetamine	Propranolol Labetalol
β₁ (Specific)	Dobutamine	Atenolol Oxprenalol Sotalol
β₂ (Specific)	Salbutamol	

of its pronounced α-effects, causes a reflex slowing of the pulse rate. The vasoconstriction causes poor tissue perfusion and reduces renal blood flow; noradrenaline is therefore only ever used in severely ill patients. Noradrenaline does possess a mild β-adrenoceptor stimulatory effect which is apparent only when the drug is given in combination with an α-adrenoceptor blocker (e.g. phentolamine). This has been used to some effect in cardiac surgery.

Isoprenaline (Isoproterenol, Saventrine)

In contrast to noradrenaline, isoprenaline exhibits mainly the β-actions of adrenaline. It is a powerful cardiac stimulant, increasing both the pulse rate (chronotropic effect) and the force of contraction (inotropic effect). It also causes peripheral vasodilatation by relaxing smooth muscle and so may cause a fall in blood pressure. Isoprenaline may also be used in treating bronchospasm, when it may be given either by inhalation using an inhaler or a Bird ventilator, subcutaneously or sublingually. Overdose of isoprenaline results in atrial tachycardia and arrhythmias, especially ventricular ectopics, ventricular tachycardia (VT) and even ventricular fibrillation (VF).

Dopamine (Inotropin)

Dopamine acts in a similar way to isoprenaline, producing predominantly β-adrenoceptor stimulation, although it has been suggested that this drug is more effective on the peripheral blood vessels than on the heart itself because it does not cause such a severe tachycardia when given systemically. Dopamine in low doses acts on specific dopaminergic receptors within the kidney producing selective renal vasodilatation and simultaneously increasing the blood pressure to a satisfactory level, while larger doses of dopamine are used for their direct myocardial stimulant action, increasing the force of contraction and the cardiac output and therefore the blood pressure. Hence dopamine infusions are used widely in intensive care to treat such conditions. High doses of dopamine may produce peripheral vasoconstriction as a result of a small α-adrenoceptor effect. Dopamine exerts only a mild effect on bronchial smooth muscle.

Ephedrine

Ephedrine is a synthetic drug related chemically to adrenaline. It raises the blood pressure mainly by increasing heart rate and myocardial contractility although it also causes some peripheral vasoconstriction. As well as being used as a vasopressor, ephedrine is useful as a bronchodilator in patients with bronchospasm. It has also been used in the treatment of myasthenia gravis, as it improves neuromuscular conduction.

Methoxamine (Vasoxine) is a direct α_2-stimulant and acts by producing peripheral vasoconstriction. It is used to counteract the hypotension caused by spinal and epidural anaesthetic-induced vasodilatation.

Amphetamine

In general, the actions of amphetamine resemble those of ephedrine but tend to be more apparent as central nervous stimulants. Amphetamine has both α- and β-adrenoceptor stimulatory effects, producing an increase in blood pressure and heart rate. However, because of its pronounced central stimulation and abuse by drug addicts, amphetamine has now been withdrawn.

Salbutamol (Ventolin)

Salbutamol is a β-adrenoceptor stimulant with a highly selective action on bronchial muscle receptors (β_2-action). Used predominantly for the relief of bronchospasm, it may be administered by inhalation, orally or intravenously. When used by the latter route, salbutamol also produces mild cardiac stimulation and a degree of peripheral vasodilatation which has been employed with some success when treating cardiogenic shock.

Dobutamine (Dobutrex)

Dobutamine is a β_1-adrenoceptor stimulant, producing an increase in myocardial contractility. It does not cause noradrenaline release, so peripheral vasoconstriction and hypertension are not common. It is claimed to be a more specific cardiac stimulant than dopamine.

Phosphodiesterase Inhibitors (Enoximone, Milrinone)

These drugs act directly on the myocardium, increasing the force of contraction in cardiac failure. Because they act in a different way, they may be useful in critically ill patients, who are unresponsive to dobutamine.

● ADRENOCEPTOR-BLOCKING DRUGS

Drugs have now been specifically developed to block the different effects of adrenoceptor stimulation (Table 13.2). The β-effects of adrenaline can be subdivided into β_1, which are the cardiac effects, and β_2, which are the effects on the bronchi. α-Adrenoceptor-blocking drugs therefore block the α-effects of adrenaline, β_1-blockers the cardiac effects of isoprenaline, and β_2-blockers, the bronchial effects (Table 13.2).

● α-ADRENOCEPTOR-BLOCKING DRUGS

Phentolamine (Rogitine)

Phentolamine is an α-adrenoceptor-blocking drug which is also a direct myocardial stimulant. It blocks the actions of adrenaline, noradrenaline and related compounds on peripheral blood vessels, thus producing vasodilatation. This will cause a fall in blood pressure and central venous pressure and therefore extra fluid will be required to maintain the circulation. Phentolamine is used:

1. To induce vasodilatation, for example, during cardiopulmonary bypass (CPB).
2. To antagonise vasoconstriction, for example, due to cardiogenic shock.
3. As a direct myocardial stimulant, the vasodilatation being antagonised by noradrenaline.
4. To antagonise the vasoconstrictive effects of noradrenaline.
5. To control the acute hypertensive attacks in patients with phaeochromocytoma.

Phentolamine is a relatively short-acting drug, its effect lasting between 15 and 30 min after intravenous injection.

Phenoxybenzamine

This α-adrenoceptor-blocking drug exerts its effect only slowly but produces a prolonged action, decreasing slowly over 3 days. Phenoxy benzamine is usually used in the treatment of abnormal peripheral vasoconstriction and in the long-term control of phaeochromocytoma, particularly in the preoperative preparation of such patients. Phenoxy benzamine therapy requires careful intravenous fluid management to counteract the gradual fall in central venous pressure as a result of increase in the intravascular space. It may produce postural hypotension and a reflex tachycardia if the fluid volume is not accurately corrected.

● β-ADRENOCEPTOR-BLOCKING DRUGS

Propranolol (Inderal)

Propranolol is a β-adrenoceptor blocker antagonising both the β_1- and β_2-effects of isoprenaline on the heart and bronchi. It causes a fall in heart rate and cardiac output and a decrease in myocardial oxygen consumption. It may, however, cause bronchoconstriction and should not be used in asthmatics. Propranolol is used:

1. To control ectopic beats. It is more effective in the control of atrial ectopics than ventricular. It is useful in the treatment of arrhythmias due to digitalis overdose.
2. To control supraventricular tachycardia.
3. To control the tachycardia which may develop when hypotensive drugs (e.g. pentolinium) are used.
4. To control tachycardia or ventricular arrhythmias due to excess adrenaline.
5. To reduce myocardial oxygen consumption and thereby the frequency of angina.

Oxprenolol (Trasicor), Sotalol (Beta-Cardone), Atenolol (Tenormin)

These are β_1-selective adrenoceptor-blocking drugs, the principal effects of which are slowing of the heart rate with a consequent reduction in myocardial oxygen consumption. They are also used in the treatment of cardiac dysrhythmias and the control of hypertension. Oxprenolol also has some sympathomimetic action of its own and is used in treating angina and dysrhythmias.

● COMBINED α- AND β-ADRENOCEPTOR-BLOCKING DRUGS

Labetalol (Trandate)

This agent possesses both α- and β-adrenoceptor-blocking effects and has been advocated for hypertension, as not only does it reduce myocardial oxygen consumption, but it also acts as a peripheral vasodilator. However, its α-blocking effects are much milder than its β-effects and are also much shorter in duration, and for this reason the predominant effects of labetalol are similar to other $β_1$-adrenoceptor-blocking drugs. Labetalol is now widely used to produce moderate reduction in blood pressure during elective surgery. By inducing vasodilatation and minimising any reflex tachycardia, the fall in blood pressure is posturally dependent and controllable.

● ANGIOTENSIN-CONVERTING ENZYME INHIBITORS

Captopril (Capoten), Enalapril (Innovace)

This group of drugs is used in the treatment of hypertension, chiefly in patients with hypertension secondary to renal causes. They block the conversion of the vasoconstrictor angiotensin I to the active form angiotensin II, by angiotensin-converting enzyme (ACE) which occurs in the lung. Like other agents used to control blood pressure, their use should be continued during surgery. Their action is not sufficiently acute to make them suitable for elective hypotension during anaesthesia but they do enhance the hypotensive effects of volatile agents, particularly isoflurane.

● CALCIUM-CHANNEL BLOCKERS

Nifedipine (Adalat), Verapamil (Cordilox), Diltiazem (Tildiem)

These drugs, introduced for the control of cardiac dysrhythmias, are being increasingly used for the control of blood pressure and for the reduction of myocardial oxygen consumption in patients with ischaemic heart disease and angina. Like patients receiving β-adrenoceptor-blocking drugs, treatment with calcium-channel blockers should continue during surgery, although their effect may enhance the hypotensive effect of halothane and enflurane. Their speed of onset of action makes them unsuitable for intra-operative induced hypotension.

14

Pre-anaesthetic Assessment and Premedication

Only in cases of dire emergency should an anaesthetist meet the patient for the first time in the anaesthetic room. The preoperative visit benefits both the anaesthetist and the patient. It gives the anaesthetist an opportunity to check the patient's preoperative preparation, to assess the psychological and physical state, to request any further investigations the anaesthetist may consider essential to decide what anaesthetic technique to use and to discuss this and the method of postoperative analgesia with the patient and the ward nurse. It is usual to obtain informed consent at the end of the interview.

● PERUSAL OF NOTES

The patient's notes should provide the anaesthetist with most of the information needed. They should contain not only the patient's history and clinical examination but also the results of any haematological, biochemical and radiological examinations. The investigations will vary widely depending on the patient's physical status and the operation intended. Anaesthetic notes from previous operations are a useful guide to indicate problems previously encountered.

● INTERVIEW AND EXAMINATION OF PATIENT

Interview

Although the anaesthetist may have gathered all the required information from the notes, it is still important to speak to and examine the patient.

Not only does it provide the opportunity to repeat some of the questions and ask any others, but it also gives the further opportunity to form some degree of rapport with the patient. Questioning and examination along the following lines is the minimum that is necessary for a patient who has not already been 'clerked', but will not be wasted even if this has taken place. In some circumstances, for example, day surgery, where it may not be possible to clerk all the patients, it is useful to give all patients a questionnaire as they come to the ward or even in the out-patient clinic as they are booked for surgery.

Is your general health good? Many patients, especially younger ones, will reply in the affirmative. This encourages the anaesthetist to think that nothing particularly adverse will be disclosed by further questions.

Have you ever had any serious illnesses? This may be taken to mean anything that necessitated admission to hospital.

Have you ever had any operations or anaesthetics? By putting the question in this way, dental-chair anaesthetics, which many patients do not regard as operations, will not be missed. The operations, their dates and whereabouts should be listed as it may be possible to obtain the anaesthetic notes if not already available.

Were you told of any problems associated with any of your anaesthetics? This may reveal a history of avoidable complications (e.g. suxamethonium pains or even the occasional suxamethonium apnoea). More commonly the patient may give a history of distressing nausea or vomiting after the operation and it may be possible to identify some causative agent.

Do you know of any family history of problems with anaesthetics, or operations? While this question seldom produces an affirmative answer, if it is not asked routinely the anaesthetist may miss the possibility of the patient having one of the hereditarily transmitted conditions such as abnormal pseudocholinesterase or malignant hyperpyrexia which have such serious anaesthetic implications (Chapter 15).

Do you have any pain in your legs or chest on taking exercise? This question is asked to elicit a history of claudication or angina. It is the first question in evaluating cardiorespiratory function and, like many of the later questions, if answered in the affirmative it is followed by further questioning to find out how long the patient has had the symptom, how readily it comes on, if the patient knows anything that will get rid of it, etc.

How easily do you get short of breath? Can the patient walk up a flight of stairs or a hill reasonably briskly without having to stop for breath, or are they out of breath at the top? Can the patient sleep lying down or do they need several pillows to avoid feeling breathless?

Do your ankles swell?

Do you have a cough? If the answer is in the affirmative it is important to enquire about the colour, quantity and consistency of the sputum.

Do you smoke? A patient who smokes may show signs of an irritable respiratory tract under the anaesthetic but, more importantly, is much more likely to suffer respiratory complications postoperatively.

Do you suffer from indigestion? An affirmative answer should be followed by more detailed questioning about the presence and nature of abdominal pain and history of acid regurgitation.

Do you have hay fever? While not itself a life-endangering disease, hay fever indicates that the patient has an allergic tendency.

Do you have asthma? This disease covers all ranges of severity and the patient will often be on medication either in tablet form or by inhaler. The treatment may have to be prescribed for the period of the operation, and the premedication and anaesthetic agents used can be chosen to some extent to try to avoid bronchospasm if general anaesthesia is to be given.

Do you have any allergies? The commonest allergies are probably to antibiotics, but many drugs, as well as other stimuli, may be incriminated (e.g. dogs, cats and horses). It is most important to enquire carefully about drug allergies and determine their nature. A distinction must also be made between true allergy and intolerance.

Are you on any regular medication? The answer indicates to the anaesthetist the condition from which the patient is suffering and whether to stop or continue the medication.

Do you drink wine or spirits? Patients who drink alcohol regularly and excessively often have an alarming resistance to general anaesthetic agents.

Do you have any false teeth? Enquiries should also be made about crowns or elaborate dental work. It is wise to ascertain whether there is anything else artificial about the patient (e.g. a false eye, wig, or a false limb). The patient is unlikely to come to the operating theatre wearing a false limb, but may wear a wig or false eye without mentioning it. These latter objects may prove disconcerting during anaesthesia, especially if the false eye is relied on to provide information about the depth of anaesthesia!

This list of questions needs much modification from patient to patient; questions about angina and claudication would be inappropriate for a young child.

Examination of Patient

Constraints on time prevent the anaesthetist examining each patient in detail. The interview gives him/her a good idea of the extent to which he should perform this examination. Of particular interest to the anaesthetist are the respiratory and cardiovascular systems, but equally important are examination of the upper airway, jaw and neck movements, sites for venous access and the spine if spinal or epidural anaesthesia is planned. These findings are commonly summarised in the patients' notes or on the anaesthetic chart. It is usual for the anaesthetist to grade the physical status of the patient and the American Society of Anesthesiologists' (ASA) classification is shown in Table 14.1. This type of grading helps anaesthetists to convey their findings, forms a system of audit and is also useful for medicolegal purposes.

● EXPLANATION AND CONSENT

After the interview and examination the anaesthetist should complete the preoperative visit by discussing with the patient points relating to the anaesthesia and surgery. Night sedation is first discussed and if necessary prescribed, and then the patient told what, if any, food or drink will be allowed on the day of the operation. The anaesthetist should then describe in what way anaesthesia will be induced in the anaesthetic room, where the patient is likely to wake up, what pain is likely to be felt from the operation and what methods will be available to relieve it. At the end of the visit the anaesthetist obtains verbal or written informed consent and writes orders for fasting, premedication and any other drug therapy.

Table 14.1 ASA classification of physical status

Class	Physical status
I	A healthy patient with no systemic disease
II	A patient with mild to moderate systemic disease not limiting activity, e.g. mild asthma, treated hypertension, smoker
III	A patient with severe systemic disease limiting activity, e.g. chronic obstructive airway disease with dyspnoea on exertion
IV	A patient with severe systemic disease which is a constant threat to life, e.g. chronic obstructive airway disease with dyspnoea at rest
V	A moribund patient who is unlikely to survive 24 h with or without surgery
E	The letter E is prefixed for any of the above having an emergency operation

● PREMEDICATION

The term 'premedication' was first used by McMechan in 1920. Premedication aims at psychological preparation and use of pharmacological agents to attain specific responses in patients presenting for surgery. The psychological preparation involves the preoperative visit by the anaesthetist and has already been discussed above. Some of the desired drug responses might include relief of anxiety, drying of secretions and prevention of vomiting and are discussed in detail below.

● AIMS OF PREMEDICATION AND DRUGS USED

Reduction of Anxiety

The most important factor in reducing patient anxiety is not the administration of drugs but the preoperative visit by the anaesthetist. Nevertheless, many patients prefer to have some sedation before arriving in the anaesthetic room and a variety of drugs are used for this purpose. The degree of sedation (or, indeed, whether it is advisable at all) depends on many factors, including the general state of the patient, whether the case is an emergency, whether the anaesthetic is to deliver a baby, how important it is that the patient regains consciousness quickly after the anaesthetic and whether the patient is intending to go home the same day. Drugs used to allay anxiety include:

Benzodiazepines

These include diazepam, lorazepam, temazepam and midazolam. They have, in addition to their sedative and tranquillising properties, an amnesic action and are effective orally. Lorazepam has a long duration of action and hence the time of administration is not very important. Temazepam, in contrast, is short acting and is useful for short procedures. Midazolam can be given intravenously in adults and orally or even intranasally in children. Their main disadvantages are that they are unreliable and do not produce any analgesia.

Opioid Analgesics

These include morphine, pethidine and papaveretum which is now rarely used. They are powerful sedatives and also produce euphoria. Pethidine additionally is a bronchodilator and is therefore appropriate in asthmatics. Opioids are useful in combination with hyoscine before major surgery. They are less routinely used nowadays because they can cause respiratory and cardiovascular depression, nausea and vomiting and because they have to be given by injection.

Antihistamines

Many of these are phenothiazine derivatives and those used in premedication include promethazine, promazine and trimeprazine. Apart from their antihistaminic action these drugs (a) produce sedation, (b) potentiate and prolong the action of opioids, (c) are anti-emetic, (d) tend to dilate the bronchi, and (e) have some atropine-like action in drying salivary secretions. Their main disadvantages are that their duration of action tends to be long and they may cause hypotension and for these reasons are now rarely used.

Drying of Salivary and Bronchial Secretions

The drying up of salivary secretions has long been considered as one of the main purposes of premedication. Drugs that have this action are called 'antisialogogues'. These agents also tend to have a similar effect on bronchial secretions.

Antisialogogue drugs were introduced in the days when anaesthesia was laboriously induced by inhalational methods. Some agents (e.g. diethyl ether), if not expertly administered, could cause copious outpouring of secretions. This made it difficult to get the patient down to deeper planes of anaesthesia and the whole procedure could be stormy, tedious and frightening. Some patients find the dry mouth caused by the premedication uncomfortable by the time they arrive in the anaesthetic room and, in the postoperative period, this antisialogogue effect may for a time make sputum viscid and difficult to expectorate. The introduction of intravenous anaesthetic agents, short-acting opioids and muscle relaxants has made the induction of anaesthesia speedier and smoother. In modern anaesthetic conditions, antisialogogues are less frequently used than formerly. A useful indication though is when the anaesthetic technique involves performing a fibreoptic intubation in an 'awake' patient. Here a dry mouth helps in the penetration of local anaesthetic drugs used for topical anaesthesia of the upper airway and prevents their dilution by the saliva. Drugs used for drying secretions include:

Atropine Sulphate

Atropine, probably the commonest agent used to dry secretions, has been in use since before the end of the nineteenth century. Its theoretical disadvantage is that it is a central nervous system stimulant, but this effect is not usually impressive. It may cause tachycardia and hence is not a popular antisialogogue drug.

Hyoscine Hydrobromide

This other commonly used antisialogogue differs from atropine in being a central nervous system depressant, causing drowsiness and amnesia. It is also an anti-emetic. With an opioid analgesic such as morphine, it provides much better pre-anaesthetic sedation than atropine, and is a more powerful drying agent than atropine. For these reasons it is the drug of choice.

Glycopyrrolate

This synthetic, long-acting anticholinergic drug was introduced in 1960. It has an equivalent drying action to that of atropine, but produces less tachycardia and does not stimulate the central nervous system. It is very quickly effective when given intravenously.

Prevention of Vagal Reflexes

The term 'vagal inhibition' is often used to describe a condition in which there is overaction of the cardiac vagus resulting in bradycardia or even asystole. Many different surgical and anaesthetic stimuli are thought to be capable of providing the afferent side of this reflex arc, including traction on any intra-abdominal mesentery, dilatation of the anus, traction on the extra-ocular eye muscles and stimulation of the upper respiratory tract with a laryngoscope, tracheal tube, sucker, or even high concentrations of anaesthetic vapours. It is more likely to happen if the patient already has a bradycardia as is often associated with the taking of β-adrenergic blocking drugs or other antihypertensive treatment, or the administration of volatile agents. It is also more likely if there is some associated predisposing factor, especially hypoxia or hypercarbia.

Atropine or glycopyrrolate administered subcutaneously or intramuscularly, in doses usually used for premedication, produces blood levels that are so low as to be almost ineffective in blocking these vagal reflexes. Hence most anaesthetists would give these drugs intravenously during anaesthesia to prevent or treat bradycardia.

Aid to Anaesthesia

All general anaesthesia consists of narcosis, analgesia and muscular relaxation (Chapter 1). The analgesia provided by an opioid given in the premedication thus forms part of the anaesthetic. There are other ways in which opioids may help to provide smooth general anaesthesia: (a) by reducing twitching and hiccoughs associated with some intravenous induction agents; (b) by reducing the tachypnoea produced by some volatile agents, for example, halothane and enflurane; and (c) by making awareness under light muscle relaxant anaesthesia less likely. However, most drugs providing sedation in premedication have a fairly long action and they are likely to have an effect long after the anaesthetic has been discontinued. This must be borne in mind if a rapid return to full consciousness is essential.

Prevention of Nausea and Vomiting

Nausea and vomiting are distressing to the patient after any operation and most anaesthetists now prefer to include an anti-emetic in the premedication to prevent nausea and vomiting. The drugs used are discussed in Chapter 12.

Prevention of Acid Aspiration (Mendelson's Syndrome)

There are a group of patients who are at risk of aspiration of stomach contents during induction of anaesthesia (e.g. emergency, trauma, obstetrics). The risk of lung damage is reduced if drugs are given to reduce the amount of acid in the stomach or to decrease the acidity of the contents already present in the stomach. The following drugs are used.

H_2 Receptor Blocking Drugs

These drugs work by inhibiting the H_2 receptors necessary in the manufacture of hydrochloric acid in the stomach. Examples include cimetidine and ranidine, the latter being the more popular drug given orally in a dose of 150 mg.

Alkalis

These are substances which when given orally will mix with the stomach contents and decrease their acidity by increasing their pH. The commonest example is a clear antacid, sodium citrate (see Chapter 38).

Prevention of Pain

The concept of 'pre-emptive analgesia' means giving analgesics before the painful stimulus is applied in the belief that the resulting stimulus will result in less pain. This view is not universally held but many anaesthetists include analgesic drugs as premedicants and these include:

Opioid Analgesics

These have already been discussed (see above).

Non-steroidal Anti-inflammatory Drugs (NSAIDs)

These include aspirin and related drugs, the most popular being diclofenac, ketorolac and ibuprofen. They may be given orally (or in the case of diclofenac as a suppository) before surgery. They inhibit the synthesis of prostaglandins and help to reduce mediators of pain and inflammation. They may not be fully effective on their own but reduce the dose of opioids and hence their side-effects.

Other Uses for Premedication

Occasionally other drugs are given with the premedication, although they are not usually regarded as true premedicant agents. These include steroids in patients who are already on (or have recently been on) steroid therapy, bronchodilators in asthmatics, insulin in diabetics and antibiotics in patients with valvular heart disease to prevent subacute bacterial endocarditis.

EMLA Cream 5% (see also Chapter 39)

This agent, introduced by Astra in 1986, is the first cream which when applied to the surface of the skin reliably reduces or even abolishes the pain of needle puncture. The technique is to apply a thick layer of the cream for at least 60 min beneath an occlusive and waterproof dressing. Its greatest use is in the 1–15 year age group, although it may be used and is effective in older patients.

Amitop – Amethocaine Hydrochloride gel (see also Chapter 39)

This gel is 4% amethocaine, a local anaesthetic with a slightly faster action than EMLA cream and a duration of action of about 4 h. It is applied like EMLA cream and has similar uses.

● PREMEDICATION FOR DIFFERENT AGE GROUPS

It is emphasised that the following is only one of many possible schemes of premedication, that there is much permissible overlap between the age groups and that adjustments should be made for particular factors, for example, debilitated patients or emergencies.

Neonate to 1 Year

Subcutaneous or intramuscular atropine or glycopyrrolate alone is commonly given to this age group 1 h before operation. Some anaesthetists avoid giving atropine to neonates. This is certainly advisable if they have a pyrexia, as atropine's action in preventing sweating tends to raise the temperature further.

1–15 Years

Since the advent of EMLA cream, intravenous induction is common in this age group. Hence antisialogogues and sedatives are usually avoided and one of the parents and a ward nurse are encouraged to accompany the child until induced. If required, sedation can be achieved by oral benzodiazepines, for example, midazolam.

Newer methods of administering drugs include the use of intranasal midazolam and the fentanyl 'lollipop' which has a fruity taste and is given to the child to suck.

16–65 Years

The 'adult' premedication mixtures of papaveretum and hyoscine, or pethidine and hyoscine, have now gone out of favour except for major surgery, and have been replaced by oral benzodiazepines, for example, diazepam 10–20 mg, temazepam 20–30 mg or lorazepam 2–4 mg in fit young adults. These are usually combined with an oral anti-emetic, for example, metoclopramide 10 mg. Some anaesthetists routinely use an H_2 blocker, for example, ranitidine 150 mg for acid aspiration prophylaxis.

65+ Years

Because of wide variations in the ageing process, the age of 65 years is only a rough guide as to where the age group should begin. If narcotics are to be used, the dose should be reduced as the patient becomes older and more frail. In all but the most robust of patients over 70, it is probably wise to give only a small dose of short-acting benzodiazepine, for example, temazepam 10 mg, or withhold premedication altogether. Older people are in general more phlegmatic, so that the undesirability of using powerful depressant drugs coincides with a lack of the psychological need for heavy sedation.

● INTERCURRENT DRUG THERAPY

Many patients who present for anaesthesia are already on some form of medication. Apart from the significance of the condition being treated, many of the drugs may react adversely with anaesthetic agents, or produce other disconcerting effects. However, it is now established as a good working principle with most drugs that patients should be maintained on their usual medication right up to the time of operation. Provided the anaesthetist is aware of this intercurrent drug therapy and any likely interaction with anaesthetic agents, it is considered in the patient's best interests to have minimal interruption of their drug treatment. A brief discussion of some of the groups of drugs patients may be taking when presenting for anaesthesia is given below.

Antihypertensive Agents

Although fashions for particular agents or groups of agents change, anti-hypertensive drugs of one kind or another represent one of the common-est groups of drugs being taken by patients coming for anaesthesia. Because of the risk of potentiation of agents used during anaesthesia which them-selves may cause hypotension (e.g. halothane, d-tubocurarine), it was once thought that they should be stopped long enough before the anaesthetic for their effect to wear off. Very few anaesthetists now hold this view. Indeed, temporary discontinuation of treatment is now thought to be even more dangerous, with the risk of a cerebrovascular accident or myocardial infarction. During anaesthesia also, the untreated patient seems to be at increased risk, with wild swings of blood pressure, particularly high blood pressure occurring at laryngoscopy and intubation.

These patients' underlying cardiovascular status is of course poor, but provided that care is taken with anaesthetic agents which produce hypotension in their own right, and provided that a steep or sudden head-up tilt is avoided (because of the dramatic fall in blood pressure that it may cause), there seems little doubt that these patients are more safely anaesthetised if their antihypertensive therapy is continued throughout the operation.

Steroid Therapy

The therapeutic use of adrenal cortical hormones (steroids) is common in many conditions, including collagen diseases such as rheumatoid arthritis and asthma. The effect of this treatment is to suppress the secretion of adrenocorticotrophic hormone (ACTH) from the patient's own pituitary gland and, without stimulatory effect, the patient's own adrenal cortex atrophies. If the patient is then exposed to some stress, such as anaesthesia and operation, the adrenal cortex may not be able to respond as normal, and acute adrenal insufficiency will occur. This may present as sudden hypotension and the patient may die unless intravenous steroids are given immediately. The suppressant effect on the adrenal cortex of therapeut-ically administered steroids may continue long after the treatment has stopped. The suppression is probably related to the dosage and duration of the therapy but may be significant after treatment for as short a period as 1 week, and the adrenal cortex may not recover completely for weeks or months. Various regimens of steroid cover have been recommended, depending on the size and duration of steroid treatment, how long has elapsed since the course of steroids finished (assuming that the patient is not still on the course), and the severity of the expected stress from the anaesthetic and operation. Sometimes the administration of 100 mg hydrocortisone sodium succinate given intramuscularly with the premedication will be adequate, while at other times the extra steroid cover, whether given parentally or orally, may have to be continued for several days.

Monoamine Oxidase Inhibitors

This group of drugs are used for depressive states. Severe, sometimes fatal reactions were reported with two entirely different groups of drugs. First, catastrophic rises in blood pressure, leading at times to acute subarachnoid haemorrhage, were seen when patients taking these drugs were given vasopressors. Secondly, pethidine in conjunction with monoamine oxidase inhibitors (MAOIs) at times produced profound collapse, hypotension and death. It is also recommended that patients on MAOIs should avoid certain foods, including Bovril, Oxo and other meat extracts, cheese, Marmite, yoghurt, pickled herrings and red wine.

Barbiturates and propofol are safe. Morphine and other opioids are probably safer than pethidine but they should be used with the utmost caution. The residual effects of MAOIs linger for a considerable time and traditionally it was recommended that if possible they should be stopped for 3 weeks before anaesthesia. This view has now changed because patients may relapse into depression by stopping these drugs. Instead it is recommended that safer drugs be used.

Tricyclic Antidepressants

These antidepressants (e.g. amitriptyline, clomipramine, dothiepin) are probably the commonest group of drugs in use at present. They may potentiate the cardiovascular effects of adrenaline and noradrenaline, causing hypertension and cardiac arrhythmias especially following the use of sympathomimetic drugs.

Sedatives and Tranquillisers

Almost any of the drugs in this huge group (e.g. phenobarbitone, diazepam) may have some (although not usually dangerous) effects on anaesthesia. In summary, where patients are on a fairly acute course of one of these drugs there is a tendency for their sedative effects to summate with that of general anaesthesia, while if the treatment is long term the patients tend to be resistant to the effects of general anaesthesia. This statement applies also to the tricyclic antidepressants and indeed to most psychotropic agents.

Oral Contraceptives and Hormone Replacement Therapy

Oral contraceptive drugs, especially those containing oestrogen, increase the risk of venous thrombosis and pulmonary embolism. It is recommended that they should be stopped for 4–6 weeks prior to surgery where there is a risk, for example, moderate or major surgery and for surgery on the legs. When this is not possible (e.g. in an emergency), then full pharmacological and mechanical measures to prevent thromboembolism should be instituted.

The situation is less clear with regard to hormone replacement therapy and it is generally accepted that this should not be stopped prior to surgery. However, pharmacological and mechanical prophylaxis should be instituted in these women.

● THE PREOPERATIVE ASSESSMENT CLINIC

The concept of a preoperative anaesthetic assessment clinic, in which patients can be assessed and the above types of problems clarified before their admission to hospital, is an excellent one. Investigations and treatment can be carried out where required as an out-patient so that the possibility of delaying the operation after admission can be reduced and the patient prepared optimally for the anaesthetic and surgery. Unfortunately, few anaesthetic departments can cope with the work involved if all patients are referred to the clinic as soon as they are booked on the surgical waiting list. Many hospitals now have clinics for selective 'high-risk' patients to which patients are referred. A scheme which works very well for day surgery patients is to ask the patients to fill in a questionnaire that allows the surgeon to decide suitability or otherwise for day surgery.

15

Anaesthesia and Intercurrent Diseases

•Cardiovascular diseases •Respiratory diseases •Obesity •Neurological and neuromuscular disorders •Epilepsy •Parkinson's disease •Malignant hyperpyrexia (malignant hyperthermia) •Serum hepatitis (hepatitis B antigen; Australia antigen) •Acquired immune deficiency syndrome (AIDS) •Sickle-cell haemoglobinopathies •Atypical pseudocholinesterases •Porphyrias •Rheumatoid arthritis

With an ageing population the incidence of intercurrent illness in patients presenting for surgery is increasing. Most common are diseases of the cardiovascular and respiratory systems. Endocrine disorders are discussed in Chapter 16. Here, a variety of diseases – some quite common, some quite rare – are collected. Many of these conditions are inherited; some are of unknown aetiology. The importance of some of them lies in the fact that, in their presence, the administration of an anaesthetic which would be perfectly reasonable in a normal person may have serious, or even fatal consequences.

● CARDIOVASCULAR DISEASES

Diseases of the cardiovascular system which may produce problems in the perioperative period include:

Hypertension

The main problem in the hypertensive patient is the lability of the blood pressure, so that in response to relatively minor stimuli, disproportionate rises and falls may occur. To a degree these fluctuations are reduced if the hypertension is treated with either calcium antagonists, β-blockers or angiotensin-converting enzyme (ACE) inhibitors and these should be continued up to the day of surgery. Antihypertensive therapy may also inter-act with anaesthetics, particularly volatile agents, for example, isoflurane.

In general the diastolic blood pressure is the more important, since anxiety will elevate systolic pressure. Good premedication with a sedative and possibly a drug such as atenolol is useful in the anxious, untreated patient.

Ischaemic Heart Disease and Angina

In these conditions, myocardial ischaemia results from a relative imbalance between oxygen supply and demand and patients are frequently treated with calcium antagonists such as nifedipine and also glyceryl trinitrate by patch or sublingually. The main determinants of oxygen demand are the heart rate and blood pressure, since these control myocardial work and therefore oxygen consumption. Oxygen is supplied to the heart muscle via the coronary arteries, flow only occurring when the myocardium is resting, i.e. during diastole. An increase in heart rate or hypertension will increase oxygen demand, while severe hypotension will reduce coronary perfusion. Care must be taken to minimise any rise in oxygen demand and to ensure an adequate supply of oxygenated blood. Drug therapy should again be continued perioperatively and changes in the ST segments of the electrocardiogram (ECG) will indicate the onset of ischaemia.

Myocardial Infarction

This is the most severe presentation of ischaemic heart disease and if recent is a relative contraindication to elective surgery. If a patient has had a heart attack within the previous 3 months, they have a 50% likelihood of reinfarction perioperatively. This is made worse by associated hypertension and dysrhythmias.

Valvular Heart Disease

The heart valves can be either stenotic or incompetent and may also be relatively fixed and unable to move freely. A stenosed valve, usually the mitral or aortic, will severely restrict blood flow and therefore any required increase in cardiac output. For this reason any anaesthetic technique which may produce hypotension such as an epidural or spinal is contraindicated as are large and potentially hypotensive doses of volatile agents. Mitral valve disease and particularly incompetence (leaking) is associated with cardiac failure.

Cardiac Failure

This may affect either the right or left side of the heart or both. Both result in an inadequate forward pumping of blood with a resultant back pressure and the development of fluid overload and oedema. In general, right-sided failure is associated with peripheral oedema of the ankles and a large liver, while left heart failure presents as pulmonary oedema. Symptoms include atrial fibrillation, often treated with digoxin, oedema, treated with diuretics, and breathlessness, particularly on lying flat (orthopnoea). Treatment should again be continued perioperatively, but patients in obvious cardiac failure should be controlled prior to operation.

Conduction Defects

Ventricular ectopic beats are common and unless frequent (>4/min) do not cause problems. Their incidence is made worse by a high carbon dioxide concentration or hypoxia and also by adrenaline in the presence of volatile agents such as halothane. If occurring frequently, they can be suppressed by a small dose of intravenous lignocaine.

Heart block is the inefficient conduction of impulses from atrium to ventricle or through the ventricles themselves along the bundle of His. In first-degree block, the PR interval is prolonged, in second-degree, some impulses do not pass on from the atrioventricular node and third-degree (complete) block is associated with a slow ventricular rhythm. Heart block is associated with relatively inefficient contraction and a low cardiac output. Inhalational anaesthesia may cause the degree of block to worsen and symptoms to increase. This may require emergency pacing.

Pacemakers

Many patients have indwelling pacemakers to regulate cardiac rhythm in cases of heart block. In most cases they are of the 'demand' type so that they 'cut in' when required at a predetermined setting of heart rate. In theory their rate of discharge can be affected by the use of diathermy so that the earth electrode should be as far away from the pacemaker as possible. Bipolar diathermy is better than monopolar. Usually the worst that can happen is that the pacemaker 'trips' into a faster rate, but this could induce myocardial ischaemia.

● RESPIRATORY DISEASES

Common Cold (Upper Respiratory Tract Infection)

In many cases, minor surgery can proceed quite safely in patients with a mild head cold, provided they feel well enough and are not febrile. The main risks involve transmission of the infection to the lungs and bronchi and therefore endotracheal intubation would be contraindicated, but use of a face mask or laryngeal mask airway (LMA) and spontaneous ventilation is probably all right.

Acute Bronchitis, Chest Infection (Lower Respiratory Tract Infection)

This is associated with cough and purulent sputum, and is more frequent in smokers. Here the risks are that inadequate postoperative coughing due to postoperative pain, etc., will prevent normal recovery and may lead to pneumonia and so all elective surgery should be delayed. Preoperative preparation should include physiotherapy and bronchodilators if necessary until the patient has recovered.

Chronic Bronchitis and Emphysema

Postoperative chest complications such as pneumonia are more common in these conditions and therefore the patients should be in the best possible state preoperatively. Smoking with its associated high carbon monoxide levels and reduced ciliary activity in the lungs must be discontinued. The patients tend to have irritable airways which may produce coughing on induction and bronchospasm. They also suffer from reduced respiratory reserve which may become borderline if postoperative pain is severe and analgesia inadequate. Continuous postoperative thoracic epidural anaesthesia is very valuable in such patients following major abdominal or thoracic surgery.

Asthma

Asthmatics are usually reasonably well controlled on bronchodilators such as Ventolin (salbutamol) and Becotide (beclomethasone) together with steroids in some cases. They have irritable airways which are made worse by intubation and irritant gases, together with drugs which release histamine such as thiopentone and some neuromuscular blockers, for example, atracurium and suxamethonium. Halothane is a good bronchodilator and can be used for inhalational anaesthesia, and sevoflurane is also well tolerated. Asthmatics tend to have good and bad times of the year, particularly if associated with hay fever, and so elective surgery should be geared to these.

● OBESITY

Next to cardiovascular and respiratory disease, obesity is one of the commonest disorders occurring in patients presenting for anaesthesia. Usually it is an incidental finding, but occasionally the surgery (e.g. apronectomy, intestinal bypass) may be treatment of the obesity itself.

The anaesthetist's difficulties begin with technical ones. For example, lifting and positioning the patient may be difficult; veins may be hard to find; the airway may be awkward to maintain in patients with short, fat necks and large tongues, and endotracheal intubation may present a problem. Even the blood pressure may not be easy to take accurately because of difficulty in applying the sphygmomanometer cuff satisfactorily to an obese arm.

Obese people are susceptible to a great many other conditions. Among these are ischaemic heart disease, hypertension, bronchitis, diabetes mellitus, varicose veins, gallstones, abdominal and hiatus hernia, arthritis of the legs and increased susceptibility to industrial, household and street accidents. The cardiovascular and respiratory problems are likely to be of the greatest importance to the anaesthetist, obese patients in particular having a tendency to hypoxaemia due to splinting of the chest and abdominal walls by adipose tissue, to the increased amount of intra-abdominal fat and to alterations in the ventilation: perfusion ratio in the lungs.

Management

Most anaesthetic techniques which would normally be appropriate for the surgery being performed are acceptable, but it is important to ensure that ventilation is adequate. The main underlying principles are to use a method which ensures that the patient rapidly regains consciousness and does not suffer from residual neuromuscular blockade. Not only do obese patients have difficulty in maintaining their airways and ventilation if still drowsy or suffering from residual neuromuscular blockade, but, as respiratory and venous thrombotic complications are more likely to occur, early active movements and ambulation are also important.

● NEUROLOGICAL AND NEUROMUSCULAR DISORDERS

Myasthenia Gravis

This disease is due to an abnormality of the neuromuscular junction and is characterised by weakness of skeletal muscle, this weakness being progressive with exercise. Myasthenia gravis varies widely in its severity, its rate of onset and the number of muscles involved. The muscle weakness recovers partially with rest and with anticholinesterase drugs and, although the theory that the disease is caused by the presence of a circulating curare-like agent has now been discounted in favour of an auto-immune cause, it may help clinically to think of the condition as being caused in this way. Thus, in addition to the improvement in muscle strength in response to anticholinesterase drugs, for example, neostigmine or pyridostigmine, these patients are extremely sensitive to non-depolarising muscle relaxants but relatively resistant to depolarising relaxants.

Anaesthetic Management

Myasthenic patients are usually on long-term anticholinesterase drugs, for example, pyridostigmine. Anaesthesia may be required for incidental surgical conditions or for thymectomy, removal of the thymus gland, which is used as a treatment for certain types of myasthenia.

If possible, it is wise to avoid the use of muscle relaxants in these patients. Anaesthesia may be induced with thiopentone or propofol and, if endotracheal intubation is required, it can usually be carried out under nitrous oxide, oxygen and isoflurane, with or without topical analgesia of the larynx. A reduced dose of suxamethonium can also be used, for the reasons outlined above. If controlled respiration is needed it can usually be easily carried out with this same anaesthetic sequence. Intermittent positive pressure ventilation (IPPV) will certainly be required for thymectomy, where a sternum-splitting incision is commonly used, and if neuromuscular blockade is required, then atracurium, with its unique non-enzymatic metabolism, is the drug of choice. If respiratory function has been severely reduced preoperatively, it may be necessary to ventilate these patients electively for several days postoperatively.

Myasthenic Syndrome (Eaton–Lambert Syndrome)

This is a condition of muscle weakness usually associated with bronchogenic carcinoma, although the latter may not have been clinically diagnosed. It differs from myasthenia gravis in that the muscle weakness tends to improve with exercise rather than deteriorate. In addition, patients tend to be sensitive both to depolarising and to non-depolarising relaxants.

Dystrophia Myotonica

This is an inherited disease with onset usually in the patient's early 30s. The weakness of the muscles which occurs is associated with difficulty in relaxing after contraction. This may be seen as difficulty in relaxing the grip after a handshake or after clenching the fist to facilitate venepuncture. Associated features are baldness, cataracts, testicular atrophy and cardiomyopathy. The myotonia or muscular contraction may be accentuated by suxamethonium, which should therefore be avoided. Non-depolarising agents may be used, but may not be effective in producing muscular relaxation. Thiopentone has been reported as causing profound respiratory depression and regional techniques or volatile agent-based inhalational anaesthesia seem the safest methods of anaesthesia.

Multiple Sclerosis

Although the effects of general anaesthesia on this neurological condition have not been carefully evaluated there is no anaesthetic technique which is known to have a definite, detrimental effect on this disease, with the possible exception of thiopentone. Even central nerve-blocking techniques (e.g. epidural analgesia) have been performed without worsening the condition. However, in advanced cases there may be much muscle wasting, and it is likely that small doses of anaesthetic and analgesic drugs will go a long way. In addition, the autonomic nervous system may be involved in the condition (autonomic neuropathy) so that the patient's blood pressure may drop in response to stresses (e.g. doses of drugs and changes in posture) which would have little or no effect on healthy individuals.

Lastly, as in any of these conditions associated with muscle weakness, patients may have difficulty in coughing up sputum after operation and are consequently prone to chest infections.

● EPILEPSY

Patients on anti-epileptic drugs should be maintained on them until pre-anaesthetic starvation, and given them again as soon as possible postoperatively. Most general anaesthetics tend to have a sedative effect on the central nervous system, but several agents, especially methohexitone, ketamine and enflurane, have been shown to produce convulsions and should not be used. While thiopentone is probably the induction agent of choice, the use of propofol (Diprivan) is still not clear since it is used as a sedative infusion to control fitting and yet has been associated with convulsions occurring in epileptic patients during routine anaesthesia. It should also be remembered that as hypoglycaemia is a stimulus to convulsions, when an epileptic patient is allowed no oral intake for a considerable time because of anaesthesia or surgery, it is worth setting up an intravenous dextrose infusion.

Status Epilepticus

This continuous convulsive state can usually be treated initially with a relatively low, careful intravenous injection of thiopentone or Diazemuls (diazepam). If the convulsions return they may be treated with an intravenous infusion of diazepam, thiopentone or phenytoin. The hypoxic and self-destructive physical effects of the convulsions may be controlled with suxamethonium and in the longer term by vecuronium, but it must be remembered that the electrical over-activity in the brain continues and in addition to the muscle relaxant, anti-epileptic drugs must be used.

● PARKINSON'S DISEASE

This condition is associated not only with involuntary tremor and a shuffling gait but also with an immobile face which may belie a still active brain.

Early treatment consisted mostly of atropine-like drugs and antihistamines, but now levodopa is widely used, this being converted to dopamine in the brain. Under general anaesthesia this drug tends to produce lability of the blood pressure and cardiac dysrhythmias. For this reason, volatile agents should be avoided and, as levodopa has a relatively short action, it should be stopped for 6–12 h before anaesthesia.

● MALIGNANT HYPERPYREXIA (MALIGNANT HYPERTHERMIA)

Although it must have existed before that date, this condition was first described in 1962 as a result of an investigation of the family of a patient who nearly died of hyperpyrexia under general anaesthesia. Findings showed that out of 37 relatives who had been given general anaesthesia, 10 had died. Other similar cases and family histories were soon reported from around the world and it became clear that the condition was inherited. The apparent sudden appearance of the disease was no doubt due not only to the fact that the condition had not previously been recognised as a clinical entity, but also to the fact that two of the most powerful triggers to the condition, namely suxamethonium and halothane, were becoming increasingly popular in anaesthetic practice at about that time.

Malignant hyperpyrexia, which is believed to be due to an abnormality of the muscle-fibre membrane, may be triggered by various pharmacological agents including lignocaine, atropine, diazepam, pancuronium and the phenothiazines, or simply by stress, but easily the most powerful triggering agents are suxamethonium and halothane. Hence it is probably the prime example of an intercurrent condition where administering normally acceptable anaesthetic agents may do devastating harm.

The first sign of the condition may be a failure to relax after suxamethonium, or even increased muscle rigidity. The patient's temperature then rises rapidly, an increase of several degrees Celsius per hour being possible. The patient becomes hot and flushed with a tachycardia. As metabolism outstrips the oxygen supply, cyanosis appears, respiratory and metabolic acidosis produce a profound fall in pH and the serum potassium rises rapidly. Death is common in the severe, untreated case.

Treatment

Earlier treatment was largely symptomatic, with the infusion of cold sodium bicarbonate to combat metabolic acidosis, insulin and glucose to try to restore serum potassium and surface cooling, steroids and procaine in an attempt to relax muscle rigidity. While sometimes successful, procaine was occasionally required in doses likely to produce cardiovascular collapse.

As malignant hyperpyrexia is to some extent dose related, discontinuation of any possible trigger agents may also help.

Dantrolene sodium (Dantrium), a skeletal muscle relaxant, has been shown to be remarkably effective in preventing or treating malignant hyperpyrexia in pigs (some strains of which are extremely susceptible to the condition) and to have a similar life-saving effect in man. To be effective in severe cases, dantrolene should be given within 30 min to 1 h of the onset of the condition. It is now available in the UK and although relatively expensive, it has a shelf-life of 3 years.

● SERUM HEPATITIS (HEPATITIS B ANTIGEN; AUSTRALIA ANTIGEN)

The viral hepatitis referred to by the above names (see also Chapter 46) varies in severity from a subclinical infection to fatal liver failure. Its importance lies not in any particular difficulty in anaesthetising these patients, but in the risk of infecting theatre personnel. Spread is mainly blood borne, but may also be transmitted by body secretions or close physical contact. Serum testing can identify degrees of infectivity and, in the cases of highest risk, disposable gloves and gowns should be used when handling patients. For further details of how to deal with these cases, referral should be made to local hospital policy. For personnel inadvertently contaminated an antiserum is available, but all anaesthetic staff should now be fully immunised.

Hepatitis C

This condition, formerly known as non-A, non-B hepatitis, has now become a clinical problem. Although not as infectious or serious as hepatitis B, hepatitis C-positive hospital staff must be prevented from carrying out exposure-prone clinical procedures, and surgeons may need to be restricted to carrying out body surface surgery. Unfortunately at present, there is no reliable treatment or immunisation available for hepatitis C except for prolonged β-interferon therapy.

● ACQUIRED IMMUNE DEFICIENCY SYNDROME (AIDS)

While this is both numerically, and from the infectivity aspect, a less serious problem than serum hepatitis B in the UK, several factors have led to the government making energetic efforts to disseminate information about prevention of spread of this disease. These features include the high mortality rate (probably 100%) in those infected who develop symptoms, the absence (at present) of any cure or antiserum, and the fact that the virus is sexually transmitted (both homosexually and heterosexually), with a consequent explosive potential for its spread.

The virus can be isolated from blood, semen, tears, saliva and breast milk, but is transmitted principally by sexual intercourse, or transfusion or inoculation by infected blood or blood products. Vomit, sputum, urine, faeces and pus are possibly dangerous if contaminated with blood. The virus is not transmitted by ordinary physical contact, so the risk of infection of theatre personnel is significantly less than with serum hepatitis, precautions being concentrated on the disposal or disinfection of articles, for example, needles, syringes, theatre instruments and drapes contaminated by spilt blood.

● SICKLE-CELL HAEMOGLOBINOPATHIES

This heading covers many genetically transmitted conditions where the patient has an abnormal haemoglobin. Normal haemoglobin is referred to as haemoglobin A. In sickle-cell disease the abnormal haemoglobin is referred to as haemoglobin S (HbS). In sickle-cell anaemia an abnormal gene is inherited from both parents (the homozygous state) so that nearly all the haemoglobin is abnormal, and the condition is also referred to as HbSS. In sickle-cell trait, the abnormal gene is inherited from only one parent (the heterozygous state), so there is a mixture of normal and abnormal haemoglobin. This condition is referred to as HbAS.

Under certain circumstances, which include hypoxia, hypercarbia, hypothermia and acidosis, the HbS may distort and rupture the red blood cells. The distorted cells (called 'sickle' cells) form aggregates in the smaller blood vessels causing infarction in many organs, or the rupture of the red blood cells leads to haemolytic anaemia. Sickling may occur under anaesthesia, especially if hypoxia, hypercarbia, hypothermia or hypotension is allowed to occur. This is much more likely in the case of sickle-cell anaemia than the trait, where lesser amounts of abnormal haemoglobin are present.

● ATYPICAL PSEUDOCHOLINESTERASES

The apnoea which may result when suxamethonium is given to patients with inherited, abnormal pseudocholinesterases is discussed in Chapter 11. If a patient is found to have this abnormal enzyme it is important to test close relatives to discover whether they are similarly affected.

● PORPHYRIAS

The porphyrins are pigments produced in the liver and bone marrow and involved in the synthesis of haem. Disorders in the metabolism of porphyrins are called 'porphyrias' and result in overproduction of some of the porphyrins or their precursors. There are several porphyrias, but only acute intermittent porphyria will be considered here.

Acute Intermittent Porphyria

This inherited condition often presents in young adults. There may be acute onset of abdominal pain, which may be mistaken for acute appendicitis; there is often a peripheral neuropathy with paraesthesia and weakness of trunk and limb muscles, which may cause respiratory embarrassment. There may also be tachycardia and hypertension. During an attack the urine turns dark on standing due to a high concentration of porphobilinogen. An acute attack of porphyria may be triggered by any of the barbiturates, which are absolutely contraindicated in this condition.

● RHEUMATOID ARTHRITIS

This is a general systemic disease which in its acute phase may show tachycardia, fever and anaemia. Typically, the small joints of the fingers and toes are the first to become affected, but other joints are frequently involved and are of interest to the anaesthetist. Such joints include the temporomandibular joint and the joints of the cervical spine where stiffness may lead to difficulty in intubation, and the costovertebral joints where limitation of movement may lead to a reduction in vital capacity and a tendency to postoperative pneumonia. Rheumatoid arthritis may affect the lung tissue itself (rheumatoid lung) and is also associated with chronic anaemia. Lastly, patients with rheumatoid arthritis may be on, or have recently taken, a course of steroids.

16

Anaesthesia and Endocrine Disease

•Thyroid gland •Adrenal (suprarenal) gland •Pituitary gland •Parathyroid glands •Pancreas

The endocrine glands consist of the pituitary, thyroid, parathyroids, adrenals, ovaries, testes and the endocrine (insulin-producing) part of the pancreas. The pituitary gland synthesises several 'trophic' hormones that are responsible for controlling the output from the other endocrine glands. These glands produce several hormones which control many of the physiological and metabolic functions of the body. For this reason, reduced or excessive activity of any of them may produce severe metabolic disturbance as seen, for example, in thyrotoxicosis or diabetes. The endocrine glands present anaesthetic problems in two situations: first, when a patient undergoing elective surgery is coincidentally suffering from an endocrine disorder and is receiving treatment; and, secondly, when the endocrine disorder itself is to be treated surgically by removal of part or all of the gland.

● THYROID GLAND

Hyperthyroidism

Unless emergency surgery is indicated, it is wise to avoid anaesthetising a patient with untreated hyperthyroidism or thyrotoxicosis, either for thyroidectomy or for a coincidental condition. Preoperative restoration of normal thyroid function is obtained by using antithyroid drugs, for example, carbimazole (neo-mercazole), and then iodine is given immediately preoperatively to decrease the vascularity of the gland. Symptomatic treatment of hyperthyroidism often includes β-adrenoceptor blockade to reduce the tachycardia, and general sedation to reduce hyperexcitability and shaking. If the patient must be anaesthetised in a hyperthyroid state, the anaesthetic should be a deep one with adequate preoperative sedation and effective β-blockade.

Hypothyroidism

This is usually a chronic condition which either arises spontaneously or results from excessive treatment of hyperthyroidism by radioactive iodine irradiation or surgery. As the thyroid gland controls metabolic activity (basal metabolic rate), underactivity of the gland causes a patient to be sluggish and prone to hypothermia, hypoglycaemia, muscle weakness and coma. They may also suffer from respiratory depression and may only metabolise drugs slowly. Satisfactory treatment is obtained by chronic administration of thyroxine, but hypothyroidism may occur, for example, when the patient suffers coincidental intestinal obstruction and fails to absorb their thyroxine. In this case, the patient may appear tired or listless but it may only be when they fail to wake up from an anaesthetic that hypothyroidism is suspected. In this case it is essential to give T_3 (triiodothyronine), which acts more rapidly than T_4 (thyroxine) to restore normal thyroid activity.

Thyroid crisis

After partial thyroidectomy in a thyrotoxic patient, a thyroid crisis occasionally occurs, this being a severe increase in the symptoms of hyperthyroidism. It is important to keep the patient cool and sedated and to control their hypertension and tachycardia, which is usually achieved with β-blockade and, if necessary, digoxin to prevent the development of congestive cardiac failure. The overactive remaining thyroid tissue is treated with intravenous iodine and carbimazole or thiouracil.

● ADRENAL (SUPRARENAL) GLAND

The adrenal glands are divided into the cortex, which secretes cortisol and aldosterone, and the medulla, which is part of the sympathetic nervous system and responsible for secreting adrenaline and noradrenaline.

Hyperadrenalism – Primary Cortical (Conn's Syndrome)

This rare condition is associated with a high serum aldosterone concentration and therefore a high sodium and low serum potassium in the blood. The patients also suffer from hypertension and impaired renal function. Anaesthesia for removing what is usually a benign cortical adenoma must take account of the metabolic problems in a similar way to anaesthetising patients in renal failure. Preoperative treatment with spironolactone, an aldosterone antagonist, may return the blood pressure and serum electrolyte concentrations to normal.

Hyperadrenalism – Secondary Cortical (Cushing's Disease)

Excess pituitary production of adrenocorticotrophic hormone (ACTH) leads to excessive activity of the adrenal cortex, producing, in particular, glucocorticoids, for example, cortisol. This produces sodium retention, oedema and hypertension together with other changes which resemble the side-effects of steroid therapy, for example, 'moon-face' and striae.

Hypoadrenalism – Primary Cortical (Addison's Disease)

In this condition atrophy of the adrenal cortex and medulla occurs and the patients become pigmented, weak and hypotensive and sometimes have considerable electrolyte disorders. Preoperative treatment with hydrocortisone and fludrocortisone is necessary to restore their metabolic balance before surgery.

Hypoadrenalism – Secondary Cortical

This usually occurs in patients who are or have recently been on steroid therapy. The side-effects of steroid therapy are important, and include euphoria, a thrombotic tendency, delayed wound healing, mild glycosuria, sodium and water retention and osteoporosis. Anaesthesia itself is only a moderate stress unless accidental hypothermia occurs or the operation is prolonged. Normal steroid cover with hydrocortisone (Chapter 14) is satisfactory for patients who are receiving or who have recently received steroid therapy, mineralocorticoid (fludrocortisone) cover not usually being necessary.

Medullary Hyperadrenalism (Phaeochromocytoma)

Tumours of the medullary portion of the adrenal gland are rare but nevertheless present considerable anaesthetic problems. A phaeochromocytoma is a tumour of chromaffin tissue which may be either benign or malignant, single or multiple. It may occur anywhere along the sympathetic chain as well as in the adrenal gland itself. As sympathetic tissue is involved, there is excessive production of noradrenaline and adrenaline. The patients usually present with paroxysmal hypertension and sweating, together with headache and palpitations. Preoperative control of wild fluctuations of blood pressure with both α- and β-adrenergic blockade is essential to provide a smooth anaesthetic. Failure to do this may produce such severe rises in blood pressure that a cerebrovascular accident may occur. Death may also result from ventricular arrhythmias.

Bilateral Adrenalectomy

This is usually carried out as a further operation in the treatment of disseminated breast cancer and, apart from needing to maintain the patient on steroid cover postoperatively, the main anaesthetic problems are that the patients are often frail with numerous bone secondaries, pleural effusions and electrolyte disorders.

● PITUITARY GLAND

Hyperpituitarism

Although the pituitary gland produces several trophic hormones it is chiefly disorders of the production of growth hormone which may present anaesthetic difficulties. Overproduction of growth hormone in adults leads to acromegaly with considerable overgrowth of the jaws, tongue, pharynx and larynx, and thickening of the vocal cords. The hands become spade-like and the skin may be extremely tough. It may be difficult to anaesthetise and intubate these patients, usually for mechanical reasons, and care must be taken not to precipitate respiratory obstruction only to find intubating the patient impossible. Once anaesthetised, patients with acromegaly do not present severe anaesthetic problems, but they are prone to obstruction and hypoxia in the recovery room and careful postoperative observation is essential.

Hypopituitarism

Reduced pituitary activity is associated with a reduction in the production of growth hormone together with other trophic hormones, resulting in lethargy and a low basal metabolic rate. These patients may be exceptionally sensitive to barbiturates and narcotic analgesics and general anaesthesia may precipitate coma in patients with severe metabolic disorders. Reduced levels of ACTH and thyroid stimulating hormone (TSH) may produce secondary effects due to failure of hormone production of the relevant glands.

● PARATHYROID GLANDS

Hyperparathyroidism

The parathyroid glands control the blood calcium concentration, which is essential for normal nerve and cardiac conduction. Parathormone, the hormone secreted by the parathyroids, increases the mobilisation of calcium from bone and in hyperparathyroidism, a high serum calcium may be associated with metabolic disorders requiring treatment with diuretics and calcitonin. The cause is usually a parathyroid adenoma requiring surgical removal; this condition is particularly common in patients with renal failure on dialysis.

Hypoparathyroidism

Hypoparathyroidism is usually a complication of thyroidectomy, the glands being removed inadvertently with the thyroid. A reduced serum concentration of calcium may be accompanied by muscle spasms and tetany, the treatment being intravenous calcium gluconate. Anaesthesia in patients with parathyroid disorders does not usually present any additional difficulties to those encountered with the thyroidectomy except that many of the patients may be in renal failure, the cause of their parathyroid disorder.

● PANCREAS

The endocrine portion of the pancreas secretes insulin and glucagon from the β- and α-cells of the islets of Langerhans, respectively. These two hormones are responsible for controlling blood sugar and diabetes mellitus is probably the commonest endocrine disorder likely to produce anaesthetic difficulties.

Management of Diabetic Patients during Anaesthesia and Surgery

In most cases, diabetes does not cause problems if the anaesthetist accepts that the patients are essentially normal people with impaired or absent insulin production. If their diabetes is well under control preoperatively there is no reason why it should not remain so throughout the operation. Patients should arrive in the anaesthetic room not only with a normal or slightly raised blood sugar level but also with normal glycogen stores, glycogen being stored in the liver and used to maintain a normal blood sugar level. It is important therefore that they are starved for the minimum time preoperatively and are operated on at the beginning of the list at a predetermined time.

Preoperative knowledge of the stability of their diabetic regimen is essential and in many cases little or no additional treatment is required. Diet-controlled diabetics can simply be starved preoperatively in the normal way, as the only problem likely to develop is hyperglycaemia. To err on the side of hyperglycaemia is a far safer way of conducting the anaesthetic. Patients on oral hypoglycaemic drugs should stop these 1–2 days before surgery and will therefore tend to become hyperglycaemic. For more major surgery, with prolonged postoperative intravenous therapy and stress, it may be necessary to introduce a temporary regimen with soluble insulin.

Those on insulin should be controlled by whatever regimen is necessary, depending on the urgency of the operation, the degree of control of the diabetes and the expected postoperative course. Most insulin-dependent diabetics tend to be maintained on a regimen of short-acting soluble insulin (Actrapid) and a longer-acting insulin preparation ('-tard'). These are frequently given in combinations such as Mixtard.

In general, patients who are undergoing a short operation may simply omit their morning dose of short-acting insulin and their breakfast, knowing that they will be eating later in the day. In major surgery, however, it is essential not only to maintain a normal blood sugar level but also to ensure that glucose passes into the cells where it can be used for metabolism; this can be achieved only by simultaneous administration of glucose and insulin. In this event a reduced morning dose of insulin together with a 5% dextrose infusion is usual. In more complicated cases, or when the diabetes is out of control, it is most satisfactory to change the patient on to a sliding scale of soluble (Actrapid) insulin controlled on 4-hourly blood or urine glucose estimations. Frequent measurements of blood sugar and intravenous administration of glucose and insulin are probably the best and most accurate way of controlling diabetes during anaesthesia.

More recently, slow intravenous insulin infusions have been successfully used to treat diabetic hyperglycaemia and these are becoming widely used for intra-operative control of diabetics undergoing major surgery, in conjunction with an intravenous glucose infusion.

In the Alberti regimen, 10 units of Actrapid insulin and 10 mmol potassium chloride are added to 500 ml 10% dextrose which is then infused over 4 h. This fail-safe system means that variations in infusion rate cannot produce an imbalance of glucose and insulin or hypokalaemia.

17

Intravenous Techniques: Central Venous Pressure

•Technique and equipment •Complications •Central venous pressure

The hypodermic syringe is usually believed to have been invented in 1853 by Pravaz of Lyons. A year later a syringe and a needle were introduced by Alexander Wood, a Scotsman, and over subsequent years various anaesthetic agents were injected intravenously, including chloral hydrate, chloroform and ether. In 1924 the first barbiturate was given intravenously, and in 1935 the most famous intravenous anaesthetic agent of them all, thiopentone, was introduced in the USA. Reusable metal intravenous cannulae began to be replaced by the disposable plastic variety in the mid-1950s. Improvements in their quality, changes in the versatility of their design and the variety of substances of which they are made have been continuing ever since. The original, reusable hypodermic needles, which had to be sharpened periodically, have been completely replaced by disposable needles.

The common uses of intravenous techniques are for taking venous samples, for administering drugs (in particular for inducing and maintaining anaesthesia), for the transfusion of blood or infusion of other fluids, for various radiological procedures, for central venous pressure measurement and for catheterisation of the right side of the heart. For long-term intravenous feeding a central venous line is almost essential.

● TECHNIQUE AND EQUIPMENT

The commonest sites for venepuncture are the superficial veins of the dorsum of the hand or of the forearm. The veins on the back of the hand are often the easiest to use, but for cannulation for intravenous infusion a straighter vein on the forearm tends to be less temperamental. It is essential that the lighting be good and preferably oblique as it tends to make the veins more obvious. The venous outflow from the arm should be occluded by a tourniquet or by an assistant squeezing the arm. The nearer the venepuncture is performed to the venous obstruction, the more distended and easier to see and palpate will the vein be.

Having occluded the venous outflow, various techniques may be used to make the vein more obvious. These include lightly tapping the vein with the fingers (firm slapping may be painful), actively or passively clenching the patient's fingers, allowing the arm to hang below the level of the heart, or occasionally by applying warmth over the intended venepuncture site. The junction of two veins, if convenient, is the best site for venepuncture because the vein is less likely to escape from the probing needle. It is also wise to pierce the skin and vein in two separate movements because the vein is less likely to be transfixed by the jerking movement which tends to accompany the passage of the needle or cannula through the skin. Needles should always be advanced at least several millimetres up the lumen of the vein to ensure that the entire needle bevel remains within the vein during injection. Blood should always be aspirated before injection. Similarly, cannulae should be advanced a few millimetres before removing the needle as it is possible for the latter to be within the vein and blood to be aspirated while the shoulder of the cannula has not yet passed through the vein wall into the lumen.

Other useful veins, particularly in emergencies, are the external jugular vein which tends to fill when the patient is placed head-down, and the veins in the antecubital fossa. The veins on the medial side of the latter site should not be used routinely because there is an appreciable risk of injection into the brachial artery or of damaging the median nerve. However, it may be a useful site for rapid infusion in a hypovolaemic patient until other more convenient veins appear as the circulating blood volume is restored.

Other useful injection sites, especially in babies, are the scalp, the front of the wrist and the saphenous vein in front of the medial malleolus at the ankle. If possible, the legs should be avoided for infusions in adults because of the risk of unpleasant thrombophlebitis.

Types of Equipment

Winged Needles

These needles have two flexible plastic wings attached to the shank of the needle and a length of flexible tubing which ends in either a female Luer adapter or a rubber bung (e.g. 'Butterfly'). The wings serve as a needle-holder and as an aid to secure taping of the needle after venepuncture. These needles were popular for induction and intermittent injections during anaesthesia, but even if securely fixed in position they retain the disadvantage of cutting out of the vein; hence they have been largely replaced by cannulae.

Cannulae and Catheters

These are made of various substances including polyvinyl chloride (PVC), nylon, silastic, polyethylene, polypropylene and Teflon, or other materials may be Teflon coated. The difference between a cannula and a catheter is simply one of length, anything under about 12 cm being considered a cannula.

The cannula is a 'needle-inside' device (e.g. 'Venflon'). Catheters may also be manufactured in this way, but have the disadvantage that the longer the catheter, the longer and more unwieldy the needle it contains. In addition, it cannot be supplied with a stilette to aid insertion, as the needle is already inside the catheter.

Another common type of catheter is the 'catheter-inside-needle' design (e.g. 'Drum-cartridge'). This is more convenient to insert, and is usually advanced still containing a stilette. The serious disadvantage of this design is that should the catheter ever be withdrawn relative to the needle, it is possible to shear off the distal part of the catheter against the bevel of the needle and the fragment may migrate centrally in the vein as an embolus.

A third type of catheter is inserted through a cannula (e.g. 'Cavafix'). The cannula is inserted over a needle in the usual way, and after withdrawing the needle the catheter is inserted through the cannula.

The final type of catheter is supplied alone and is intended for insertion by surgical cut-down.

Seldinger Technique

This technique was originally devised for the insertion of catheters into veins or arteries for radiological investigations. A needle or cannula is used to insert a flexible guidewire into the chosen vein. The needle is then removed and a tapered dilator threaded over the guidewire to enlarge the hole in the vein. The dilator is then removed and a large cannula threaded over the guidewire which in turn is then removed. This cannula can then be used to pass a variety of catheters, for example, triple lumen or Swan-Ganz, for anaesthetic or intensive care purposes.

● COMPLICATIONS

Complications of intravenous techniques range from trivial to life-endangering. Minor problems include haematoma formation at the injection site and the development of temporary erythema or weals along the line of the vein due to a localised allergic reaction to the substance injected.

A more unpleasant complication of venepuncture is inflammation of the vein (phlebitis). Sooner or later this occurs with any prolonged venous cannulation and is caused by a combination of the irritating effect of infused fluids (e.g. potassium or antibiotics) on the vein wall and bacterial action caused by bacteria entering through the puncture site in the skin. Fluids administered into a central venous catheter are rapidly diluted by the large volume of blood, so that their irritant action is greatly reduced, and if care is taken to maintain the puncture site sterile, these central venous lines may remain *in situ* for weeks.

When phlebitis occurs, apart from the redness and tenderness of the overlying skin the vein rapidly becomes blocked by thrombi (thrombophlebitis). Fortunately, these thrombi are firmly attached to the vein wall by the inflammation, so seldom give rise to emboli. However, if the blockage occurs in a major vein (e.g. femoral) this alone may lead to disability owing to the oedema produced in the limb.

Embolism of catheter fragments caused by faulty technique has already been mentioned. Catheter embolism may also occur if the shaft of a cannula or catheter separates from the hub due to faulty bonding of the two parts – a much less likely occurrence with improved methods of manufacture.

Air embolism may occur when entry is made into a vein where the pressure is subatmospheric. For this reason patients should be placed head-down to raise the pressure in the neck veins before performing venous cannulation. Air may also gain entry to the venous system with some methods of pressure transfusion, but not with the methods whereby the infusion bag is squeezed from outside (Fenwal, Tycos pressure infusers) because infusion automatically stops when the bag is empty.

Transmission of viruses, for example, hepatitis B and C and human immunodeficiency virus (HIV), are the biggest threat to personnel performing the above procedures and hospitals have policies to safeguard staff against these. Such precautions include wearing disposable gloves, not resheathing needles, and using special equipment, for example, vacuum-containing tubes to draw blood.

● CENTRAL VENOUS PRESSURE

In recent years the measurement of central venous pressure has become an important aid in managing seriously ill and especially hypovolaemic patients. The veins concerned are the large intrathoracic veins leading to the right side of the heart, i.e. the superior and inferior venae cavae.

To understand central venous pressure it helps to consider the circulation as being divided into three parts: (a) the venous system, which returns the blood down a pressure gradient from the periphery to (b) the heart, which pumps the blood out into (c), the arterial system, which provides a varying peripheral resistance. It also makes it easier to consider the left ventricle as being the heart's pump and the right side of the heart and pulmonary circulation simply as part of the venous system leading to it, i.e. the reservoir.

The normal central venous pressure is 0–12 cmH$_2$O, measured from the point at which the mid-axillary line crosses the fourth intercostal space with the patient supine. In the presence of hypovolaemia, the venous return and the central venous pressure fall. The body attempts to maintain the blood pressure by venoconstriction to reduce venous pooling and improve venous turn, and by vasoconstriction on the arterial side to increase peripheral resistance. Only after these compensatory mechanisms have failed does the blood pressure fall. Thus the central venous pressure is a more sensitive index of reduced blood volume than blood pressure. It is safe to infuse fluids quickly provided that the central venous pressure does not rise above normal limits.

Conversely, the central venous pressure tends to rise above normal in overtransfusion. It also rises when the pump, i.e. the heart, fails. Common examples of this condition are a heart weakened by acute or chronic myocardial ischaemia, or compromised by depressant anaesthetic agents such as thiopentone or halothane. Clearly, these two groups of factors causing a rise in central venous pressure may be interrelated, it being much easier to overtransfuse a weak heart.

Central Venous Pressure Catheter Techniques

The various routes by which catheters may be inserted into the central veins are shown in Figure 17.1 and summarised below with some of the advantages and disadvantages of the various approaches. The complications described above for catheters apply, of course, catheter embolisation being a real danger with some types of equipment. Care must be taken to avoid infection, it being wise to insert the catheter with a full aseptic technique, to apply an antibiotic locally to the injection site and to apply a transparent occlusive dressing, which should be changed regularly.

The ideal position for the catheter tip is in the superior vena cava. A catheter which has stopped too peripherally, i.e. outside the thoracic cavity, will give an incorrect reading, while a catheter which has been inserted too far may perforate the wall of the right atrium. If the catheter is advanced even further it may enter the right ventricle, which has a much higher pressure. A rough guide to the length of catheter to be inserted may be gained by holding another catheter (or the catheter's stilette) against the patient's skin along the line of the vein that has been used. Even so, accurate confirmation of the position of the catheter tip can be made only by X-ray examination of the chest.

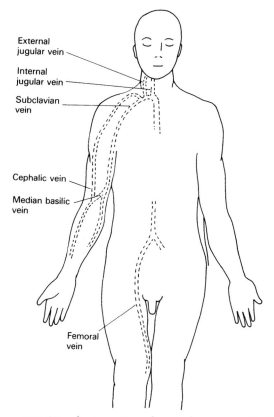

Figure 17.1 Sites for insertion of central venous catheters.

Methods of Central Venous Catheterisation

Veins in the Arm

The veins in the ante cubital fossa are normally used, the approach through the median basilic vein on the medial aspect of the elbow being more likely to prove successful than the cephalic vein on the outer aspect of the antecubital fossa. All the arm veins require long catheters which makes them less likely to be successful than a more central approach, but, as they are free from some of the serious complications of the direct approaches to the neck veins (e.g. pneumothorax), they should usually be the first choice.

External Jugular Vein

With the patient slightly head-down, venepuncture of this vein may be easy. However, for an approach so close to the central veins, this method is unfortunately accompanied by a rather high failure rate in accurate placement of the catheter, since the vein kinks as it passes into the thoracic cavity.

Subclavian Vein

The patient should be placed head-down to distend the vein and to prevent air embolism. Supraclavicular and infraclavicular techniques are used. They have the highest success rates, but also the highest incidence of pneumothorax.

Internal Jugular Vein

The patient is placed head-down and the skin pierced at the apex of a triangle formed by the two heads of the sternocleidomastoid muscle lateral to the artery. This approach also has a high success rate and pneumothorax is less likely. However, there is some risk of producing a haematoma if the neighbouring carotid artery is pierced, and on the left side damage to the thoracic duct may result in chylothorax.

Femoral Vein

The femoral vein should be avoided if possible for central venous catheterisation because the incidence of thrombophlebitis and oedema of the leg is high when this site is used.

18

Airway Management in Anaesthesia

•Face masks •Artificial airways •Tracheal intubation •Indications for tracheal intubation •Intubation equipment •Complications of tracheal intubation •Difficult airway management

The supply of anaesthetic gases to the anaesthetic machine is discussed in Chapter 7 and their transport from its outlet to the patient in Chapter 8. The muscles of the upper airway relax under general anaesthesia. This may cause the upper airway to obstruct, thereby hampering the supply of oxygen and anaesthetic gases to the patient. There is also a risk of regurgitation and aspiration of gastric contents under anaesthetic (see Chapter 24). One of the fundamental responsibilities of the anaesthetist is to maintain a clear, unobstructed airway and protect the lungs from soiling by gastric contents. This chapter discusses some of the equipment and techniques that are used to achieve one or both of these aims.

● FACE MASKS (Fig. 18.1)

Face masks have a body with an inflatable cuff to facilitate an airtight seal around the mouth and nose. A hole in the body of the mask connects it to an angle piece and the breathing system. Currently used masks are clear so that it is possible to see if the patient vomits, a distinct advantage over the previously used black, opaque antistatic rubber masks. These masks are disposable and available in various sizes and a comprehensive choice should be available in every anaesthetic room.

● ARTIFICIAL AIRWAYS

'Airways' are artificial aids introduced through the mouth or nose to help the anaesthetist maintain an unobstructed passage of gases to and from the patient and to also aspirate secretions from the pharynx.

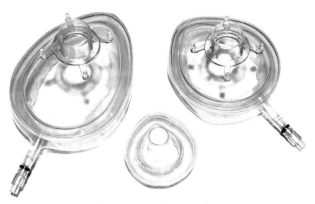

Figure 18.1 Face masks.

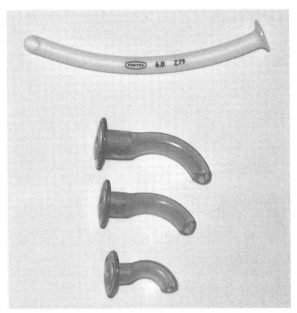

Figure 18.2 Guedel oropharyngeal airway (bottom). Nasopharyngeal airway (top).

Oropharyngeal Airways

The most common example is the Guedel oropharyngeal airway illustrated in Figure 18.2. It is a flattened tube with a broad flange at its proximal end designed to prevent it slipping into the patient's mouth, a curved 'body' which lies on the tongue and a narrow distal end. These airways are made of polyvinyl chloride (PVC), are disposable, are available in various sizes and are easy to introduce when the patient is deeply anaesthetised. They may cause damage to the teeth if introduced when the patient is lightly anaesthetised, or during emergence from anaesthesia.

Nasopharyngeal Airways

These are curved tubes with a small flange at the 'nasal' end and a bevelled 'pharyngeal' end that lies in the pharynx (Fig. 18.2). A safety pin is commonly attached to this flange to prevent the airway slipping into the nostril. They are made of different materials including PVC, red rubber or silastic and are available in various sizes. A good guide to selecting the appropriate size is to choose an airway with a diameter that roughly is similar to the patient's little finger. Unlike oropharyngeal airways, they are easily tolerated by lightly anaesthetised patients and are very useful in patients with difficult airways during both induction and recovery from anaesthesia. They prevent damage to teeth and suction of secretions is more effectively achieved through them, but because the nasal mucosa is very vascular they may cause bleeding when inserted. Nasal airways (and also nasogastric tubes and nasotracheal tubes) are contraindicated in patients who have had a fracture of the base of their skull.

Cuffed Oropharyngeal Airway

A modification of the Guedel airway has been described where a cuff can be inflated around the tubular portion of the device to provide an airtight seal in the pharynx and a 15 mm connector at its proximal end to connect it to an anaesthetic breathing system (Fig. 18.3). Unlike a face mask–Guedel airway combination which requires the anaesthetist constantly to support the jaw, with the cuffed oropharyngeal airway (COPA) a 'hands free' system is possible. The COPA is mainly used in spontaneously breathing patients. It is available in various sizes and is disposable. Although attractive in design, its use has not become very popular.

Laryngeal Mask Airway (Fig. 18.4)

This device was invented in 1983 by Dr Archie Brain, a British anaesthetist. It was designed with the idea of providing a patent airway with a device which could be inserted without an instrument (such as a laryngoscope) and which would lie above the vocal cords rather than below them as in the case of a tracheal tube.

The first prototype was made with a mini facemask attached to a cut tracheal tube allowing the 'mask' to sit in the hypopharynx and above the laryngeal inlet and the tube to be connected to an anaesthetic breathing system. The commercial version has a 'cup' with an inflatable cuff

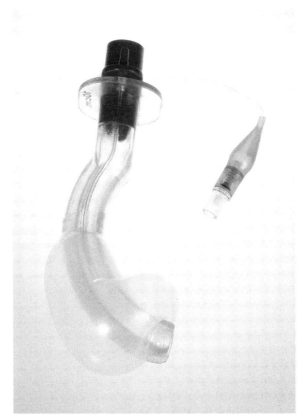

Figure 18.3 Cuffed oropharyngeal airway.

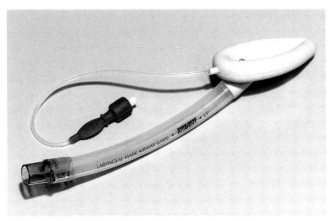

Figure 18.4 Standard laryngeal mask airway.

surrounding it and connected to a flexible stem, the proximal end of which has a 15 mm standard connector designed to fit to an anaesthetic breathing system. The cuff of the laryngeal mask airway (LMA) which lies above the vocal cords when inflated does not, however, prevent aspiration of gastric contents, unlike the cuff of the tracheal tube which when inflated provides an airtight seal in the trachea.

The LMA is made of silicone rubber and is available in various sizes so that it can be used in patients of all ages and sizes. It is reusable after sterilisation by autoclaving. It is now the most commonly used airway device in anaesthetic practice. It frees the anaesthetist to perform other tasks, it causes less morbidity compared to a tracheal tube and can be left *in situ* postoperatively until the patient is literally awake when it can be safely removed by the recovery staff. Its use can be quickly and easily learnt even by paramedical staff. It can be safely used both in spontaneously breathing patients and in those undergoing controlled ventilation provided the inflation pressures are <25 cmH$_2$O. It is frequently effective in maintaining oxygenation in a patient with a difficult airway. It can also be used as a conduit to pass a tracheal tube into the lungs through its stem although the intubating LMA (see below) is more appropriate for this use. The LMA does not prevent aspiration of gastric contents into the trachea and its use is not recommended in patients at risk of this complication.

Modifications of the standard LMA described above are also available and include a single-use disposable variety – the LMA UNIQUE®, a reinforced design with a flexometallic stem for use in head and neck surgery and more recently the LMA PRO-SEAL®. This latter device is designed to provide a higher seal and has a double tube arrangement, the second tube acting as a drain tube for gastric secretions and also allowing for easy passage of a nasogastric tube. This arrangement is thought to prevent gastric insufflation and it is likely that this device would be of use when a longer duration of intermittent positive pressure ventilation (IPPV) with an LMA is required.

Intubating Laryngeal Mask Airway (Fig. 18.5)

As the name suggests, the intubating laryngeal mask airway (ILMA) is specifically designed to facilitate the placement of a tracheal tube. Its design overcomes some of the limitations of a standard LMA as an intubation device. The principal features of this device are an anatomically curved, rigid airway tube (unlike the flexible stem of a standard LMA) with an integral guiding handle. It is possible to connect this tube to a breathing system and it also allows tracheal tubes of up to 8 mm internal diameter to be passed through it. An epiglottic elevating bar elevates the epiglottis during tracheal tube insertion thereby improving success rates and

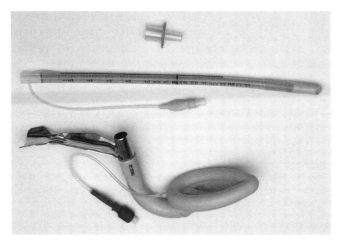

Figure 18.5 Intubating laryngeal mask airway with dedicated tracheal tube.

avoiding trauma. To avoid the problems of railroading with ordinary tubes, a proprietary tracheal tube is also supplied with the device. This is made of silicone, is reinforced and comes with a detachable 15 mm connector and a special conical tip that avoids impingement on the vocal cords or arytenoids thereby reducing the chances of trauma and improving the success rate. A tracheal tube pusher allows the removal of the ILMA once intubation is complete. Unlike the standard LMA which requires the anaesthetists' fingers to manipulate its position in the mouth, the ILMA cup can be manipulated by moving its handle outside the patient's mouth – a distinct advantage in difficult cases. A high success rate of intubation has been achieved with this device in patients with both a normal and difficult airway. Intubation can be achieved either by a blind technique or by visual guidance using a flexible fibrescope. The ILMA is available in various sizes and is reusable after autoclaving. Some disadvantages include the fact that this device cannot be used in patients who have limited mouth opening and it cannot be used for placement of nasal tubes. Its high costs also preclude its routine use.

● TRACHEAL INTUBATION

The first uses of tracheal intubation were in the treatment of asphyxia neonatorum and in cases of drowning. For these purposes, in 1754, Benjamin Pugh, a Chelmsford surgeon, designed a tube made from a coiled wire covered with soft leather, and in 1788, Charles Kite, a surgeon from Gravesend, designed a curved metal cannula which he used in several cases of apparent drowning in the River Thames. These earlier tubes were introduced blindly into the larynx, usually with the help of the operator's finger.

In 1880 anaesthesia was administered for the first time through a tracheal tube. The next main advance in tracheal intubation was the invention of the first laryngoscope by Kirstein in 1895, but the instrument was somewhat primitive and did not gain widespread popularity. Not until an improved laryngoscope was designed by Chevalier Jackson in 1920 did intubation under direct vision become a more widespread technique. Added impetus to the popular use of tracheal intubation occurred in the First World War, which resulted in a great many casualties requiring surgery to the head and neck. During this period Magill introduced the orotracheal tube with an inflatable cuff.

● INDICATIONS FOR TRACHEAL INTUBATION

There is some variation among individual anaesthetists as to exactly which patient they consider requires intubation, but the following are typical indications.

For Head and Neck Operations or Remoteness from Patient

For most operations on the head and neck, and especially for those on the upper respiratory tract, tracheal intubation is desirable or even essential.

On other occasions it may be desirable that the anaesthetist keeps some distance away from the patient. This might happen, for instance, in anaesthesia for X-ray procedures where, to avoid excessive irradiation, it is essential that the anaesthetist be remote from the patient.

To Prevent Aspiration of Gastric Contents into the Lungs

Under general anaesthesia the respiratory tract is completely safe from contamination by gastric contents only when a tracheal tube has been passed and its cuff inflated. For this reason tracheal intubation is indicated in most emergency anaesthesia.

When Intermittent Positive-pressure Ventilation is to be Used

It is difficult and dangerous to ventilate a patient with a face mask for any length of time, there always being the possibility of regurgitation, especially if the stomach is inadvertently inflated. Many anaesthetists now use an LMA for this purpose especially when the procedure is short and there is no risk of regurgitation and aspiration of gastric contents.

When the Airway is Difficult

In some patients it may be difficult or impossible to maintain an airway for any length of time with a mask. The degree of difficulty varies in different patients. The patient's position may also make using a mask difficult, for example, the prone position.

For Ill Patients, or With Complicated Anaesthetic Techniques

Where perfect control of the airway is essential at all times it is better to use tracheal intubation. Examples of this include the very frail or ill patient, or when some special technique is being used, for example, hypotensive anaesthesia.

For Resuscitation

The apnoeic patient is most effectively and safely ventilated through a tracheal tube, although simpler methods, such as mouth-to-mouth respiration or ventilation with a face mask, are usually effective if equipment for intubation is not to hand. An LMA is also recommended for this purpose.

In longer term intensive care, nasotracheal or orotracheal intubation may be continued for several days while the problem of whether the patient requires a tracheostomy is resolved.

● INTUBATION EQUIPMENT

Familiarity with the equipment required for tracheal intubation is best learned in the anaesthetic room. The following is intended as a general introduction.

Laryngoscopes

Laryngoscopes consist of a handle and a detachable blade usually made of metal. Batteries in the handle illuminate a tiny bulb, screwed into a socket on the blade, allowing the laryngoscope to be used to pass a tracheal tube into the larynx under direct vision.

Traditional laryngoscope blades are of two types, the straight-bladed type (Fig. 18.6a) and the curved-bladed type (Fig. 18.6b), the Macintosh. The essential difference is that with the straight-bladed type it is intended that

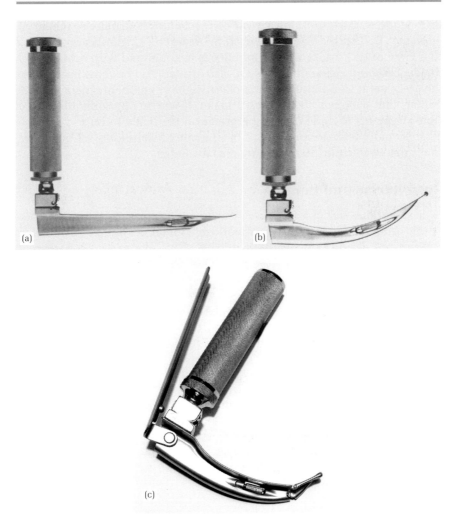

Figure 18.6 (a) Straight-bladed laryngoscope (Soper pattern). (b) Macintosh laryngoscope. (c) McCoy laryngoscope.

the laryngoscope blade be passed underneath the epiglottis, which it lifts forwards. The Macintosh blade, in contrast, is designed for passing into the vallecula, i.e. in front of the epiglottis, which is indirectly lifted forwards by pressure against the root of the tongue. Many different shapes and sizes of blades have been described, mainly designed to aid in specific situations, for example, the Oxford blade with a 'C' shape for intubating patients with cleft palate, the polio and the McCoy blades for use in difficult intubation. The McCoy blade (Fig. 18.6c) has a hinged tip which can be lifted up by pressing a lever connected to the handle of the laryngoscope. The hinged tip can be used to lift up the epiglottis and improve the view of the larynx when difficulty is encountered with a Macintosh blade. Different sizes of handles are also available and a short handle may be very useful to aid intubation in obese patients and in pregnant patients when the enlarged breasts can make laryngoscopy difficult. Other improvements include clipping a prism on the blade to improve vision. Traditionally laryngoscopes have been made of stainless steel but nowadays disposable plastic blades are also available.

Introducers and Bougies

It is sometimes difficult to place a tracheal tube correctly when the vocal cords are not fully visualised. A malleable metal introducer can then be introduced into the tracheal tube and its shape altered to aid passage of the tube into the larynx. A more popular and useful device is a long gum-elastic bougie (Eschmann type) which has a bent tip (Fig. 18.7). A lubricated bougie can be introduced through the vocal cords on its own while performing laryngoscopy. A tracheal tube is then railroaded onto the bougie and into the trachea. A 'light wand' is a device which can be introduced into the tracheal tube and its tip lighted to aid intubation.

Magill Intubating Forceps (Fig. 18.8)

These forceps are useful in directing a tracheal tube into the larynx or a nasogastric tube into the oesophagus. Their design allows the anaesthetist to use the laryngoscope with the left hand while holding the forceps in the right hand. The angle in the forceps between the handles and the jaws allows them to be used with the handles out of the direct line of sight.

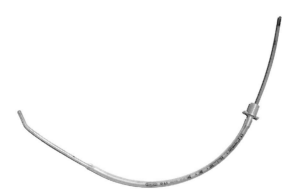

Figure 18.7 Gum-elastic bougie through a tracheal tube.

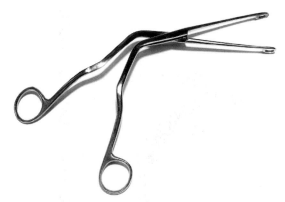

Figure 18.8 Magill intubating forceps.

Flexible Fibreoptic Laryngoscope (Fig. 18.9)

The most recent development in intubating equipment is the availability of a fibreoptic instrument where both light and image can be transmitted along flexible fibreoptic bundles encased in an insertion cord which has a movable tip at its distal end. This tip can be manipulated by a lever situated on the proximal section or 'body' of the instrument. Light is carried from a light source via light transmission fibreoptic bundles to illuminate the object. Light is then reflected onto an objective lens situated at the tip of the fibrescope from where it travels along the image transmission bundles. An eyepiece lens also situated on the body allows the operator to view the image which has been transmitted from the tip of the fibrescope. In this way the 'eye' is at the tip of the instrument, making continuous visualisation of the airway possible at all times. The intention is to pass the instrument (with a tracheal tube loaded on the insertion cord) into the nose or mouth and under direct vision manipulate its tip through the pharynx and larynx and into the trachea. The tracheal tube is then railroaded over the fibreoptic laryngoscope into the trachea.

Fibreoptic intubation is particularly useful for securing the airway in patients who might be difficult to intubate with conventional laryngoscopy. The flexible fibreoptic laryngoscope has many advantages over conventional laryngoscopes. Its flexibility allows manoeuvring under direct vision even in the patient with a difficult airway anatomy, it is applicable for both oral and nasal intubation, is less traumatic and can be used in patients of all age groups. Local anaesthetic can be 'sprayed' through a working channel in the insertion cord thereby allowing topical anaesthesia of the upper airway during an 'awake' intubation. It is also possible to check the position of the tube as soon as intubation is accomplished. This is a distinct advantage over conventional laryngoscopy.

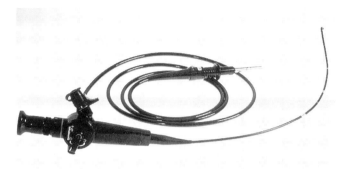

Figure 18.9 Flexible fibreoptic laryngoscope.

A flexible fibrescope can also be connected to a camera control unit and the image seen on a closed circuit television screen (Fig. 18.10). This greatly facilitates teaching of the technique and images can also be stored on video tapes for future reference. With modern technology a battery powered intubating fibrescope has become available in which the light source is a simple lithium camera battery in a casing (Fig. 18.11a). This is interchangeable with the universal light cord which can be operated by mains power (Fig. 18.11b). This facility has made the fibrescope a truly portable piece of equipment allowing its use in many areas. Anaesthetists always viewed mastering fibreoptic techniques as a difficult task. Fortunately there are now several departments offering structured training in their use.

Other uses of flexible fibrescopes include checking the position of double-lumen tubes used in thoracic anaesthesia and for examining the respiratory tract in intensive care.

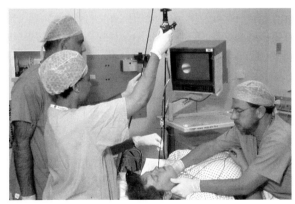

Figure 18.10 Flexible fibreoptic laryngoscope with camera and closed-circuit television.

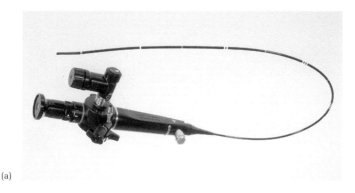

(a)

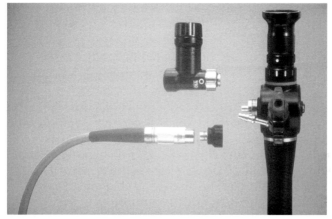

(b)

Figure 18.11 (a) Battery powered flexible fibreoptic laryngoscope. (b) Battery casing and mains light source are interchangeable.

Tracheal Tubes

Traditionally, tracheal tubes were made of red rubber but now tracheal and tracheostomy tubes made of PVC are standard. Advantages claimed for tubes made of PVC include disposability, reduced irritant effect on the tracheal mucosa and, in long-term use, the provision of 'low-pressure' cuffs, which exert less pressure on the tracheal mucosa and are less likely to cause mucosal damage.

The Magill-type Tracheal Tube

The commonest type of tube is the Magill pattern made of PVC (Fig. 18.12). It is a tube with a circular lumen whose size denotes the internal diameter in millimetres. It is curved with a proximal end that can be connected to

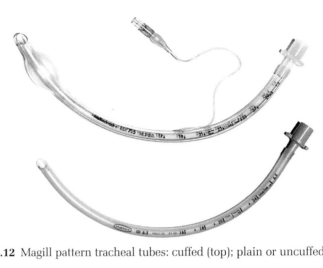

Figure 18.12 Magill pattern tracheal tubes: cuffed (top); plain or uncuffed (bottom).

an anaesthetic breathing system by a standard 15 mm connector and a distal end which has a bevel to the left. Some tubes have an additional hole at the distal end called a Murphy's eye which maintains ventilation should the original hole become obstructed. Sizes larger than 5 mm have a cuff which can be inflated through an inflating tube and a pilot balloon. These tubes may be used for both orotracheal and nasotracheal intubation. They are available in a standard length and have to be cut to the appropriate size. The main disadvantage of this tube is that it is prone to kink and may pass into the right main bronchus if it is too long.

Latex Armoured Tracheal Tube

The earlier tubes of this type were also called 'flexo-metallic', being made by repeatedly dipping a wire spiral in latex rubber. The spiral is now usually made of nylon; the reinforced part is virtually unkinkable but, as they are relatively expensive and difficult to insert without an introducer, they tend to be reserved for procedures where kinking of a tracheal tube is more likely (e.g. neurosurgical anaesthesia).

RAE Tubes

These are preformed tubes available for oral (Fig. 18.13, top) and nasal (Fig. 18.13, bottom) intubation. The oral (or south-facing) tube faces the toes and is useful in operations on the head and neck because it conforms to the shape of the upper airway and moves all the connections away from

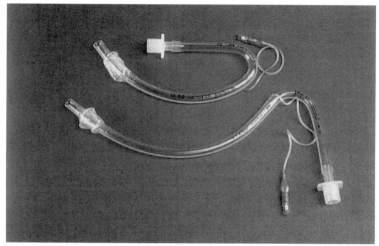

Figure 18.13 Oral RAE tube (top). Nasal RAE tube (bottom).

the site of surgery. The nasal (or north-facing) tube is useful for operations where the surgeon needs access to structures in the oral cavity.

Other special tubes include paediatric tubes (Chapter 37), metal tubes for laser surgery (Chapter 25) and endobronchial tubes for thoracic surgery (Chapter 34).

● COMPLICATIONS OF TRACHEAL INTUBATION

It is clear from the list of indications given earlier in the chapter that in some circumstances endotracheal anaesthesia is considered mandatory. It is important to remember that the passage of a tracheal tube does not guarantee trouble-free anaesthesia. There is a formidable list of minor and major sequelae and, while serious complications are rare, they can lead to the death of the patient. The following are some of the sequelae of endotracheal anaesthesia.

Complications Arising During Intubation

Oesophageal and Endobronchial Intubation

Potentially, the most serious complication which can arise is that the tracheal tube is not introduced into the larynx at all, but is passed behind the larynx into the pharynx and oesophagus. A good rule for the anaesthetist to follow is: 'if in doubt, take it out' and ensure that the patient is adequately oxygenated before the next attempt at intubation. The presence of end-tidal carbon dioxide is the surest sign that the tube is in the trachea and carbon dioxide monitors are now mandatory where intubation is practised. Auscultation of the chest is useful, but transmitted sounds from the oesophagus may deceive the anaesthetist. Oesophageal intubation detector devices, to detect if the tube is in the oesophagus, are less commonly used.

Endobronchial intubation implies that the tube is lying in one main bronchus, usually the right. Should this happen, one lung is preferentially ventilated while the other collapses, resulting in hypoxia and hypercarbia. Auscultation of the chest on both sides will identify the problem. It is prevented by cutting the tube to the appropriate length and by making sure only a small length of tube is passed after the tip enters the vocal cords. The tube should be secured once its correct positioning has been identified.

Trauma During Laryngoscopy

Damage may occur to lips, teeth, parts of the mouth, pharynx or larynx. These injuries may cause discomfort, or may be frankly dangerous – for example, in the case of teeth passing into the bronchi, or oedema or haematoma of the larynx causing respiratory obstruction.

Trauma During Insertion of Tracheal Tube

Injury may be caused by the tracheal tube, or by a protruding introducer (especially a metal one) used to aid its insertion. A nasotracheal tube may perforate the nasopharyngeal mucosa causing a false passage that may ultimately lead to retropharyngeal abscess or mediastinitis.

Trauma to the larynx may lead to surgical emphysema of the neck or mediastinum or even to pneumothorax.

Cardiac Arrhythmias

Disturbances of cardiac rhythm at intubation are probably due to afferent impulses travelling up the vagus nerve and producing reflex excitation of the vagus or sympathetic system. Thus a wide variety of arrhythmias are seen, ranging from sinus bradycardia and atrial or ventricular extrasystoles to asystole or ventricular fibrillation. These disturbances are usually transient but may be serious, especially if associated with other adverse factors such as hypoxia, hypercarbia or hyperkalaemia. Intravenous atropine will block the vagal excitatory effects, but may accentuate the sympathetic effects. The sympathomimetic response can be harmful in some patients and may be prevented by administering intravenously a large dose of short-acting opioid, a β-blocker such as esmolol or lignocaine before laryngoscopy.

Complications During Endotracheal Anaesthesia

These are usually caused by mechanical faults or failures and include foreign bodies within the lumen of tubes or connectors, kinking tubes, or obstruction caused by cuff defects. An overinflated tracheal tube cuff may herniate downwards over the end of the tube and cause respiratory obstruction. Many of these faults have been almost eliminated by improved manufacturing techniques and routine monitoring.

Complications Occurring During Extubation

Cardiac arrhythmias may again occur at extubation or during tracheal suction. Laryngeal spasm of varying degree is not uncommon at extubation.

Complications Occurring After Extubation

Sore throat is the commonest complication of tracheal intubation and occurs to some extent in about half the patients intubated. Laryngitis is much less common and pronounced laryngeal oedema is rare, except in children where the use of too large a tube may lead to enough oedema to cause obstruction in these small airways. Even more rarely, a granuloma of the vocal cords may follow endotracheal intubation.

This list should serve as a reminder that although with better training of anaesthetists and more refined manufacturing of equipment the incidence of severe complications of endotracheal anaesthesia is low, the risk of minor complications is appreciable even in the best hands. These factors should always be borne in mind before deciding to perform endotracheal intubation.

● DIFFICULT AIRWAY MANAGEMENT

A difficult airway is one where a trained anaesthetist finds it difficult to maintain a patent airway with a mask and/or tracheal tube.

Normal Laryngoscopy and Intubation

Tracheal intubation with a Macintosh laryngoscope requires that the axis of the mouth, pharynx and trachea be brought in a straight line of vision. This is achieved by placing the patient's head and neck in the ideal intubating or popularly known 'sniffing the morning air' position. This position involves placing a pillow under the head so that the lower part of the neck is flexed to bring the pharynx and trachea in alignment (Fig. 18.14b). The head is then extended on the neck to bring the mouth, pharynx and trachea in alignment (Fig. 18.14c). The mouth is then maximally opened to insert the laryngoscope blade from the right side thus displacing the tongue to the left. The tip of the blade is then advanced behind the base of the tongue which is elevated until the epiglottis is seen. The tip is further advanced into the vallecula, anterior to the base of the epiglottis, which is then lifted forwards to reveal the vocal cords. The tracheal tube is then placed under direct vision through the vocal cords.

Causes of Difficult Intubation

It is clear from the above description that tracheal intubation will be difficult when any one or more of the above steps cannot be achieved easily. Most difficulties arise as a result of anatomical abnormalities of neck mobility (e.g. rheumatoid arthritis), limitation of mouth opening or intraoral pathology due to infection, tumour, trauma, burns, surgery or radiotherapy. Other associated conditions where difficulties in tracheal intubation arise are pregnancy (see Chapter 38), obesity, short neck, prominent maxillary teeth, high arched palate and large goitre. Some examples of patients in whom a difficult airway can be expected are shown in Figure 18.15a–d.

Evaluation of the Airway

A careful history and examination of the patient and in particular a full evaluation of the airway are required to ascertain the nature of airway difficulties. Where gross distortion of the airway is present, the difficulties are obvious. Various bedside tests to determine whether laryngoscopy with a conventional blade will be difficult have been described, and should be performed routinely before every anaesthetic. These tests include checking head and neck movement, ability to open the mouth adequately and also to bring the lower jaw in front of the upper jaw. The Mallampati (or its modification by Samsoon and Young) test is an indirect method of determining the size of the tongue in relation to the size of the pharyngeal cavity. It involves asking the patient to open their mouth and without phonating protrude their tongue out. The assessor inspects the pharyngeal structures visible and a score is allocated depending on which structures are visible (Fig. 18.16). Most anaesthetists would consider that patients with a class III or IV airway would have a difficult laryngoscopy. The distance between the tip of the mandible and the anterior aspect of the thyroid cartilage (thryromental distance) if <6 cm is also indicative of possible difficulties in intubation. It must be emphasised that these tests may predict difficult intubation which turns out to be easy (false positive) or easy intubation which turns out to be difficult (false negative). The

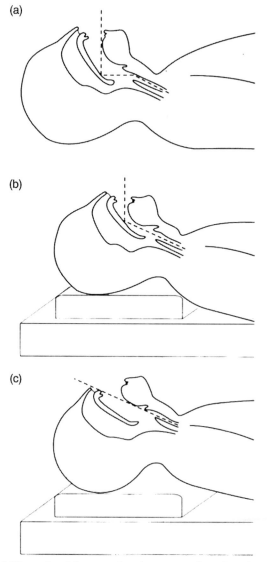

Figure 18.14 (a) The axis of the mouth, pharynx and trachea in supine position. (b) Flexion of lower part of cervical spine brings pharynx and trachea in alignment. (c) Extension of the head on neck brings the axis of mouth, pharynx and trachea in alignment. (Figure from *Difficulties in Tracheal Intubation* by Latto I.P., Vaughan R.S., 2nd edn, W.B. Saunders Company Ltd, with permission.)

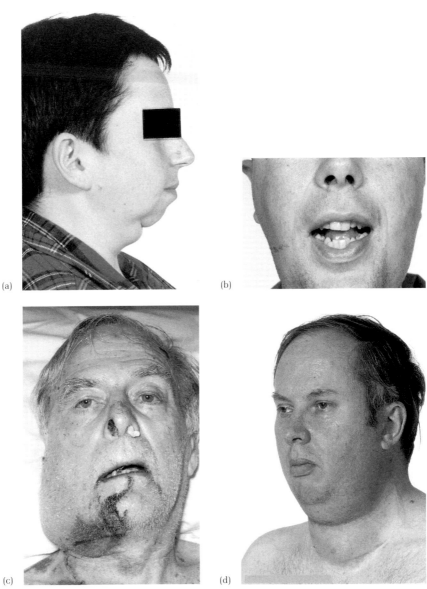

(a)

(b)

(c)

(d)

Figure 18.15 Some examples of patients with anticipated difficult intubation. (a) Rheumatoid arthritis. (b) Temporomandibular joint ankylosis (limited mouth opening). (c) Surgery and radiotherapy after oral cancer. (d) Big retrosternal thyroid goitre.

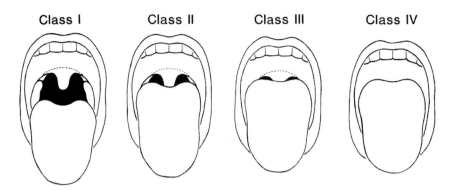

Figure 18.16 Modified Mallampati (Samsoon–Young) classification to predict difficult laryngoscopy. (From *Anaesthesia* 1987; 42: 487–90, with permission from Blackwell Science): Class I, soft palate, fauces, uvula and both pillars; Class II, soft palate, uvula and fauces; Class III, soft palate, base of uvula; Class IV, only soft palate visible.

anaesthetist should therefore always be prepared for the unexpected difficulty.

Management

Anticipated Difficult Airway

When difficulties are anticipated, it is generally considered safer for the patient if the airway is secured before induction of general anaesthesia. This technique is often referred to as an 'awake' intubation. Its advantages are that an 'awake' patient maintains their own airway, oxygenation and ventilation are not a problem and there is no risk of aspiration of gastric contents. The safety factor is that the patient is safe, i.e. no bridges are burned even if the technique fails. Intubation in an 'awake' patient does not literally mean that patients are completely awake. Most patients can be and should be given sedation so that they are comfortable and do not remember the procedure. Meticulous topical anaesthesia of the upper airway with local anaesthetic is also provided. General anaesthesia is induced only after the intubation is complete and the position of the tube has been verified in the trachea. In the past awake intubation was performed by a 'blind' technique usually through the nasal route. Nowadays, the flexible fibreoptic laryngoscope has made this a very acceptable technique with a very high success rate (Fig. 18.17a–c).

There may be instances (e.g. children, adults with learning difficulties) where awake intubation is desired but not feasible. In these instances

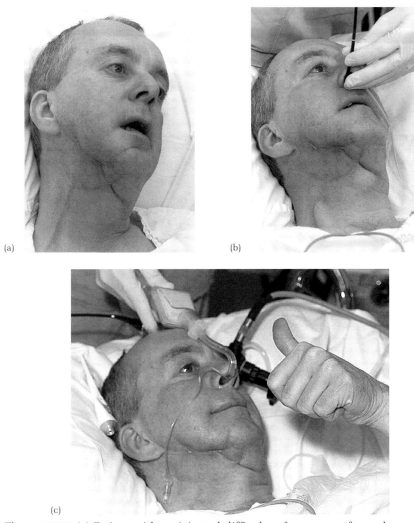

(a)

(b)

(c)

Figure 18.17 (a) Patient with anticipated difficulty after surgery for oral cancer. (b) Awake nasal fibreoptic intubation in progress. (c) Awake fibreoptic intubation accomplished.

decisions should be made about the best way to induce anaesthesia (intravenous or inhalation), achieve ventilation and intubation. Many devices have been described with which tracheal intubation can be achieved in these patients. Some of these include different laryngoscope blades (straight, polio, McCoy), flexible fibreoptic laryngoscope and intubating LMA. The anaesthetist should always use techniques with which they are familiar.

Whatever technique is used, it is always safe to work out a back-up plan (Plan B) if the first plan (Plan A) fails. This back-up plan may include senior help, additional equipment and assistance or even a surgeon standing by to perform a tracheostomy.

Unanticipated Difficulties

The priority is to maintain oxygenation and ventilation when unanticipated difficulties occur after induction of anaesthesia and muscle paralysis. This can be achieved with a face mask and an oropharyngeal/nasopharyngeal airway or with an LMA. Before any more attempts are made at laryngoscopy, the head and neck position should be checked. Often external pressure applied on the larynx by an assistant may improve the view. A gum elastic bougie or introducer or a different blade may also be used to get a better view. It is important in this situation to avoid excessive trauma, bleeding and swelling that result from repetitive attempts at intubation. Fatalities have occurred when a perfectly easy ventilation situation has been turned into a nightmare scenario of being unable to ventilate because repeated intubation attempts have caused trauma and oedema of the upper airway. An anaesthetist experienced in using the flexible fibrescope may be able to achieve intubation successfully in this situation without causing undue trauma. Another option is to use an LMA or even better still an ILMA as a conduit for intubation (see under LMA/ILMA above). In some cases it is safer to awaken the patient and perform an 'awake' intubation (see above).

Can't Ventilate, Can't Intubate

Very rarely but most frighteningly, a patient may not only be difficult to intubate but also be difficult to ventilate with a face mask. It can also result from the trauma of repeated attempts at intubation (see above). In this scenario it is recommended that an LMA be used to provide rescue ventilation. A device called the Combitube has also been advocated in this scenario but is not popular in the UK. It must be remembered that the LMA is a supraglottic (above the vocal cords) device and may not be useful in patients with airway obstruction below the cords. If an LMA fails, then immediate oxygenation should be provided by a route below the vocal cords. The simplest way is to perform a needle cricothyroidotomy. This is

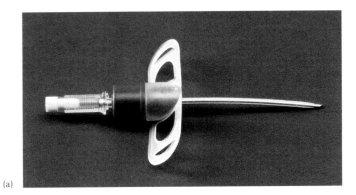

(a)

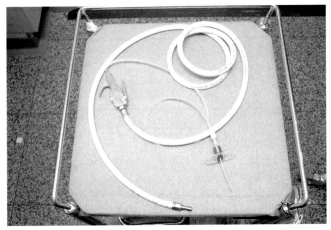

(b)

Figure 18.18 Cricothyroidotomy and transtracheal jet ventilation. (a) Ravussin cricothyroidotomy needle and cannula. (b) Cannula connected to jet ventilator.

a puncture in the cricothyroid membrane (connecting the cricoid and thyroid cartilage). Although any intravenous cannula can be used for this purpose, a dedicated device such as the one shown in Figure 18.18a is preferable and should be available in all areas where anaesthetics are given. Once the puncture is made, the needle is removed and the cannula is connected to a jet ventilation device such as a Sander's injector (Fig. 18.18b). Surgical tracheostomy should be considered only as a last resort.

Difficult Intubation Trolley

It is important that there should be in or near each anaesthetic room a choice of special items of equipment in a clearly labelled 'Difficult Intubation Trolley'. The following is by no means a comprehensive list of possible contents, but gives an idea of some useful items: a selection of oral and nasal airways, a selection of standard and intubating laryngeal mask airways; Magill intubating forceps, straight and McCoy laryngoscope blades; short handle, long gum-elastic bougie; cricothyroidotomy set and a jet ventilation device. In addition, a flexible fibreoptic laryngoscope should be readily available and each theatre area should have a sterile tracheostomy set ready for use.

19

Principles of Ventilators

'All anaesthetists are bag-squeezers'
'All ventilators are bag-squeezers'
'Therefore all anaesthetists are ventilators or all ventilators are anaesthetists!'

When an intubated patient is ventilated by hand with an Ambu bag there are two main variables in the pattern of ventilation: (a) the rate at which the bag is squeezed and (b) the depth to which it is squeezed, corresponding to the respiratory rate and the tidal volume. It is also possible to produce a fast or a slow inspiration by rapid or slow compression of the bag, so the inspiratory flow rate may be considered to be a third but somewhat minor variable. Expiration, however, is a passive phase in virtually all methods of artificial ventilation, depending only on the elastic recoil of the patient's lungs.

● REQUIREMENTS OF VENTILATION

Power for Inflation

Ventilators require some source of power, which may be either gas pressure or an electric motor. The gas used may be either compressed air, in which case this is used only to power the ventilator and plays no part in ventilating the patient's alveoli, or oxygen in various concentrations at either high or low pressure. Some ventilators (e.g. the Bird, Oxylog) effectively interrupt the high-pressure oxygen pipeline supply at intervals, thereby inflating the lungs. Low-pressure gas from an anaesthetic machine may be used continuously to fill a reservoir bellows which intermittently empties into an inflation bellows, thereby ventilating the patient; for example, the Manley ventilator.

Power for Cycling

There are four essential phases of ventilation: inspiration; inspiration to expiration cycling; expiration; and expiration to inspiration cycling. Each ventilator requires a method of cycling from one phase to the other and this is usually achieved electromechanically.

Patient Requirements

Whatever the method of ventilation used, the patient's requirements are simply those of fresh-gas flow – it is only while gas is flowing that the alveoli are expanded and gas exchange is achieved.

The commonest form of artificial ventilation uses the principle of intermittent positive pressure – that is to say, fresh gas is driven into the lungs under positive pressure, and leaves the lungs passively as a result of the elastic recoil. During normal breathing, inspiration is produced by creating negative intrathoracic pressure due to expansion of the rib cage, which is the opposite of the positive pressure produced during artificial ventilation. This may have serious effects on the cardiovascular system, because the negative pressure created in normal breathing helps to draw blood back into the chest, increasing the venous return and therefore the cardiac output. Intermittent positive pressure produces the opposite effect and therefore often causes a small but significant fall in cardiac output.

● VENTILATOR TYPES

As inspiration is the fundamental phase of any ventilator, it is possible to divide the different types of ventilators into two main groups, depending on how they produce inspiration.

Pressure Generators (Manley)

These rely on compression of a bellows by a weight, usually resting on a hinged bracket above the bag (Fig. 19.1). When the weight is allowed to drop freely the bellows are compressed, the rate of compression depending on the resistance to inflation produced by the patient. As this resistance rises, the weight applied to the bellows must be increased to maintain the same inflation rate, and therefore this type of ventilator is suitable only for patients with relatively normal lungs. Those with stiff lungs (low compliance) or high airways resistance are usually unsuitable for a pressure generator, because if the resistance offered to ventilation is too high the bellows will hardly be compressed at all and the tidal volume will be inadequate.

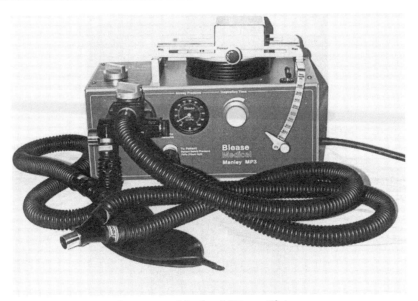

Figure 19.1 Manley MP3 ventilator.

Flow Generators

Many different ventilators can be included in this group, but they possess the same fundamental property, i.e. they are powerful enough to overcome lungs with low compliance or high airways resistance so that gas flow into such patients is maintained constant due to the reserves of power available in the ventilators. Flow generators may be subdivided into two main types:

1. Those using high gas pressure. This can be applied either directly or indirectly to the airway.
   (a) Direct application means that the high-pressure gas is actually the fresh gas passing into the lungs, the flow being intermittently interrupted (e.g. Bird, Harlow, Oxylog ventilators).
   (b) Indirect use of high-pressure gas as a driving force. In this case the high-pressure gas is used to compress a bellows, which contains the fresh gas, for example, 'bag-in-bottle' ventilators such as the Ohmeda and Nuffield 400. The power of the driving gas, which could be compressed air, is such that the ventilator behaves as a flow generator.
   In the Penlon Nuffield 200 ventilator (Fig. 19.2), the high-pressure driving gas is cycled via a fluid logic switching system and the ventilator is connected to the expiratory limb of a coaxial circuit, for example, Bain

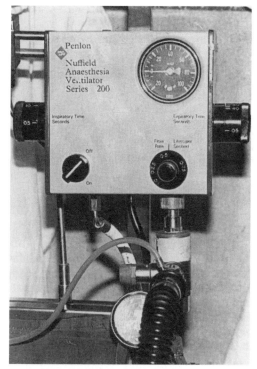

Figure 19.2 Nuffield 200 ventilator.

or Lack (Chapter 8). Fresh gas enters the inspiratory limb of the circuit as normal and therefore the gas driving the ventilator never actually reaches the patient, provided the fresh-gas flow is adequate. Alternatively, a flow generator, such as the Nuffield 200, can be incorporated into a 'bag-in-a-bottle' closed-circuit system (Fig. 19.3).

In the case of the Servo 900C (Fig. 19.4), the ventilator functions at a gas pressure of 414 kPa (60 psi). The compressed gas expels fresh gas from a bellows, the power of the gas pressure being more than sufficient to overcome any airway resistance. Other examples of flow generators used in critical care units include the Servo 300 (Fig. 19.5) and the Drager Evita 4 (Fig. 19.6).

2. Those using a powerful motor to produce constant gas flow. In this situation the ventilator is equipped with a sufficiently powerful motor to produce a constant gas flow irrespective of the resistance offered by the lungs (e.g. Cape and Engström ventilators).

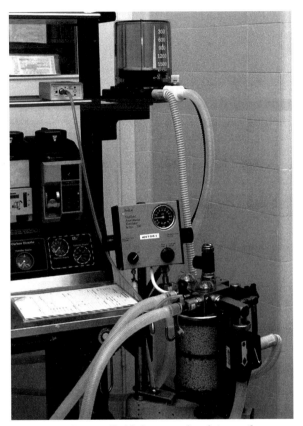

Figure 19.3 Penlon Nuffield 'bag-in-a-bottle' ventilator system.

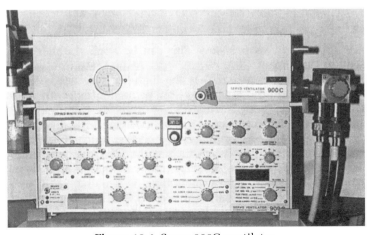

Figure 19.4 Servo 900C ventilator.

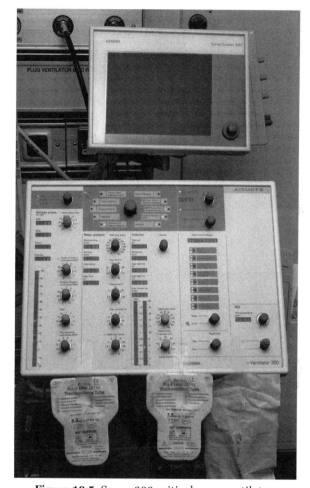

Figure 19.5 Servo 300 critical care ventilator.

● GAS FLOW DURING INSPIRATION

In summary, we can subdivide gas flow during inspiration into two types depending upon the ventilator used.

Pressure Generator

Here the flow into the lungs depends upon the compliance of the lung and the airways resistance. As the resistance to inflation produced by these factors rises, gas flow falls if constant pressure is applied. This type of ventilator is perfectly satisfactory for general use and is inadequate when the

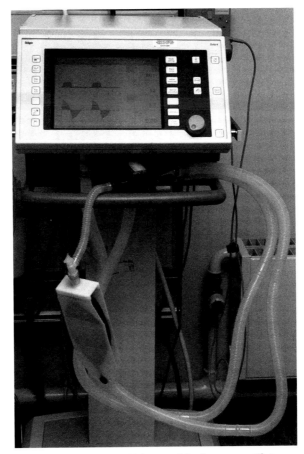

Figure 19.6 Drager Evita 4 critical care ventilator.

maximum possible generated pressure is not able to overcome the resistance offered by the lung.

Flow Generator

Here the flow into the lungs is maintained constant, the inflation pressure produced by the ventilator being more than adequate to overcome any resistance offered by the lung.

Gas flow into the lungs occurs while there is a pressure difference between the airway and the thoracic cavity which equals oesophageal pressure. The variations occurring in gas flow into the lungs in various conditions and types of ventilator are illustrated in Figure 19.7. This confirms that when using a pressure generator, in a patient with low lung

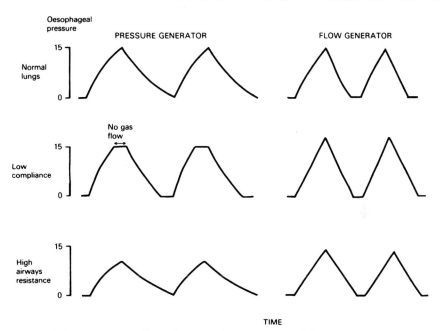

Figure 19.7 Gas flow diagrams for pressure and flow generators.

compliance, as the ventilator pressure rises rapidly and quickly equals the resistance of the lung, gas flow ceases when the inspiratory phase continues for a fixed length of time. This does not occur with a flow generator. In the case of high airways resistance, gas flow into the lungs is continuously impeded, preventing the intrapulmonary pressure rising to equal the ventilator pressure before the inspiratory phase has finished. In this case therefore the tidal volume falls, although less so for the flow than for the pressure generators.

Inspiratory time

A short inspiratory time leads to increased physiological dead space. This occurs because the length of inspiration controls the degree of gas exchange and mixing which occurs in the alveoli. If inadequate time is allowed for this to occur, a number of alveoli will not take part in gas exchange and therefore remain as dead space. This is known as physiological dead space in contrast to the anatomical dead space of the conducting airways, which does not vary with ventilation. A long inspiratory time, however, does not improve gas distribution and merely allows the intrathoracic pressure to be elevated for an excessive time, resulting in further impairment of venous return and reduction in cardiac output.

● EFFECT OF LEAKS OR OBSTRUCTION IN VENTILATOR CIRCUITS

Pressure Generator

Obstruction

The bellows cease to move as pressure is inadequate.

Leak

The bellows empty quickly and the patient is not inflated. The ventilator sounds different.

Flow Generator

Obstruction

The pressure gauge shows an increase in airway pressure and the tidal volume falls. Pressure 'blow-off' occurs if obstruction is complete.

Leak

There is no change in ventilator operation, but the gauge pressure and tidal volume fall.

● CYCLING

Cycling is the term given to the mechanism built into the ventilator which allows the inspiratory phase to change to the expiratory phase and back to inspiration, and may be subdivided into several types depending on the mechanism used.

Time-cycling

This is the commonest method used and essentially means that the change from inspiration to expiration, or the reverse, is produced by a timing mechanism that is not influenced by changes in the patient's lungs. The commonest form of time-cycling is an electromechanical method which occurs, for example, in the Cape and Engström ventilators. It works in similar fashion to the time clock in a central heating system with a revolving disc driven by an electric motor which trips a switch to initiate and terminate both inspiration and expiration. A complete revolution of this disc represents one complete respiratory cycle.

Some ventilators also use time-cycling, operated electrically by a solenoid switch (e.g. the Barnet ventilator). This mechanism is far less common.

Pressure-cycling (Pressure Control)

This method is used both in the Oxylog and Bird ventilators, i.e. those ventilators which allow inflation of the patient by intermittent interruption of a high-pressure gas source. In pressure-cycling, inspiration continues until the pressure in the lungs – which rises as more air enters them – reaches a predetermined value at which the ventilator cycles to expiration. When the pressure falls to zero again, the ventilator cycles back to a further inspiratory phase.

Volume-cycling (Volume Control)

Although some ventilators may appear to deliver a predetermined volume (e.g. the Cape, Servo 900C) this in fact is time cycled in the sense that the ventilator is so powerful that whatever tidal volume is set it will be delivered within a predetermined time. True volume-cycling means that the ventilator will not cycle until the preset tidal volume has been delivered, even if this takes many seconds in cases of high airways resistance. Volume-cycling is therefore relatively uncommon and unsatisfactory.

Flow-cycling

Some ventilators (e.g. the Bennett) are flow cycled, meaning that they will cycle when no flow exists, either at the end of inspiration or at the end of expiration. Although this method is used on relatively few ventilators at present, it is still very satisfactory in some situations, particularly since a no-flow situation in the chest is of no benefit to the patient and merely dams back venous return.

Patient-cycling (Triggering)

Here the ventilator will cycle to the inspiratory phase when the patient generates a negative pressure by voluntary inspiration. When a predetermined pressure has been reached the ventilator will augment the patient's inspiratory effort and produce inflation; hence this is a variable control which may be used to encourage patients to wean from a ventilator or when they hypoventilate to any extent. The Bird ventilator is one which includes a patient-triggering system and is often used by physiotherapists to encourage patients to breathe deeply.

● THE IDEAL VENTILATOR

It is apparent therefore that the ideal ventilator for normal lungs in most conditions can be described simply as a 'bag-squeezer'. Such ventilators are cheap and easy to operate but are often unsuitable for ventilating patients with lung disease. Such patients with stiff lungs (low compliance) or high airways resistance require a ventilator with adequate reserves of power. This is usually one in which the tidal volume is preset and one which is able to produce a constant gas flow to deliver whatever tidal volume is set within a fixed inspiratory time.

● VENTILATOR TERMINOLOGY

Inspiration/Expiration Ratio

On many ventilators this is a preset value, usually of 1 : 2, so that inspiration is half as long as expiration. This is satisfactory for most patients, although in some with obstructive airways disease expiration may need to be prolonged to allow adequate emptying of the lungs between breaths. In children, and especially neonates, this ratio usually approaches 1 : 1, but the cardiovascular consequences of this must not be forgotten. The inspiration/expiration (I/E) ratio can also be varied in some ventilators by changes in inspiratory and expiratory time and flow rate, for example, Nuffield 200.

Intermittent Mandatory Ventilation

This technique is popular in weaning patients from ventilators. Essentially it means that the patient receives a number of predetermined breaths per minute, usually about six, in between which they are able to breathe for themselves. The patients usually settle down to a rhythm, for example, two of their own breaths to one ventilator breath and so on. The interval between mandatory breaths may be steadily increased allowing patients to take over more of the respiratory function for themselves. In synchronised intermittent mandatory ventilation (SIMV) the ventilator constantly adjusts its ventilation rate to synchronise with the patient's own respiration.

Minute Mandatory Ventilation (MMV)

In contrast to intermittent mandatory ventilation (IMV), this technique depends on the fact that the patient is required to breathe a predetermined volume of gas per minute. If this is done without help from a ventilator, no ventilation occurs. If, however, the patient is unable to exchange the amount of gas required, the ventilator will supplement his breathing with four to six large breaths a minute to make up the difference in the overall gas exchange.

Positive End-expiratory Pressure

Positive end-expiratory pressure (PEEP) maintains a continuously raised intrathoracic pressure during the expiratory pause, usually in the region of 5–10 cmH$_2$O. Normal expiration occurs, brought about by the elastic recoil of the lungs, but instead of the intrathoracic pressure falling to zero it is maintained slightly above this level. This is intended to keep the alveoli expanded and filled with the gas mixture, which is oxygen enriched. PEEP therefore increases gas transfer across the alveoli and consequently arterial blood oxygenation. It may also be used to prevent fluid leak across the alveolar capillary membrane which occurs in pulmonary oedema. Nevertheless, the haemodynamic effects of PEEP must not be forgotten, because continually raised intrathoracic pressure prevents venous return and may therefore reduce cardiac output.

Minute-volume Divider

This term is used to describe ventilators which operate via the low-pressure gas source from the anaesthetic machine (e.g. Manley). The minute volume of gases entering the ventilator is preset on the rotameters of the anaesthetic machine. Having adjusted the tidal volume on the ventilator and predetermined the minute volume, the number of breaths per minute is automatically determined by dividing the minute volume by the tidal volume. Thus the ventilator acts as a minute-volume divider.

Servo Ventilator

A servo (self-adjusting) system (e.g. Siemens-Elema Servo 900C, Fig. 19.4; Servo 300, Fig. 19.5; Dräger Evita 4, Fig. 19.6) is one in which, in the case of a ventilator, an abnormally small breath is compensated for automatically by a corresponding increase in the volume of the next breath. The servo ventilator contains a system for measuring both inspiratory and expiratory gas flow and therefore volume. Predetermined minute- and tidal-volume settings on the machine are continuously monitored automatically. If the expired volume is inadequate the ventilator automatically compensates for this by temporarily increasing the tidal volume, so that the overall preset minute volume is achieved.

'Bag-in-a-bottle' Ventilator

This principle is now extensively used, with the increasing use of closed-circuit anaesthesia. This employs low inspiratory gas flow rates to minimise both pollution and the expense of the newer volatile anaesthetic agents. The fresh-gas flow passes into the low flow circuit of which the bellows is an integral part. The bellows in the bottle is then compressed externally, by air pumped into the bottle, but outside the bellows, by the ventilator, for example, Penlon Nuffield 200. Thus the air from the ventilator does not ventilate the patient directly and just squeezes the contents of the bellows into the lungs (Fig. 19.3).

Continuous Positive Airway Pressure and Pressure Support Modes

Although continuous positive airway pressure (CPAP) is available on most intensive care ventilators, for example, Servo 900 series, its use is only applicable to spontaneous ventilation in an intubated patient. In the expiratory phase, CPAP produces a similar effect to PEEP, but the presence of a constantly elevated airway pressure during inspiration provides a small amount of assistance to supplement the patient's own inspiratory effort.

This is in contrast to the pressure support mode where the patient's own inspiratory effort is supplemented by a preset inspiratory assistance from the ventilator. Unlike patient triggering, however, the tidal volume is determined by the magnitude of the patient's effort rather than by a predetermined ventilator setting.

20

Monitoring During Anaesthesia

Although it is essential for the anaesthetist to remain in close contact with the patient during induction, maintenance and recovery from anaesthesia, more complex anaesthetic techniques and the relative increase in the number of very ill patients being anaesthetised both require more complex monitoring equipment. If the anaesthetist can remain in physical contact with the patient throughout the anaesthetic, a good assessment is continually available of pulse, blood pressure, peripheral perfusion and general adequacy of anaesthesia. In many cases, however, due to the type of surgery being performed, this contact is only partial and additional equipment is necessary.

● MEASUREMENT OF CARDIAC RATE AND RHYTHM

Electrocardiographic (ECG) monitoring is discussed in detail in Chapter 22, but it is also important to include this under the general heading of monitoring equipment. The ECG reflects changes in the electrical activity of the heart as impulses are transmitted through the excitable cardiac muscle, which then contracts. Although, in routine 12-lead ECG recording, different positions of the electrodes allow diagnosis of changing electrical activity in various parts of the heart, ECG monitoring during anaesthesia uses one chest lead (commonly CM5, chest, manubrium, V5) which gives a satisfactory display of all aspects of the cardiac cycle. In this lead three electrodes are used, the right arm (red) over the manubrium sternum, the right leg (yellow) over the left shoulder and the left arm (black) in the fifth intercostal space in the midclavicular line, the setting on the ECG machine being turned to lead I. It is also possible to obtain a reasonable ECG by laying the patient on an electrode mat, but only if they are supine.

It is important to emphasise that ECG recording merely reflects electrical activity, and gives no indication of peripheral blood flow. ECG machines are usually coupled to a rate meter giving an indication of the pulse rate.

Pulse rate can also be measured using a pulse meter, an instrument which depends on a light-sensitive photoelectric cell. The sensing device clips on to either the fingertip or earlobe, both of which normally have a good blood supply. The sensor contains a small light beam which shines through the fingertip or earlobe, changes in light intensity being sensed by the photoelectric cell. As blood flows into the fingertip, the light intensity will be reduced in a pulsatile manner. This change in intensity can then be assessed simply in terms of heart rate or can be displayed on an oscilloscope as a waveform reflecting blood flow. This is usually now performed in conjunction with oxygen saturation measurements, as pulse oximetry. Measurement of peripheral flow, however, is severely reduced in vasoconstriction and this method is reliable only when blood pressure and flow are reasonably normal.

● MEASUREMENT OF BLOOD PRESSURE

Accurate blood pressure measurement is an essential part of anaesthetic monitoring. Although palpation of the radial pulse gives an indication of satisfactory blood pressure, it is not possible to measure changes. Systemic blood pressure measurement involves either indirect intermittent recording or direct continuous measurement using an intra-arterial cannula.

Indirect Arterial Monitoring

The cuff method of measuring arterial blood pressure has been adapted in several forms for use during anaesthesia, particularly when access to the brachial pulse is impossible. In its simplest form, a single blood pressure cuff and stethoscope taped over the brachial artery allow auscultation of the Korotkov sounds corresponding to systolic and diastolic blood pressure in the conventional way. It is also possible to obtain an estimation of systolic blood pressure by using a pulse meter on the fingertip and a single cuff, systolic pressure being indicated when the pulse meter output ceases after inflation of the cuff, or reappears on deflating the cuff.

Indirect monitoring using the cuff principle has been adapted for anaesthetic use. Most methods are semi-automatic or automatic adaptations of the oscillotonometer involving different methods of recording arterial pulsation from the sensing cuff.

Oscillotonometer

This method is now rarely used. It consists of two inflatable cuffs enclosed in a single outer cuff which is placed around the upper arm. The upper of the two cuffs, or occluding cuff, corresponds to a normal blood pressure cuff, and the lower one, which is narrower than the upper, is the sensing cuff corresponding to a palpating finger or stethoscope. This method is relatively inaccurate at the extremes of blood pressure but is reliable at systolic blood pressures between 60 and 160 mmHg.

Other Indirect Cuff Methods, Based upon the Oscillotonometer Principle

The Arteriosonde uses a small transducer (see below) instead of a sensing cuff which has to be placed over the brachial artery, while the Dinamap (Figs 20.1 and 20.2) uses a single cuff for both occlusion and sensing, whose

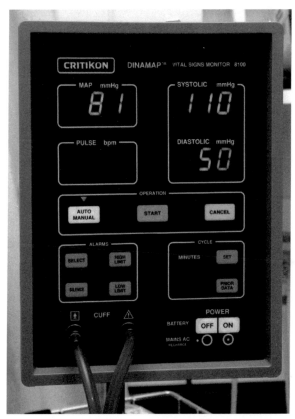

Figure 20.1 Dinamap vital signs automatic blood pressure monitor.

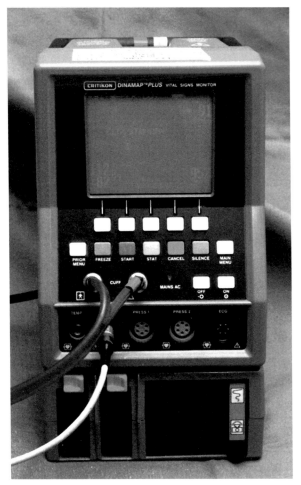

Figure 20.2 Dinamap Plus vital signs automatic blood pressure monitor.

changing pressure is then transmitted via a transducer. All these methods have similar limitations to the oscillotonometer. The Dinamap can measure at very frequent intervals in the 'stat' mode and can be useful at induction before an indwelling arterial cannula is introduced.

Direct Intravascular Pressure Monitoring

Intravascular pressure, whether venous, systemic arterial or pulmonary, can be measured with the same system provided that the instruments used are adjusted to respond to a suitable pressure range. Arterial pressure monitoring involves placing a cannula in a suitable artery, usually radial

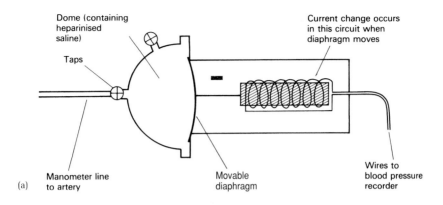

Dome (containing heparinised saline)

Taps

Current change occurs in this circuit when diaphragm moves

Wires to blood pressure recorder

(a) Manometer line to artery

Movable diaphragm

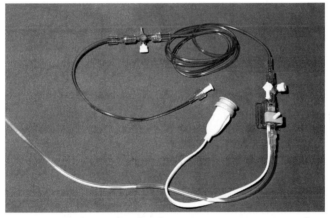

(b)

Figure 20.3 (a) Transducer. (b) Blood pressure monitoring transducer.

or brachial, and the transmission of the arterial pulse via a length of non-distensible manometer tubing to a method of pressure display. In its simplest form the pressure line may be connected to a pressure gauge or mercury manometer, provided that there is an air gap in the tube between the saline and the mercury. Although simple, this method is not suitable for demonstrating pulsatile arterial flow, but merely gives a damped recording, providing an accurate measurement of mean arterial blood pressure.

Connecting the pressure tubing to a transducer and then to an oscilloscope will provide dynamic measurement of blood pressure. A transducer is simply a device that changes energy from one form into another, in this case, changing pulsatile movement of a column of fluid into electrical energy (Fig. 20.3a and b).

Changes of pressure within the column of fluid cause movement of the diaphragm in the transducer and set up an electrical current which can then be transmitted and displayed on the oscilloscope. Inevitably, arterial blood pressure monitoring is more accurate, particularly at the extremes of blood pressure, than any indirect form. Provided that the technique is used only when indicated, and arterial lines are only left in place for as long as they are needed and then removed, the morbidity is extremely low. Dangers, however, result from prolonged arterial cannulation, particularly in patients with peripheral vasoconstriction and also the inadvertent intra-arterial injection of certain drugs, particularly thiopentone.

● MEASUREMENT OF CENTRAL VENOUS PRESSURE

The techniques of central venous cannulation have already been discussed in Chapter 17. As in direct arterial monitoring, central venous pressure can be displayed on a transducer and oscilloscope. However, the relatively low pressures found in the venous system also permit the use of a fluid column to show venous pressure. Provided that the central venous cannula is in the chest (preferably in the right atrium), by connecting it to a column of fluid and zeroing the column at the level of the heart, the height of the fluid above zero will equal the pressure in the right atrium. Again, this method cannot respond to beat-by-beat change in pressure but gives an accurate measurement of mean central venous pressure. Balloon catheters (Swan-Ganz) are sometimes floated into the right atrium and then to the right ventricle and pulmonary artery to give a measurement of pulmonary artery blood pressure. As this is higher than central venous pressure it is necessary to use a transducer and oscilloscope (the 0–60 scale) to display the pressure, usually in the region of 25 mmHg systolic.

● MEASUREMENT OF EXPIRED GAS FLOW

This is usually measured electronically as an integral part of the ventilator. A sensor (pneumotachograph) in the anaesthetic circuit provides breath-by-breath measurement of tidal volume, minute volume and respiratory rate.

● MEASUREMENT OF TEMPERATURE

Temperature monitoring is widely used, particularly during prolonged anaesthesia. Different temperature-sensing devices are available for use in various sites such as the skin, oesophagus, rectum and eardrum. They are all either thermistors or thermocouples, producing changes in electrical activity in response to temperature variation. The temperature can then be displayed on a gauge or by digital readout. It is useful to measure simultaneously both central temperature (usually either rectal or oesophageal) and skin temperature. Skin temperature reflects peripheral perfusion and the difference between central and peripheral temperatures indicates the degree of vasoconstriction or vasodilatation, which may be important in assessing the adequacy of fluid replacement and metabolic state of the patient.

● MEASUREMENT OF OXYGEN (OXIMETRY)

Within the Anaesthetic Circuit

Several devices are available for measuring the oxygen percentage in a gas mixture within the anaesthetic circuit. Those in clinical use utilise a fuel cell the electrical output of which is dependent upon the concentration of oxygen to which it is exposed. They also contain high and low alarms to increase their usefulness and are frequently now incorporated into standard anaesthetic machines. They do, however, only measure the oxygen within the circuit and not within the patient.

Within Blood

Although blood gas measurement is the definitive method by which oxygen concentration is estimated, it is invasive and only provides intermittent results (Chapter 2). Indwelling arterial oxygen electrodes are being developed to provide continuous estimation, but are not yet routinely available. Continuous non-invasive measurement of oxygen saturation, using pulse oximetry (Fig. 20.4), is now universally employed. Unlike the fuel cell within the anaesthetic circuit, the measurement made is of the patient's oxygenation. The method used is an adaptation of the finger plethysmograph trace, which depends upon shining a light, of particular wavelength, through the finger and detecting the change in transmitted light related to the degree of oxygenation of pulsatile arterial blood. The wavelength used allows the maximum difference in light absorption between oxygenated and reduced haemoglobin. Pulse oximeters are accurate down to saturations of 70% but since they can make measurements on very small quantities of blood, should not be relied upon as an index of adequacy of blood flow. Errors in measurement occur with cold, peripheral vasoconstriction and in the earlier models, skin pigmentation and nail varnish.

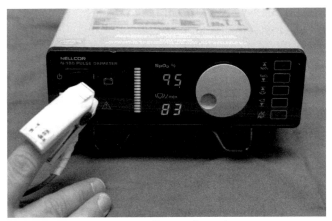

Figure 20.4 Nellcor pulse oximeter.

● MEASUREMENT OF CARBON DIOXIDE (CAPNOGRAPHY)

Measurement of the percentage concentration of carbon dioxide (CO_2) in expired air at the end of normal expiration is equivalent to the alveolar and therefore arterial CO_2 concentration. End-tidal CO_2 analysers depend upon the absorption of infra-red light by CO_2 – the higher the absorption, the less light is transmitted. They provide accurate, non-invasive, breath-by-breath measurement and as such monitor the adequacy of ventilation.

They do not measure oxygenation at the same time, although many instruments are now combined oximeters and CO_2 analysers.

● VOLATILE AGENT MONITORING

With the increasing use of circle anaesthetic breathing systems, largely designed to work at low flows and conserve expensive anaesthetic gases and vapours, it has become essential to know the concentration of agents within the system. 'Agent' monitors are now available, usually working on an adsorption principle which must be precalibrated, to monitor breath-by-breath concentrations of volatile agents such as halothane, enflurane and isoflurane. Although relatively expensive, their cost is more than offset by savings made in the quantity of agents used, apart from the reduced levels of theatre pollution.

● INTEGRATED PATIENT MONITORING SYSTEMS

Whenever possible, many monitoring parameters such as ECG, indirect and direct arterial blood pressure, central venous pressure, oxygen saturation,

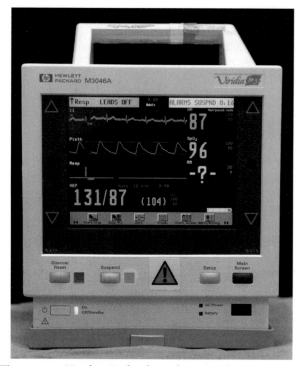

Figure 20.5 Hewlett-Packard Viridia critical care monitor.

end-tidal carbon dioxide, agent monitoring and temperature are incorporated into integrated systems which can be used in theatre or critical care areas. There are many advantages, not only of cost, but also versatility, interchangeable modules, compact size and design, and an integrated alarm system. Examples of these include the Hewlett-Packard Viridia (Fig. 20.5), the Hewlett-Packard Merlin system (Fig. 20.6) and Datex (Fig. 20.7).

● MEASUREMENT OF CARDIAC OUTPUT

Although cardiac output measurement is not used routinely except during cardiopulmonary bypass, its use in severely ill patients is increasing. Measurement involves the injection of a known quantity of either green dye or ice-cold saline into the right atrium and measuring either the dilution of the dye or the change in temperature of the blood in response to the cold saline injection after passing through the heart. The cardiac output is obtained by measuring the degree of dilution of the dye and then calculating the volume of blood into which a fixed quantity of dye must

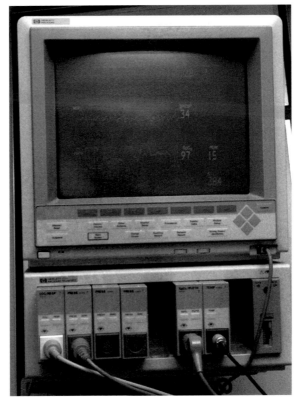

Figure 20.6 Hewlett-Packard Merlin critical care monitoring system.

have diffused to obtain this dilution. Similar calculations apply to the use of ice-cold saline, the temperature change being sensed by a thermistor at the tip of a specially adapted Swan-Ganz catheter and the result passed to a dedicated cardiac output computer.

● VENTILATOR ALARMS

Ventilator alarms have now become routinely incorporated into most ventilator circuits on anaesthetic machines, if not into the ventilators themselves (e.g. Servo 900, Chapter 22). Those used in theatre such as the Penlon IDP Alarm (Fig. 20.8) are pressure sensitive and contain both high (60 cmH$_2$O) and low (12 cmH$_2$O) settings. There is also a time delay in the region of 12 s built in to allow for the use of very slow respiratory rates. They are usually activated simply by being plugged in and can be tested by pressurising the anaesthetic circuit.

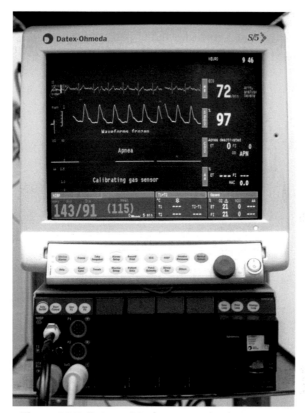

Figure 20.7 Datex critical care monitoring system.

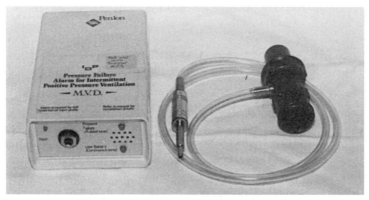

Figure 20.8 Penlon IDP ventilator alarm.

21

Complications of Anaesthesia: The Recovery Room

•Respiratory system •Cardiovascular system •Awareness •Peripheral nerve injuries •Ophthalmic complications •Skin complications •Hypothermia •Hypersensitivity to anaesthetic drugs •Recovery from anaesthesia

The possible complications of anaesthesia are numerous, varying from minor and commonplace to serious and bizarre. The possible causes fall into various groups, for example, anaesthetic equipment like laryngoscopes, endotracheal tubes, cannulae and needles inevitably produce a variety of complications. Another group is associated with the use of various anaesthetic agents, for example, muscle relaxants. Some complications are more closely associated with the surgery than with anaesthesia, although it is not unusual for anaesthesia to be blamed: this group includes postoperative respiratory complications and venous thrombotic and embolic phenomena. Lastly, a group of complications – important because most of them are avoidable – arise simply because the patient is rendered unconscious. This is because anaesthesia is responsible for the patient losing various protective reflexes and it is the anaesthetist's responsibility to look after these functions. These protective reflexes are found in various systems, for example, the respiratory system, the eyes and the peripheral nervous system. From the extensive choice, this chapter selects some of the commoner and some of the more avoidable complications and sequelae.

● RESPIRATORY SYSTEM

Obstruction

This is probably the commonest respiratory complication which may occur at any level of the respiratory tract and for many different reasons.

With the mouth closed, breathing occurs through the nose. If for some reason the nasal airway is obstructed, breathing can occur only if the lips are separated. Thus there tends to be some degree of respiratory obstruction unless an oropharyngeal airway is used. It should be noted that in edentulous people the unsupported lips are much more mobile and the upper lip can be pulled right over the external nares when attempts are made to improve the airway by pulling the jaw forward. As the lips are also together, breathing is then completely obstructed.

Obstruction at pharyngeal level is most commonly due to the tongue falling back against the posterior wall of the pharynx. This occurs because the tongue is largely composed of muscle fibres, some of which arise from the mandible. The latter falls backwards as the unconscious patient relaxes, and the tongue goes with it. Extension of the head (and with it the mandible) frequently restores the airway, but there are times when this can be done only by pressing the thumbs or fingers directly behind the angle of the mandible and lifting it forwards.

Obstruction from the level of the larynx downwards is usually due to complications associated with endotracheal tubes, laryngeal or bronchospasm or to soiling of the respiratory tract with blood, vomit or secretions. Endotracheal tubes may be kinked or compressed at any level, including the nose and nasopharynx. Occlusion of the distal end of the tube may occur if the bevel is pressed against the tracheal wall or if an overinflated cuff herniates over the end of the tube. Various problems associated with the faulty manufacture of endotracheal tubes and their cuffs have been reported in the past, but happily these are much less common with modern manufacturing standards.

Laryngeal spasm and bronchospasm may be precipitated by many factors, and are much more common in patients with an irritable respiratory tract (e.g. heavy smokers, bronchitics and asthmatics). Common stimuli include the sudden inspiration of too high a concentration of almost any volatile anaesthetic, or reflex spasm occurring in response to a surgical stimulus at too light a plane of anaesthesia. The spasm usually resolves when the stimulus is removed. In recalcitrant cases laryngeal spasm (which is impossible, of course, if an endotracheal tube is *in situ*) will respond to a muscle relaxant because the laryngeal muscles responsible for this spasm are striated muscle. Bronchospasm may be slower to subside and may require bronchodilators.

Pre-existing Respiratory Disease and Anaesthesia

Pre-existing respiratory disease causes concern less often under general anaesthesia than might be expected. While laryngeal spasm or bronchospasm may be worrying, few intubated patients have much trouble during anaesthesia. This is not surprising because the ultimate treatment for respiratory failure nowadays is endotracheal intubation and ventilation.

The dangerous time for a patient with respiratory disease is in the post-operative period. The pain of the surgical incision, especially if it is an upper abdominal one, tends to make breathing shallow and coughing inefficient. Sputum retention tends to occur and atelectasis follows as the air is absorbed from the lung distal to the blocked bronchi. In the earlier days of anaesthesia these problems were accentuated by the prolonged drowsiness which followed deep levels of anaesthesia. With modern anaesthetic techniques these complications must be regarded as associated with the surgery rather than with the anaesthetic.

Hypoxia

Varying degrees of hypoxia may occur in association with many complications of anaesthesia. Even in normal circumstances, however, there is a tendency for hypoxia to occur during anaesthesia, and this may continue into the postoperative period. While being most severe after abdominal operations, it nevertheless occurs to some extent after quite simple procedures and is believed to be caused by underventilation of the dependent parts of the lung.

A much shorter period of hypoxia occurs after any nitrous oxide-based anaesthetic and is called 'diffusion hypoxia' (p. 56). After the nitrous oxide has been turned off, large quantities of it leave the body through the alveoli. With the recovering patient breathing oxygen or worse still air, the alveoli contain oxygen, nitrogen and nitrous oxide, together with carbon dioxide and water vapour. In this situation, the concentration of oxygen is inevitably reduced, leading to hypoxia. This probably lasts <10 min and is of no great significance in a healthy patient, but may add to the problems of the ill or debilitated patient who should always be given added oxygen during this period.

● CARDIOVASCULAR SYSTEM

The commonest cardiovascular complications of anaesthesia are dysrhythmias and hypotension. A great variety of abnormal rhythms can occur under anaesthesia and some of these are described in more detail in Chapter 22. Not all dysrhythmias are serious, and the anaesthetist's main concern is whether they are or are likely to become life-endangering. Hypotension is never far away under general anaesthesia, as most anaesthetic agents tend to produce some degree of depression of the heart and peripheral vasomotor tone either directly or by their depressant action on the brain. With a fit patient under light anaesthesia, compensation is usually complete with a normal blood pressure. However, at deeper levels of anaesthesia or in older or debilitated patients, some degree of fall in blood pressure is common.

Predisposing Factors

Various factors make dysrhythmias or hypertension more likely to occur under anaesthesia. These factors summate, and as some of them are avoidable it is important that by careful choice and execution of anaesthetic technique the anaesthetist reduces to a minimum the likelihood of these complications.

Pre-existing Cardiovascular Disease

The patient with cardiovascular disease is susceptible to complications during anaesthesia. The disease may be discovered at the preoperative visit, but this is not always so. It is wise to expect that every elderly patient has a relatively compromised cardiovascular system.

Anaesthetic Agents

Some volatile anaesthetic agents, especially halothane, have the propensity to produce dysrhythmias, some of them potentially serious. Halothane and enflurane are particularly likely to produce hypotension.

Increased Catecholamine Levels

Serious ventricular dysrhythmias are likely to occur in the presence of high circulating levels of catecholamines. These catecholamines, of which adrenaline is the most likely to produce dysrhythmias, may be exogenous (i.e. injected) or endogenous (i.e. produced within the body).

Hypoxia and Hypercarbia

Both these factors tend to increase the incidence of dysrhythmias. They are usually due to faults in anaesthetic technique.

Direct or Reflex Stimulation

Direct stimulation of the heart at cardiac surgery or during operations nearby may produce abnormalities of cardiac rhythm. More commonly, dysrhythmias occur reflexly in response to stimulation of other areas of the body (e.g. the pharynx, the larynx, intra-abdominal mesenteries or traction on the extraocular eye muscles).

An example of several of these factors summating might be the administration of an adrenaline-containing local anaesthetic solution to a patient spontaneously breathing a high concentration of halothane. (This technique is nearly always associated with some degree of hypercarbia.) The exogenously administered adrenaline, the halothane and the hypercarbia would combine to produce ideal conditions for generating serious ventricular dysrhythmia.

Air Embolism

Air may occasionally gain entry to the arterial side of the cardiovascular system at open heart surgery. More frequently it enters the venous side, the commonest situation being when a vein is opened in an area where the venous pressure is low. This most commonly occurs at neurosurgical operations or other operations on the head and neck when the operation site is above the level of the heart. It can occur at other times, for example, accidentally, at intravenous infusion. The air passes to the right ventricle where it is churned into froth. If of sufficient degree this may obstruct the pulmonary circulation. The air may also pass through the lungs or patent intracardiac defects and cause embolisation of the coronary or cerebral circulation.

Deep Vein Thrombosis and Pulmonary Embolism

Pulmonary emboli arise as fragments of thrombus occurring usually in the veins of the legs or pelvis. Neither venous thrombi nor pulmonary emboli usually occur during the anaesthetic, but they may occur 3–14 days afterwards. Hence these complications are the province of the whole surgical team rather than the anaesthetist. Although the exact 'trigger' to the formation of venous thrombi is unknown, some of the factors associated with a high incidence are known and a certain amount of prophylaxis is possible. The incidence is highest in the middle-aged and elderly, with prolonged bed rest, after major and prolonged surgery especially of the lower abdomen, pelvis and hip joint, and in patients with known coronary artery disease. In patients at risk it may be possible to improve venous return by raising the foot of the operating table or bed postoperatively, and pressure on the calves may be prevented by raising them off the surface of the operating table by sponge rubber supports under the heels. Venous pooling may be prevented by elastic (TED) stockings.

More active prevention includes subcutaneous heparin 5000 units 8-hourly for about 5 days starting 2 h preoperatively, low molecular weight heparin (Clexane 20–40 mg), subcutaneously once daily, or 500 ml intravenous dextran 70 daily until the patient is mobile. Intermittent pneumatic calf compression using 'Flotron' leggings (Fig. 3.3) is the most widely used active mechanical method of venous thrombosis prevention and is very effective.

Although complications associated with anaesthesia may occur in many of the systems of the body, those discussed below belong to the group arising due to the loss of the patient's protective reflexes under anaesthesia.

● AWARENESS

The effectiveness and widespread use of the neuromuscular-blocking agents has led to a new problem of general anaesthesia, unknown in the old 'single-agent anaesthesia' days: the problem of 'awareness' under anaesthesia. A patient under muscle-relaxant anaesthesia may, if the anaesthesia is too light, be returning to consciousness but, because of muscle paralysis, be unable to communicate with the anaesthetist. The sense of hearing is usually the last to go on induction of anaesthesia and the first to return as anaesthesia lightens. Many of the reported cases of awareness are of conversations heard during the anaesthetic. Although pain is seldom complained of (probably a tribute to the efficacy of nitrous oxide as an analgesic) these incidents can be distressing to the patient and every anaesthetist must do his utmost to avoid them. It is now known that if only nitrous oxide and oxygen are used to maintain anaesthesia, even heavy premedication does not eliminate the possibility of awareness and, except in the case of very ill patients, an intravenous or inhalational adjuvant should be added to the anaesthetic. Even then, awareness is possible especially with intravenous adjuvants which are usually given as periodic increments rather than as a continuous infusion, so it is still possible for anaesthesia to become dangerously light as the time for the next increment approaches.

● PERIPHERAL NERVE INJURIES

Injuries to peripheral nerves may arise as a result of compression against bony points or by tourniquets, from stretching of nerve trunks or plexuses in abnormal positions, by injection of irritant solutions (e.g. thiopentone) around nerves, or due to hypotension causing ischaemia. Examples of nerves susceptible to pressure injuries include the radial nerve as it winds around the shaft of the humerus, the ulnar nerve as it runs behind the medial epicondyle of the humerus, and the lateral popliteal nerve as it runs across the neck of the fibula. Traction injury probably occurs most commonly to the brachial plexus. The nerve most likely to be damaged by thiopentone injection is the median nerve in the antecubital fossa. For this reason, most anaesthetists induce anaesthesia through a cannula introduced into the veins on the dorsum of the hand.

● OPHTHALMIC COMPLICATIONS

The part of the eye most commonly damaged under anaesthesia is the cornea, which may ulcerate if it dries out as a result of the eye staying open during the anaesthetic, or it may become abraded by irritant vapours or antiseptic solutions. Central retinal artery thrombosis is a rare complication of anaesthesia and probably occurs only where there is hypotension in a patient already suffering from vascular disease.

Postoperative pain around the supra-orbital nerve has been reported and is probably due to prolonged pressure by a catheter mount over this nerve.

● SKIN COMPLICATIONS

Ulceration of the skin over bony prominences (typically the sacrum) is always a danger in old or debilitated patients. This is more a problem of intensive care units, but is worth bearing in mind in such patients in the operating theatre, especially if surgery is prolonged.

● HYPOTHERMIA

Significant falls in body temperature under anaesthesia are most likely to occur at the extremes of age, being particularly important in the neonate. The rate of fall in temperature is related to the temperature of the operating theatre. In normal adult patients heat loss is unlikely to be serious, provided that the theatre temperature is kept above 21°C. Active warm air circulating blankets are now widely available and should be used wherever possible during prolonged operations (Fig. 21.1). Other causes of pronounced heat loss are the administration of large volumes of refrigerated fluids, especially blood, and irrigation of hollow viscera by fluids at temperatures <37°C, for example, the bladder during transurethral prostatectomy.

Postoperatively, hypothermia may cause shivering with a distinct increase in metabolic rate and therefore in oxygen requirement. The patient feels uncomfortable and vasoconstricts. The shivering commonly occurring after halothane and isoflurane anaesthesia does not seem to be associated with significant falls in temperature and is part of a generalised muscular spasticity. The masseteric spasm – frequently part of this syndrome – may be so fierce that if an oral airway is in place at this time the incisor teeth may be loosened.

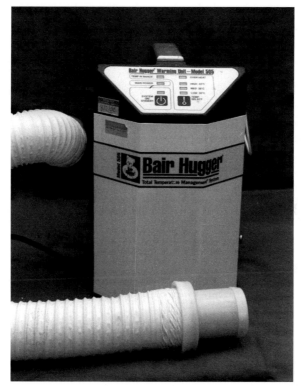

Figure 21.1 'Bair Hugger' warm air circulating system.

● HYPERSENSITIVITY TO ANAESTHETIC DRUGS

This became increasingly important with the extensive use of the intravenous induction agent Althesin, which has since been withdrawn. It was a relatively frequent problem (1 in 400 administrations), particularly when the drug was given repeatedly over a short space of time. All drugs given intravenously have the potential to cause adverse reactions either nonspecifically, related to the pH of the drug, preservatives or histamine release, or specifically as part of an immune-mediated response. The intravenous route bypasses all the normal protective mechanisms of the body such as skin, mucous membranes, gut, etc., making the occurrence of severe reactions relatively common and unpredictable.

Of the intravenous induction agents currently available, neither etomidate, propofol (Diprivan) nor ketamine has been specifically associated with hypersensitivity reactions. The incidence of reactions to thiopentone is approximately 1 in 20 000 and to methohexitone 1 in 7000, although when these do occur, they are often severe, associated with bronchospasm and cardiovascular collapse. Neuromuscular-blocking drugs, particularly suxamethonium, atracurium and d-tubocurarine, are frequently associated with non-specific histamine release, producing flushing, tachycardia, hypotension and sometimes bronchospasm. Others, such as pancuronium, vecuronium and rocuronium, are much less of a problem.

The initial treatment of hypersensitivity reactions should include intravenous fluids to correct the relative hypovolaemia and intravenous or subcutaneous adrenaline together possibly with antihistamines, for example, chlorpheniramine (Piriton), to antagonise the effects of excessive histamine release and anaphylactic shock.

RECOVERY FROM ANAESTHESIA

The Recovery Room

The period of recovery from anaesthesia is undoubtedly one of the most dangerous times during a surgical patient's stay in hospital. Many factors contribute to this danger. The patients have to regain their protective reflexes, especially those protecting the respiratory tract. As anaesthesia lightens, vomiting is likely and, with regurgitation an ever-present danger, it is a wise rule to turn all patients onto their side as they recover from anaesthesia, or before extubation if an endotracheal tube has been used. Only rarely does the surgery make this impossible, for example, when traction has been set up by means of a Steinmann pin through the tibia, or after facial surgery. Other adverse factors include possible hypoxia or hypercarbia as the patient tends to breath-hold in light planes of anaesthesia, or breathe inadequately as spontaneous respiration returns after muscle-relaxant anaesthesia. Extubation and pharyngeal suction may provoke serious dysrhythmias, especially if any of the above factors are present. Cardiac arrest may occur, but surrounded by trained medical and nursing staff and with resuscitation equipment at hand, there is a good chance of success if resuscitative measures are instituted promptly.

Before the advent of dedicated recovery rooms, the standard of patient care after leaving the operating theatre fell dramatically. The patient was often transported semi-conscious and with inadequate nursing supervision straight back to the ward. There was an appreciable incidence of morbidity and even mortality on the journey from operating theatre to ward, and even care of the recovering patient in the ward was sometimes inadequate. A recovery room is included in the design of all new theatre suites, and many old theatres have been modified to include them. These units aim to provide an area where the patient may recover consciousness under the supervision of trained nurses with all the necessary resuscitation equipment and with the anaesthetist nearby. The pulse rate, blood pressure, respiration, oxygen saturation and temperature should be measured and charted and the recovery room personnel should also be expert at supervising other postoperative aspects of surgery, for example, managing continuous bladder irrigation after prostatectomy.

While all recovery rooms should keep patients until they have regained their protective reflexes and achieved cardiovascular stability, whether the patient stays longer depends on the site and staffing of the recovery room. Most recovery rooms look after patients for only an hour or two at the most, but there is no doubt that longer-stay recovery wards have their advantages, for example, for postoperative epidural analgesia (Chapter 42). The argument that recovery areas deprive ward nurses of experience in postoperative patient care is no longer acceptable; student nurses can be rotated through recovery wards where in a short time they will gain much better experience than they would obtain in months in a general surgical ward. The widespread introduction of recovery rooms in recent years has undoubtedly done much to increase safety for surgical patients.

22

Interpretation of the Electrocardiogram

•Preoperative ECG interpretation •Intra-operative ECG interpretation
•Common intra-operative arrhythmias and their treatment

Although electrocardiography (ECG) is a specialist subject in itself, the use of monitoring and the simple interpretation of arrhythmias are extremely important in anaesthetic practice. There is little excuse for failing to monitor the ECG continuously during anaesthesia and although this is simply a record of the electrical activity of the heart and does not reflect peripheral blood flow, abnormalities may give an early indication of problems during anaesthesia.

When excitable tissue, either nerve or muscle, is activated to produce either contraction or impulse transmission, this is effected by a change in permeability of the cell membrane, allowing sodium ions to flow in and potassium ions to flow out of the cell. This depolarisation, as it is known, results in a change in electrical charge inside the cell, and is followed by a repolarisation process when the charge returns to normal. Resting cells are negatively charged with respect to the outside while depolarised cells become positive. If electrodes are placed in certain positions on the chest wall or the limbs, changes in electrical activity in the heart due to contraction are detected at the electrode as a change in charge. If this electrical activity is then demonstrated on the ECG, an upward deflection of the baseline reflects a positive change and a downward deflection a negative change, this being the basis of the ECG recording. The ECG waveform (Fig. 22.1) reflects the changes in charge occurring at different points in the cardiac cycle.

The heart lies in a fixed position in the chest, so if these changes in charge are viewed from the right arm or the left arm, for example, the appearance will differ. By using different leads it is possible to examine the different parts of the heart for abnormalities of contraction or conduction, reflecting, for example, myocardial ischaemia or heart block. The intra-operative use of ECG monitoring, however, is limited to a single lead (usually lead 2) that is designed to reflect major disturbances in rate and

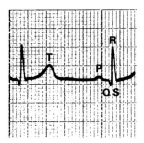

Figure 22.1 Normal ECG waveforms.

rhythm rather than to diagnose focal areas of ischaemia which requires a full 12-lead ECG.

● PREOPERATIVE ECG INTERPRETATION

Preoperative 12-lead ECG records should be obtained routinely from all patients over the age of 60 years and all those with a history of cardiac disease irrespective of age. In patients in whom cardiac problems are expected, it is important to have a preoperative baseline ECG with which to compare any postoperative change. Normal ECG interpretation includes the following.

Rate

The paper speed of a normal ECG recording is 25 mm per second, and as the small squares on the ECG paper are 1 mm, this means that the paper travels at 25 small squares (five large squares) per second; 300 large squares are therefore covered every minute, and by dividing 300 into the number of large squares between the same point (usually the R wave) of two ECG complexes, the heart rate is derived (e.g. 300/5 = heart rate of 60). This is applicable only to patients with a regular heart beat (sinus rhythm).

Cardiac Rhythm

Normal sinus rhythm is diagnosed by the presence of a P wave, reflecting atrial contraction, before each QRS complex (Fig. 22.1). This results in a regular heartbeat which will vary only slightly with respiration (sinus arrhythmia).

The normal pacemaker of the heart (the sino-atrial node) initiates impulses at a regular rate, which travels across the atrium to the atrio-ventricular (A–V) node and then down the bundle of His which divides to

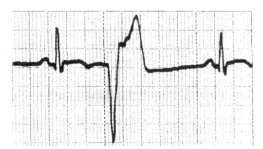

Figure 22.2 Ventricular ectopic beats.

supply the right and left ventricles. Normal ECG complexes of the type shown in Figure 22.1 reflect contractions which are initiated from the atrium (supraventricularly).

The absence of P waves preceding some or all of the cardiac complexes, which are nevertheless of a supraventricular type, indicates that the normal pacemaker is not functioning. If the rate is regular, this implies that another area of the atrium has taken over the task of pacemaker, for example, the A–V node or, if the rate is irregular without P waves and usually relatively fast, this is indicative of atrial fibrillation. A number of P waves regularly preceding each cardiac contraction indicates atrial flutter with a degree of heart block that allows only one in every three or four impulses to cross the A–V septum and pass down the bundle of His.

In nodal rhythms, the impulse rises in or near the A–V node. In this case, normal, regular QRS complexes are seen. The P waves may be either present, but the PR interval is short, or lost within the QRS complex.

Ventricular ectopic beats (Fig. 22.2) are very different in appearance from supraventricular contractions. They appear broader and are irregular, not preceded by a P wave and may occur at any stage in the resting period or, occasionally, during cardiac contraction. Regular runs of ventricular beats (ventricular tachycardia) or coupled beats (one supraventricular, one ventricular) are both indicative of conduction disturbances or myocardial ischaemia.

Conduction Defects

Heart Block

This refers to conduction defect at the A–V node preventing impulse transmission between the atria and ventricles and is of three types.

A first degree heart block is indicated on the ECG by a long PR interval (normal 0.12–0.2 s). It is usually clinically insignificant but may be due to increased vagal tone, drugs (e.g. digoxin) or myocardial ischaemia.

There are two types of second degree heart block. Type I is indicated by an increasing PR interval with successive beats until a beat is dropped and type II where a beat is dropped every or second or third beat. Type II may lead to a complete heart block.

In complete heart block the atria and ventricles have their own pacemakers, the ventricular rate being very slow. These patients may present with syncope and need a pacemaker before surgery.

Bundle Branch Block

The conduction defects in the bundle of His result in broad (>0.12 s), biphasic QRS complexes. If they occur in the right-sided leads (I and V1–V2) then the abnormality is called a right bundle branch block and is usually insignificant. A left bundle branch block is indicated by broad biphasic complexes in leads I and V4–V6. A left bundle branch block usually signifies ischaemic or valvular cardiac disease. Presence of a bundle branch block in itself is not a contraindication for anaesthesia but when associated with syncope or an increased PR interval is an indication for insertion of a pacemaker preoperatively.

Cardiac Pacemakers

Pacemakers are implanted in patients suffering consequences of arrhythmias due to both a slow and fast heart rate. Pacemaker technology has advanced a lot in the last few years but broadly two types are implanted, a fixed one where the heart is paced at a predetermined rate or a demand one where the pacemaker will activate on demand. An ECG of a patient with a pacemaker will show pacing spikes before QRS complexes. Details of the type of the pacemaker, the reasons why it was implanted and when it was checked are usually available on a Pacemaker Registration Card which all patients should carry.

Myocardial Ischaemia

Recent myocardial ischaemia is reflected by ST-segment elevation (Fig. 22.3), particularly in the chest leads, often accompanied by flattening or inversion of the T wave. Large Q waves in the chest leads are indicative of old myocardial ischaemia.

Metabolic Disturbances

Hyperkalaemia is the most important metabolic disturbance detectable on the ECG. High-peaked T waves indicate severe hyperkalaemia requiring emergency treatment with either calcium or glucose and insulin.

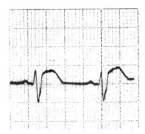

Figure 22.3 ST-segment elevation – myocardial ischaemia.

● INTRA-OPERATIVE ECG INTERPRETATION

In this situation a simple ECG monitor with three leads is used mainly as a rate and rhythm monitor, although severe changes in the appearance of the ECG complex with the leads remaining in the same position may be interpreted as myocardial ischaemia if they follow some important clinical event. It is then wise to repeat a 12-lead ECG in the immediate postoperative period. One possible way to use the ECG monitor to detect myocardial ischaemia is to use a 'modified V5 lead' – CM5 – where the right arm electrode of lead I is placed on the manubrium sterni, the left arm electrode is placed over the V5 position (left anterior axillary line in the fifth intercostal space) and the ground electrode is placed on the left shoulder. A recent advance has been the ability to process the ECG signal to provide information on the beat-to-beat (R–R) interval. This variability has been shown to be a good indicator of the balance between sympathetic and parasympathetic activity and may give a good indication of the depth of anaesthesia.

ECG monitoring during anaesthesia can be interfered with by patient movement, shivering, diathermy and dislodgment of leads.

● COMMON INTRA-OPERATIVE ARRHYTHMIAS AND THEIR TREATMENT

Disorders of Sinus Rhythm

Sinus Tachycardia

An increase in heart rate is produced as an early response to many anaesthetic problems although it may not occur in patients on β-adrenergic blockers. Common causes include inadequate anaesthesia and analgesia, hypoxia, hypercarbia and hypovolaemia. The anaesthetic technique should be examined for inadequate gas flow or oxygenation, inadequate analgesia or sedation, and also the presence of excessive blood loss requiring transfusion.

Sinus Bradycardia

This is a common arrhythmia, often produced by anaesthetic agents, particularly halothane and suxamethonium, which stimulate the vagus nerve, producing a bradycardia. Other causes of vagal stimulation are discussed in Chapter 14. It is important to remember that normal, fit patients' heart rates are far slower when they are asleep, sometimes being as slow as 40 beats per min. Although a full vagal blocking dose of intravenous atropine is 2 mg, it is often possible to increase the heart rate to an acceptable level with a very small dose of atropine (0.2–0.3 mg) or glycopyrrolate (0.2 mg). Excessively slow heart rates may also produce other arrhythmias (see below).

Supraventricular Dysrhythmias

Wandering Pacemaker and Nodal Rhythm

Not infrequently during anaesthesia, the pacemaker in the atrium shifts from the normal sino-atrial node to another area of the atrium or to the A–V node itself. If the atrial impulses are coming from varying sites in runs of three or four beats, which then change to a slightly different supraventricular complex, this is known as a wandering pacemaker. Nodal tachycardia has already been mentioned. Supraventricular arrhythmias may occur as a result of sinus bradycardia, presumably because the normal rate is insufficient to prevent additional beats occurring. For this reason they often respond well to atropine, producing a slight increase in heart rate.

Atrial Fibrillation

It is relatively uncommon for atrial fibrillation to occur during anaesthesia in a patient who is in sinus rhythm preoperatively unless the pericardium is disturbed, as, for example, during thoracic surgery. If atrial flutter or fibrillation does arise, however, it may be necessary to digitalise the patient urgently to prevent a fall in cardiac output resulting from lack of atrial contraction.

Supraventricular Tachycardia

This arrhythmia is again relatively rare during anaesthesia, but it may occur particularly if the patient is inadequately anaesthetised. Like a severe sinus tachycardia, it is sometimes controllable with additional analgesia or sedation but may require β-adrenergic blockade to reduce the heart rate.

Ventricular Arrhythmias

Ventricular Ectopics

Ventricular ectopic beats may occur in any patient, particularly if he is anxious or inadequately anaesthetised, and are frequently seen during induction when this period is monitored on the ECG. The occurrence of the occasional ventricular ectopic is probably of no importance, particularly if it is present on the preoperative ECG, but regular ectopics occurring either in groups of three or four or coupled with a supraventricular beat, are more serious. As a general rule, an incidence of more than one ventricular ectopic in five beats requires treatment and this rule may be extended if cardiac output is impaired. Ventricular ectopics may also reflect myocardial ischaemia and should be carefully evaluated. Intravenous lignocaine (50–100 mg) is usually sufficient to treat intra-operative ventricular ectopics, although, as in the case of supraventricular dysrhythmias, a change in anaesthetic technique may be required. Occasionally a lignocaine drip is necessary to abate the ventricular dysrhythmia permanently. Intravenous disopyramide may also be useful. However, both these drugs cause myocardial depression and may therefore aggravate the hypotension that frequent ectopics tend to produce, and treatment should be given only when absolutely necessary. Care should also be taken to ensure that patients are metabolically normal since hypokalaemia, in particular, may predispose to ventricular arrhythmias.

Ventricular Tachycardia and Fibrillation

The treatment of these is discussed in detail in Chapter 23.

23

Adult Cardiopulmonary Resuscitation

•Basic life support •Advanced life support: restoration of normal cardiac activity
•Ventricular fibrillation/pulseless ventricular tachycardia •Non-VF/VT rhythms
• 'Crash trolley' contents •Defibrillators

Anaesthetists and anaesthetic assistants play an important role in the management of cardiac arrest either as members of the hospital 'resuscitation' team or in the operating theatre. They also provide training and teaching of resuscitation skills. In recent years, cardiopulmonary resuscitation (CPR) has progressed to the extent that each hospital has its own resuscitation team and a training officer who trains staff in the necessary skills. Management is also standardised and recommended guidelines are published by national bodies such as Resuscitation Council (UK). These guidelines are updated regularly on their website, www.resus.org.uk

The management of every cardiac arrest falls into two parts. First, providing blood and oxygen to vital tissues by providing basic life support (BLS), and secondly establishing spontaneous heartbeat and ventilation with advanced life support (ALS).

● BASIC LIFE SUPPORT

The idea is to maintain circulation and ventilation until help arrives to institute advanced life support. Although basic equipment may be easily available when cardiac arrest occurs in the hospital, ideally all health care personnel should be proficient in BLS without additional equipment.

The sequence of BLS actions when performed without any equipment are outlined in Table 23.1. A useful mnemonic is DRS (Doctors!), where D is Danger; R, Response and S, Shout; and the A–B–C principle where A is Airway, B, Breathing and C, Circulation.

Table 23.1 Basic life support

1. Ensure that there is no Danger to the rescuer or the patient
2. Check the patient's Response to shaking and shouting
3. If there is no response then Shout for help
4. Open the Airway (head tilt and chin lift) and look, listen and feel for Breathing for 10 s
5. If there is breathing, turn the patient to the recovery position
6. If there is no breathing then send someone (if available) for assistance or go yourself if you are on your own
7. Give two effective rescue breaths by ensuring head tilt and chin lift and pinching the patient's nose, covering the patient's mouth with your own and blowing steadily into the mouth for 2 s while watching for a clear chest rise
8. Assess the patient for signs of Circulation (not >10 s) by checking the carotid pulse
9. If there is circulation then continue rescue breathing and check for circulation every minute
10. If there is no circulation then start chest compressions at a rate of 100/min. Continue to provide compressions and breaths in a ratio of 15 : 2

BLS in the Hospital

It is likely that more than one health care professional will be available making it possible for several of the above actions to be undertaken at the same time. The BLS protocol above will almost certainly not cause a return of spontaneous circulation. The priority is therefore to monitor the cardiac rhythm and defibrillate the heart. Airway management and ventilation should be started with the most appropriate equipment and expertise available. Pocket masks and airway adjuncts such as oropharyngeal airway, face mask and bag should be readily available and must be used to provide supplemental oxygen.

● ADVANCED LIFE SUPPORT: RESTORATION OF NORMAL CARDIAC ACTIVITY

The universal algorithm used for the management of cardiac arrest is shown in Figure 23.1. Heart rhythms associated with cardiac arrest can be divided into two groups:

1. Ventricular fibrillation/pulseless ventricular tachycardia (VF/VT).

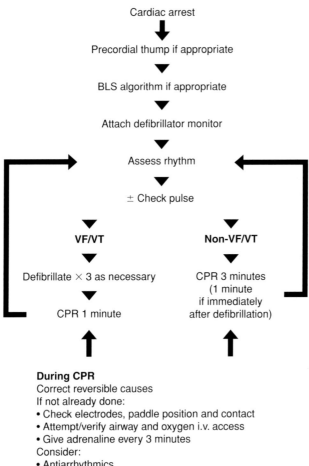

Figure 23.1 Universal algorithm for management of cardiac arrest.

2. Non-VF/VT rhythms, usually asystole or pulseless electrical activity (PEA), also known as electromechanical dissociation (EMD).

The principal difference in the management of these two groups is the need to defibrillate early in patients with VF/VT. Subsequent actions including chest compressions, airway management and ventilation, venous access, administration of adrenaline and identification and correction of contributing factors are the same for both groups (Fig. 23.1).

● VENTRICULAR FIBRILLATION/PULSELESS VENTRICULAR TACHYCARDIA

In this condition, contraction of the myocardial fibres is uncoordinated and not strong enough to produce forward flow of blood. This is the commonest rhythm in adult cardiac arrest and has the highest survival rate if rapidly and corrected by electrical defibrillation. Hence modern technology has been applied to manufacturing portable defibrillators which are being made available not only in hospitals where acute patients are treated, but also in ambulances and even in places of work. Ambulance personnel, nurses and even lay people are being trained to recognise this rhythm and treat it without wasting time. The chances of survival decline by 10% for each minute that the arrhythmia persists and myocardial energy levels are depleted. BLS slows the process but does not halt it. The priority is therefore to determine the rhythm and deliver a shock if indicated. BLS must not delay defibrillation. If the arrest was witnessed or monitored, and a defibrillator is not immediately available, a single precordial thump should be administered, as the energy delivered may be enough to defibrillate the heart.

Defibrillation

This delivers a direct current (d.c.) 'shock' (measured in joules) to the heart which produces simultaneous depolarisation of all myocardial cells. This stops the heart momentarily but then the subsequent cardiac impulse may start from the normal cardiac pacemaker (sino-atrial node) and heartbeat is restored.

Up to three shocks are given initially with energies of 200, 200 and 360 J. The rationale for starting defibrillation with a shock of 200 J is that an initial shock of this energy will cause little myocardial injury and in most recoverable situations is adequate to defibrillate the patient successfully. The second shock is also 200 J because the first shock reduces transthoracic impedance increasing the energy reaching the heart from a shock of similar energy. The third and subsequent shocks are at 360 J until a rhythm compatible with cardiac output is restored. When all three shocks are required, it is important to deliver these within 1 min.

After delivering a shock there is often a delay of a few seconds before an electrocardiographic (ECG) display of diagnostic quality is obtained. Successful defibrillation is usually followed by a few seconds of true asystole (electrical stunning); furthermore even when a rhythm normally compatible with a cardiac output is obtained, there is often a period of temporary impairment in myocardial contractility (myocardial stunning) resulting in a pulse which is weak and difficult to palpate. Therefore a diagnosis of PEA should not be made after defibrillation if the rhythm is compatible with an output but no pulse is felt. For this reason the algorithm indicates 1 min of CPR before reassessing the rhythm and making a further pulse check. During this 1 min adrenaline should not be given as it may be harmful to a patient who has had a rhythm of spontaneous circulation.

Chest Compressions, Airway and Ventilation

If VF persists after the three initial shocks then myocardial and cerebral viability must be maintained by chest compressions and ventilation of the lungs. Defibrillation still has the best chance of restoring rhythm. For 1 min CPR with a compression: ventilation ratio of 15 : 2 is undertaken and during which reversible causes should be considered and treated. A check is also made of paddle positions and contacts.

The airway is secured. Tracheal intubation provides the most reliable way but should be performed by only experienced personnel. The laryngeal mask airway (LMA) is a suitable alternative (Chapter 18). The aim is to deliver the highest possible concentration of oxygen (preferably 100%) to the lungs. Once intubated chest compressions can be continued at 100/min except when defibrillation and pulse checks are needed. Ventilation is continued at about 12 breaths/min by connecting the tube to a bag-valve assembly and an oxygen supply.

Intravenous Access and Drug Therapy

Intravenous access should be established at the earliest opportunity. Central venous access is ideal for drug delivery if expertise and equipment are available. Peripheral venous access is acceptable but the line must be flushed with at least 20 ml normal saline after each drug delivery for it to reach the heart.

Adrenaline

Adrenaline is administered in 1 mg doses by the intravenous route or 2–3 mg via the tracheal route but diluted to at least 10 ml with sterile water.

Adrenaline improves the efficacy of CPR and its α-adrenergic action causes vasoconstriction which increases myocardial and cerebral perfusion pressure. The dose is repeated every 3 min during a cardiac arrest.

Anti-arrhythmic Drugs

The role of these drugs in the treatment of VF/VT is not well established. Amiodarone can be considered to treat shock refractory cardiac arrest due to VF or pulseless VT (i.e. after three unsuccessful shocks). It should not, however, delay the delivery of a shock.

Lignocaine should not be given if the patient has received amiodarone but may be used as an alternative if amiodarone is unavailable.

Procainamide is another alternative to amiodarone and lignocaine for refractory VF.

The use of bicarbonate (50 mmol) is considered if the arterial pH is <7.1 or if the cardiac arrest is associated with tricyclic antidepressent overdose or hyperkalaemia.

It is important to ensure that the potentially reversible causes (4 Hs and 4 Ts; see below) have been eliminated as any of these can reduce the chances of successful defibrillation.

The number of times the loop is repeated during any individual resuscitation is a matter of clinical judgement and the perceived prospect of successful outcome.

● NON-VF/VT RHYTHMS

The outcome from non-VF/VT rhythms is relatively poor unless a reversible cause can be found and treated effectively. If apparent asystole or PEA occurs immediately after delivery of a shock (see above), the rhythm and pulse should be checked just after 1 min (right loop of the algorithm). If asystole or PEA is confirmed, appropriate drugs are given and a further 2 min CPR is given to complete the loop.

Asystole

It is important to make the correct diagnosis and not to miss VF. Asystole must be confirmed by:

• checking that the leads are attached correctly
• checking the gain
• viewing the rhythm through leads I and II.

Chest compressions and ventilation should be undertaken for 3 min with each loop (or 1 min if directly after a shock) during which the airway can be secured, intravenous access obtained and the first dose of adrenaline given. Atropine 3 mg intravenously or 6 mg via the tracheal tube can be given once to produce total blockade of the vagus nerve.

If the rhythm changes to VF the left side of the algorithm should be followed, otherwise CPR is continued and adrenaline given every 3 min. Reversible causes should be sought and corrected.

Pulseless Electrical Activity

This condition comprises the clinical signs of a cardiac arrest with an ECG rhythm compatible with a cardiac output. The patient's best chance of survival will be by prompt identification and treatment of any underlying cause. The potential causes are categorised in two groups (see below). Resuscitation should be continued while the causes are sought. CPR is started immediately; the airway and ventilation are managed as appropriate and intravenous access is obtained. Adrenaline 1 mg intravenously is administered every 3 min. If there is an associated bradycardia then atropine 3 mg intravenously or 6 mg via the tracheal tube may be considered.

Potentially Reversible Causes

During every cardiac arrest potential causes for which there is a specific treatment should be sought and treated. For ease of memory these are divided into two groups of four based upon the initial letter H or T.

The four Hs are:

- hypoxia
- hypovolaemia
- hypo/hyperkalaemia and metabolic disorders
- hypothermia.

The four Ts are:

- tension pneumothorax
- tamponade (cardiac)
- toxic/therapeutic disorders
- thromboembolic and mechanical obstruction.

● 'CRASH TROLLEY' CONTENTS

These trolleys may become unnecessarily complicated. In general, the following should be considered essential:

- Defibrillators and essentials such as pads, jelly, etc.
- Yankauer oropharyngeal suckers and a range of suction catheters.

- Oropharyngeal airways, LMAs, tracheal tubes and connections appropriate to the size of the patients.
- A tracheal tube introducer or bougie.
- Self-inflating bag, valve and face masks of various sizes.
- Two working laryngoscopes.
- Intravenous drip set and cannulae (it is unnecessarily confusing to have a wide range of these).
- Intravenous fluids; crystalloids and colloids.

Drug Boxes

Adrenaline and atropine are considered 'first-line' drugs and are supplied in a different coloured box. A 'second-line' drug box contains all the other drugs which may include amiodorone, lignocaine, procainamide, calcium, dopamine, frusemide, glucagon, etc., as decided by the individual hospital resuscitation team.

The trolleys should be checked each time they are used and also at weekly intervals to ensure that items such as laryngoscopes are in full working order.

● DEFIBRILLATORS (Fig. 23.2)

The defibrillators in hospitals are usually of the manual, d.c. type and are designed to pass an electric current across the heart in the form of a shock

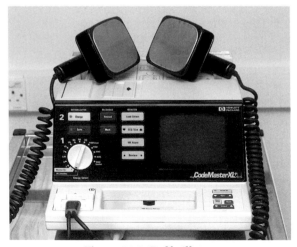

Figure 23.2 Defibrillator.

to alter the cardiac rhythm. This is most often used to convert VF back into sinus rhythm, but synchronised d.c. shock is also used to convert patients in atrial flutter or atrial fibrillation back into sinus rhythm. Switches control power on–off and magnitude of charge (measured in joules) shown on the dial. The charge and discharge buttons are placed on the paddles. Other parts include a monitor with digital heart rate display, delivered energy display, ECG source display, i.e. from the pads or separate electrodes and alarms. It is essential that the user is familiar with the layout of all the controls on the defibrillator they will use.

Procedure for Defibrillation

A short description of the procedure is included. It is vital before using the machine on patients that the rescuer is familiar with the particular model used in that hospital. The procedure is as follows:

1. Apply gel pads to the chest.
2. Turn on the defibrillator.
3. Select the energy level.
4. Assure proper placement of paddles as follows: 'sternal' pad – under the right clavicle; 'apical' pad – to the left of the nipple in the left mid-axillary line.
5. Apply about 25 lb (11 kg) pressure on the paddles.
6. Say loudly 'Stand Clear!', and make a visual check to ensure no personnel are in direct contact with the patient.
7. Remove oxygen delivery device from the patient.
8. Charge defibrillator by pressing charge buttons on the handles.
9. Deliver shock by depressing both discharge buttons on the paddles simultaneously.

Recently semi-automated defibrillators have become available which are smaller and portable. It is likely that these will become more universally available.

24

Anaesthesia for Emergency Surgery and Trauma

•Vomiting and regurgitation •Fluid and electrolyte depletion •Local and regional analgesia •Anaesthesia after major trauma

The term 'emergency' implies an urgency which prevents the full and careful preparation of the patient that would be possible and desirable before an elective procedure. Few surgical emergencies are so dire that a full history and physical examination are not possible. The degree to which laboratory and radiological investigations are considered essential in the individual case will depend upon the time available and the severity of intercurrent disease. Few anaesthetists in the UK would anaesthetise an elderly, bronchitic patient with several days' history of intestinal obstruction without full biochemical and haematological information and a chest X-ray examination, but the same anaesthetist might have to proceed without the advantage of any of these investigations if presented with a similar patient in an underdeveloped country. Conversely, to request extensive investigation on every fit, young patient who has suffered an uncomplicated limb fracture would waste time and money. Each anaesthetist and each surgical team will know the environment in which they work and should strive for as good a preoperative assessment as circumstances allow.

There are other circumstances, usually associated with uncontrollable bleeding, where there may just be time to obtain laboratory information but full resuscitation of the patient is impossible before the operation has to be carried out to save their life. Rapid transfusion of blood (which may have to be uncrossed group O Rh-negative) and other fluids may effect temporary improvement in the patient's condition, but this usually worsens again as increased blood pressure produces further bleeding. Examples of such cases are bleeding from a duodenal ulcer or badly ruptured ectopic pregnancy.

● VOMITING AND REGURGITATION

Probably the most important factor common to all emergency procedures is the possibility that the stomach will contain undigested food or fluid material which may be vomited or regurgitated into the pharynx, whence it may find its way into the lungs.

The gastric contents are usually derived from one of two sources: undigested food and alimentary canal secretions.

Undigested Food

Any patient being presented for anaesthesia may have undigested food in his stomach. Before elective procedures, all food and fluid are withheld for a long enough time for the stomach to have emptied. This period is usually taken as about 2–3 h for clear liquids and 6 h for solid food. In emergency anaesthesia there are some reasons why the stomach may not have emptied. First, the surgical treatment may be considered to be of such urgency that it is not possible to wait for several hours, and secondly (and probably more importantly), in most emergencies gastric digestion is greatly slowed or may even cease. Where the patient has had an accident, it is wise to calculate from the time the patient last ate until the time of the accident rather than from the last meal until the induction of anaesthesia.

Less obvious trauma than broken bones, for example, the psychological stress of being admitted unexpectedly to hospital and also the presence of pain and its treatment with opioid analgesics may delay gastric emptying in many patients; only in the least urgent of emergency procedures is it reasonable to regard the stomach as being empty.

Alimentary Canal Secretions

Variable amounts of liquid gastric contents are common when there is stasis in the alimentary tract, whether in the stomach itself or further down the intestine. In these circumstances, the presence of fluid in the stomach is inherent to the condition, and the situation will not improve (and indeed will probably become worse) by delaying.

Differences between Vomiting and Regurgitation

Vomiting is an active process involving contraction not only of the smooth muscle of the upper alimentary canal but also of the striated muscle of the diaphragm and abdominal muscles. It occurs only in light planes of anaesthesia which are usually seen only at induction of and emergence from anaesthesia. It cannot occur when a patient has been effectively paralysed by a neuromuscular blocking agent and cannot occur under deep anaesthesia.

Regurgitation, on the other hand, is a passive process and simply implies the flowing of fluids under the influence of gravity. It is more likely to occur under deep anaesthesia or in patients who have been given muscle relaxants. Regurgitation is normally prevented by the lower oesophageal sphincter (LOS). This is an area of high pressure at the lower end of the oesophagus. Normally LOS pressure is higher than the intragastric pressure and regurgitation does not occur. Regurgitation can occur either when the intragastric pressure is higher than the LOS pressure (e.g. in pregnancy, ascites, large abdominal masses) or when the LOS pressure itself is lowered (e.g. after induction of anaesthesia, muscle paralysis, unconsciousness). Suxamethonium fasciculations will also cause an increase in intragastric pressure. Metoclopramide increases LOS pressure.

Prevention of Inhalation of Gastric Contents

If not prevented, vomiting or regurgitation of stomach contents may result in asphyxia or aspiration pneumonitis (Mendelson's syndrome, Chapter 38). The severity of the lung damage depends on the acidity of the gastric contents. Efforts are made to reduce the amount and acidity of stomach contents by pharmacological or physical means (see below). Prevention of regurgitated contents entering the lungs is achieved by the technique of a rapid sequence (often rather inappropriately referred to as 'crash') induction.

Alkalis and H_2 Blockers

These drugs are discussed in Chapter 38. Even in emergency cases it is worth administering ranitidine intravenously because inhalation of foreign material may be a problem during emergence from as well as induction of anaesthesia.

Nasogastric and Orogastric Tubes

Where the gastric contents are thought to be liquid (as in most cases of intestinal stasis), a small tube (size 12 or 14 FG) passed into the stomach will serve to aspirate the gastric contents. The additional benefit of passing a wider bore tube when the gastric contents are expected to be solid or semi-solid is debatable, because the eyelets of even the largest tubes are easily blocked by particulate matter.

The disadvantages of these tubes are that they cannot be guaranteed to empty the stomach and, by their presence, tend to lower the LOS pressure. Opinion is divided but, having emptied the stomach, most anaesthetists would remove the tube before inducing anaesthesia.

General Anaesthesia Using Rapid Sequence ('Crash') Induction

The patient's airway is only safe under general anaesthesia when a cuffed tracheal tube is in place. The danger period is between induction of anaesthesia and inflation of the cuff on the tube. With modern anaesthetic techniques it is usually possible to reduce this period to a few seconds with the technique of rapid sequence induction.

Before inducing anaesthesia, secure access to a vein is essential. The anaesthetic equipment must be (as always) carefully checked and must include two laryngoscopes. Particular attention must be paid to the adequacy of the suction apparatus and to checking the ease with which the trolley or table can be placed in the head-down position.

It is wise to pre-oxygenate the patient for at least 3 min. This increases the amount of oxygen in the lung alveoli so that the continuing circulation of blood through the pulmonary capillaries will continue to pick up oxygen and maintain arterial Po_2 while the patient is apnoeic. Active inflation of the lungs by squeezing the reservoir bag – routine at elective procedures – is dangerous since inadvertent inflation of the stomach will increase the likelihood of regurgitation.

Anaesthesia is rapidly induced with an intravenous induction agent, the dose of which is scaled down to allow for the patient's debility, and intubation carried out with the help of suxamethonium while applying cricoid pressure (see below). Thiopentone is the induction agent with which most anaesthetists have the greatest familiarity. Carefully used, it is safe, but it should be remembered that it has a depressant effect on the myocardium.

Rapid sequence induction has only become acceptable since the introduction of cricoid pressure (Sellick's manoeuvre), which involves pressure on the cricoid cartilage to squeeze the upper end of the oesophagus against the sixth cervical vertebra, thus preventing the regurgitation of fluids into the pharynx (Fig. 24.1). The reason for using the cricoid cartilage is that it is the only complete ring of cartilage in the respiratory tract so that its firm posterior part is more effective at occluding the pharynx. In the single-handed technique cricoid pressure is applied with the forefinger and thumb of the right hand, while in the two-handed technique in addition, the left hand is placed behind the patient's neck which is then lifted forwards (Fig. 24.2). It is thought that this prevents the pressure of the right hand from undoing the flexion of the cervical spine on the thoracic spine which is the best position for laryngoscopy and intubation. Whichever technique is preferred, the pressure is maintained until the tracheal tube is passed and its cuff inflated.

It is now accepted that cricoid pressure should only be applied by a trained assistant. Training should involve practice on a weighing scale. A force of about 30 N (equivalent to 3 kg on a weighing scale) is enough to prevent regurgitation. More force than this may cause difficulties in intubation. It is also known that the LOS pressure decreases as soon as thiopentone is given and that in the awake patient cricoid pressure is uncomfortable and may provoke vomiting. For this reason light pressure of about 10 N (equal to 1 kg) should be applied in the awake patient increasing it to 30 N as the patient goes to sleep.

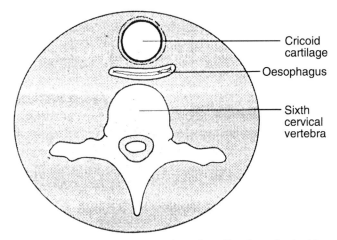

Figure 24.1 Diagrammatic representation of application of cricoid pressure.

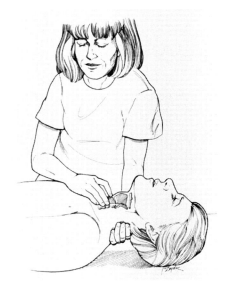

Figure 24.2 Two-handed application of cricoid pressure.

Induction of emergency cases in the steep head-up, supine position (to prevent regurgitation), or the left lateral, head-down position (hopefully to allow gastric contents to run harmlessly out of the mouth or nose) has, except in a few circumstances (see Chapter 25, Anaesthesia for Ear, Nose and Throat Surgery) gone out of fashion.

Maintenance of Anaesthesia

Maintenance of anaesthesia for abdominal emergencies is usually by controlled respiration with a non-depolarising muscle relaxant, using nitrous oxide and oxygen with a small amount of inhalational or parenteral adjuvant.

With the widespread introduction of intensive therapy units the discussion as to the possible causes of inadequate breathing at the end of operation has now become somewhat academic. It is now realised that instead of anxiously watching the still-intubated patient to decide whether their breathing is adequate, it is much safer to leave them intubated and ventilated for a few hours, during which time the problem almost invariably resolves spontaneously.

Spontaneous respiration anaesthesia is satisfactory for most peripheral operations (e.g. orthopaedic procedures) but if the patient is intubated for airway protection then it is easier to keep them lightly anaesthetised with muscle-relaxant anaesthesia and it is increasingly common to paralyse patients undergoing emergency procedures even when not strictly necessary to provide good surgical operating conditions. It is safer for the patient (and more comforting for the anaesthetist) to be in full control of protective reflexes before returning to what may be indifferent recovery facilities, especially at night.

Emergence from Anaesthesia

The likelihood of vomiting is greatest, and the risk of regurgitation has not entirely passed, as the patient is recovering consciousness. The patient should be turned on their left side, breathing oxygen and the mouth and pharynx carefully sucked out. The tracheal tube should be left in place with the cuff inflated until the patient shows signs of coughing on the tube. Extubation should be carried out with reasonably firm pressure on the reservoir bag which helps both to inflate atelectatic alveoli and to blow out any liquid which may have collected in the larynx above the tracheal tube cuff, where it is beyond the reach of the pharyngeal sucker.

● FLUID AND ELECTROLYTE DEPLETION

Many patients presenting for emergency anaesthesia are suffering from some sort of fluid and electrolyte depletion. The nature and severity of the fluid loss will depend on the cause and its duration. The fluid required may, for example, be blood in cases of haemorrhage, blood and plasma after burns and scalds, plasma in peritonitis, and various electrolyte-containing fluids with different levels of intestinal obstruction. A careful history and clinical examination of the patient will give a good idea of what is required and this is confirmed by haematological and biochemical investigation. At least partial restoration of the patient's fluid and electrolyte balance adds greatly to the safety of the whole procedure, but as mentioned earlier, resuscitation in cases of severe bleeding may be only partially successful.

● LOCAL AND REGIONAL ANALGESIA

Another approach to the problem of emergency anaesthesia is to perform the operation under local analgesia, thus eliminating the dangers of vomiting and regurgitation. For peripheral operations these techniques have much to recommend them. The fact that they are not used routinely for these procedures in the UK is probably a reflection of the fact that the usually high standard of general anaesthesia has led most patients to expect (and most anaesthetists to provide) general anaesthesia for most operations. There are signs, however, that there is an increasing use of regional techniques for emergency operations on the limbs. This may be associated with higher standards of training of anaesthetists, the description of new regional techniques and the introduction of more reliable and longer-acting local analgesic drugs, for example, bupivacaine and ropivacaine.

Central regional techniques, i.e. spinal and epidural analgesia for emergency surgery especially of the lower limbs, are an attractive option. They may be more reliable than multiple peripheral blocks, for example, combined sciatic and femoral blocks for leg operations, but any central block providing analgesia above the level of the knee, i.e. the third lumbar segment, leads to some degree of sympathetic blockade. The higher the block the more vasodilatation is produced and the less able is the body to compensate for any reduction in circulating blood volume from whatever cause.

It is now accepted that with even uncomplicated fractures of long bones of the legs there is the loss of some 500–1000 ml of blood into the surrounding tissues. Fluid replacement is therefore important before induction of spinal or epidural analgesia to prevent hypotension.

Providing spinal or epidural analgesia for abdominal surgery requires a higher block and the implications of this sort of analgesia for abdominal surgery are discussed in Chapter 30. It will be remembered that if abdominal viscera are not distended or their mesenteries pulled upon, they can normally be cut, ligated or burnt without pain. Unfortunately, this is not true for inflamed or near-gangrenous bowel, the handling of which can cause great distress. The afferent impulses are carried not only in the sympathetic nerves (which can be blocked by analgesia extending up to the fifth thoracic segment) but also in the branches of the vagus nerve. This nerve, which, as a cranial nerve, does not run within the spinal cord, is unaffected by epidural and spinal anaesthesia. Bilateral vagal block requires either a coeliac plexus block or the infiltration of local anaesthetic round the vagal trunks as they lie on the oeosophagus in the highest part of the abdomen. This area is inaccessible through most surgical incisions.

As always, the anaesthetist is safest using the techniques with which he/she is most familiar, and it is safer for the patient if a well-tried technique is employed in an emergency, rather than experimenting with some unfamiliar method.

● ANAESTHESIA AFTER MAJOR TRAUMA

Of the wide variety of causes of major trauma, road traffic accidents are the commonest, being the leading cause of death in the first four decades of life, and closely following atherosclerosis and cancer in later years of life.

Management of the trauma patient has recently undergone many changes. It is now widely accepted that the morbidity and mortality from trauma is reduced if assessment and resuscitation are started before the patient reaches hospital and that in the hospital this is continued by dedicated trauma teams who follow an organised, consistent approach to the treatment. The introduction of training programmes such as the Advanced Trauma Life Support (ATLS) course has made this approach possible. Anaesthetists are important members of hospital trauma teams. The approach of primary survey, resuscitation, secondary survey and definitive treatment recommended in the ATLS course is sum-marised below.

Primary Survey

This is a very quick (should not take more than 1 min) survey of the patient to assess the ABC, i.e. airway, breathing and circulation. The patient is assessed and resuscitated simultaneously and life-threatening conditions are dealt with.

Airway Management (and Cervical Spine Control)

The mouth and pharynx are cleared and if required an oropharyngeal airway is used to maintain an unobstructed airway. With the exception of patients with severe chest trauma, tracheal intubation following extensive injuries is confined to those patients who are unable to protect their own airway, usually as a result of unconsciousness or severe faciomaxillary damage. A patient who actively resists all efforts at intubation does not require intubation. Nevertheless, following major trauma all patients should be given supplementary oxygen whether or not they appear to need it and whether or not they are prepared to tolerate it, because the dangers of cerebral, hepatic and renal hypoxia in this condition are appreciable. Monitoring oxygen saturation with a pulse oximeter is very useful (to detect hypoxia). A hard collar is applied to the cervical spine as soon as possible.

Breathing

If the patient has been intubated, artificial ventilation is instituted if indicated. Other indications for ventilation include severe head injury, shock, pain, and in all cases where doubt exists that the patient is maintaining oxygenation. However, in severe chest injuries where pneumothorax is suspected, intermittent positive pressure ventilation (IPPV) may cause harm and bilateral chest drains should be inserted before it is instituted.

Circulation and Control of Haemorrhage

It is important to avoid hypovolaemic shock (where there is evidence of severe blood loss) by the early administration of intravenous crystalloids and colloidal plasma volume substitutes. These should be replaced as soon as possible with whole blood, since although the plasma substitutes will maintain blood pressure, they do not carry oxygen, and filling the circulation with them may prevent subsequent blood transfusion without causing fluid overload.

To the ABC it is useful to add a 'D' for disability where a quick neurological assessment is performed and 'E' for exposure where the patient is fully exposed to avoid missing any injuries.

Resuscitation

As mentioned above, resuscitation should be started simultaneously with primary survey and includes inserting large-bore intravenous cannulae, giving blood and other fluids, introducing monitoring to assess physiological functions, for example, pulse oximetry, electrocardiograph (ECG) and blood pressure.

Secondary Survey

Successful immediate resuscitation of patients suffering from major trauma must be followed by a detailed assessment of their injuries. It is vital that this is done in a logical sequence as follows.

Head Injury

Examination for skull fractures must be accompanied by assessment of the level of consciousness, of pupil size and reactivity and other evidence of raised intracranial pressure due to bleeding.

Facial Injuries

These are often extensive and may well prevent normal laryngoscopy and intubation. It is important to avoid displacing facial fractures, which is easily done during emergency intubation.

Cervical Spine Injuries

If there is any suspicion of spinal fractures it is vital that no movement occurs in this region, because transection of the cord may result in quadriplegia. The cervical spine should be immobilised with a hard collar until it is proved by X-rays that there is no significant cervical spine injury. Intubation is performed with the surgeon providing in-line traction of the cervical spine.

Chest Injuries

Injuries to the chest include those to the trachea and bronchi as a result of tear or rupture of the air passages, tears of the major thoracic vessels or heart, and injuries to the chest wall and lung. Blood in the tracheobronchial tree usually indicates direct lung trauma. Chest injuries range from isolated rib fractures – which may involve underlying lung contusion or pneumothorax – to flail chest injuries resulting from individual ribs fractured in two places. Stove-in chest is often complicated by ruptured viscera, haemopneumothorax and damage to intrathoracic structures. After immediate resuscitation it is important to establish the severity of such injuries by X-ray and computed tomographic (CT) examination and possibly angiography.

Abdominal and Pelvic Injuries

These again are usually a combination of fractures, commonly of the pelvis, together with ruptured or contused viscera, particularly the liver, the spleen and the small bowel and are best diagnosed with abdominal CT scanning. Acute gastric dilatation may occur after a severe accident and may produce abdominal swelling suggesting severe haemorrhage. Vigorous transfusion without adequate diagnostic procedures may result in pulmonary oedema even in fit young people. Rectal examination should not be forgotten.

Peripheral Fractures

It is important to assess each fracture for potential blood loss and temporary immobilisation may be adequate until after the treatment of more severe injuries. Major fractures are associated with a surprisingly large concealed blood loss, for example, femur 2–3 units, pelvis 3–4 units, tibia and fibula 1–2 units.

Definitive Treatment

This is the comprehensive management of the patient and includes continual re-evaluation, operative intervention and fracture stabilisation. A complete history is also obtained at this stage. A useful mnemonic is AMPLE, i.e. allergies, medications, past history, last meal and event of injury.

It is also important to elucidate whether the patient has received anaesthesia uneventfully in the past. If this is impossible for any reason, the patient's belongings should be checked to see if they carry a medical warning card, for example, to indicate diabetes mellitus or steroid therapy.

Subsequent treatment of patients suffering severe trauma is based on the maxim of getting everything into perspective. For example, a ruptured spleen is more important than a fractured ankle despite the fact that the peripheral fracture may be obvious while the intra-abdominal injury may be concealed. A detailed examination of the patient together with a chest X-ray, an abdominal and pelvic X-ray and any other relevant X-ray and CT examinations, for example, CT scan of the head, should be done immediately, possibly with a peritoneal lavage to exclude intraperitoneal bleeding. Detailed X-ray examination of peripheral fractures may be carried out at a later date.

Analgesia

Following major trauma, patients may suffer extreme pain and unless they are completely unconscious it is unreasonable to withhold all forms of analgesia. Intravenous opiates provide the most satisfactory and efficient form of analgesia, but their use is contraindicated in patients with head injuries or respiratory difficulty. Entonox has been used with some success in such cases, but most neurosurgeons prefer codeine phosphate for analgesia in patients with head injury to avoid masking neurological signs.

Anaesthesia and Surgery

As mentioned above, life-threatening emergencies are dealt with at the same time as resuscitation of the patient. Depending on the nature of the injury and its severity, the patient needs stabilisation either in the intensive therapy unit, in theatre or on the ward before proceeding to treat long bone or other fractures. Whenever possible it is essential for the patient to be visited preoperatively by the anaesthetist, not only to assess the extent of injuries and therefore the special measures which may be necessary during the operation, but more especially to allay the inevitable anxiety these patients have. Many patients will be in severe pain and may also be confused or semi-conscious. Premedication with analgesia has usually already been given if the patient has been treated in the casualty department, but the possibility of the patient having a full stomach may necessitate the administration of preoperative antacids. Further details of emergency anaesthesia have already been discussed above. The patient should be fully assessed along the lines described in Chapter 14.

Anaesthetic Techniques

General anaesthesia is generally advisable for the patient with moderate to severe trauma. This is because the ABC are better controlled in the anaesthetised patient. Induction of anaesthesia is as mentioned above for the patient undergoing emergency surgery.

A muscle relaxant technique with oxygen, nitrous oxide, inhalational agent and parenteral opioid adjuvants is suitable in most patients. However, some patients with only peripheral fractures are not operated on for many hours, and they may be treated as fasted patients and the technique adjusted accordingly.

Suxamethonium is contraindicated in the burned patient (Chapter 29). Local infiltration and nerve blocks are very useful for providing intra-operative and postoperative pain relief and should be used wherever possible. However, some surgeons do not permit the use of nerve blocks because the postoperative assessment of the limb becomes difficult. Opioids remain the mainstay of postoperative analgesia and patient-controlled analgesia (PCA) is quite frequently used on this group of patients (Chapter 42).

Once the patient is asleep and the injuries can be examined more closely, it is important to plan the surgical treatment according to what the patient can withstand at that time and to anticipate prolonged postoperative ventilation. Major trauma cases benefit enormously from postoperative care in an intensive care unit where their fluid balance, blood replacement and other physiological parameters can be closely monitored. Many will require a period of postoperative ventilation and the attention of many different specialists such as anaesthetist, general, orthopaedic and neurosurgeons. An intensive care unit where such treatment can be effectively coordinated is the best place to coordinate this treatment.

25

Anaesthesia for Ear, Nose and Throat Surgery

*•General considerations •Surgical access •Other general principles
•Individual operations*

● GENERAL CONSIDERATIONS

Operations on the ear, nose and throat (ENT) provide the anaesthetist with some challenging problems. The most important one is that these operations are performed in or near the upper respiratory tract and require the anaesthetist to provide the surgeon with adequate access while maintaining a patent airway and preventing blood and debris soiling the lungs.

Another problem is that the patients for these operations range from young, fit children and adults having quick tonsillectomies, grommet insertions and nose operations to the very elderly and frail having complex laryngeal operations for carcinoma. Some of the most challenging aspects of anaesthesia are seen in this branch of surgery; for example, a young, fit child having a tonsillectomy in the morning may be the most frightening anaesthetic emergency when the tonsil bed bleeds later (see below).

● SURGICAL ACCESS

There are several techniques by which the anaesthetist can provide the surgeon with good access to the operation site yet maintain oxygenation and anaesthesia.

Tracheal Intubation and LMA

Where possible, a cuffed oral tube is used, but at times a nasal tube may be indicated. In addition to the cuff a throat pack helps to protect the upper larynx from blood and secretions. Many anaesthetists now use the reinforced laryngeal mask airway (LMA, Chapter 18) for intranasal surgery in the belief that the blood and secretions will collect on the cuff of the LMA and not soil the lungs.

Insufflation Anaesthesia

This involves blowing a gaseous anaesthetic mixture into the patient's upper respiratory tract. The patient breathes spontaneously, and dilutes the mixture with an amount of air depending on his tidal and minute volume and the volume of anaesthetic mixture being provided. This was a popular method for administering nitrous oxide, oxygen and ether for tonsillectomy, the mixture usually being given via a side-tube on the Boyle–Davis gag.

A more modern version of this technique is sometimes used for laryngeal microsurgery by administering oxygen through a small tube, for example, a 12 or 14 FG suction catheter passed through the vocal cords so that the tip lies somewhere between the larynx and carina. Anaesthesia is usually maintained by a total intravenous technique with propofol and opioids instead of using volatile agents.

Deep Anaesthesia

Another way to leave the operating field clear for the surgeon is to induce anaesthesia and deepen it to a plane depending on the operation to be carried out. The face mask is then removed and the surgeon performs his task as anaesthesia is lightening. This technique was used when guillotine tonsillectomy was in fashion but is now no longer practised.

Local Analgesia

This was formerly very popular in nose and throat surgery, many operations (e.g. tonsillectomy, nasal polypectomy and even laryngectomy) being possible under regional techniques. Most modern surgeons regard most of these operations as requiring considerable heroism on the part of the patient if carried out in this way, and now request general anaesthesia. However, the upper respiratory tract is highly vascular, and to reduce bleeding it is quite common to inject vasoconstrictor solutions, or to apply topical vasoconstrictor agents, for example, cocaine solution 5–10%. Some operations, especially on the larynx, may be carried out under general anaesthesia with, in addition, the topical spraying of a local analgesic solution on the operation site. The larynx is extremely sensitive, and this technique allows the use of lighter general anaesthesia.

● OTHER GENERAL PRINCIPLES

Premedication for nose and throat operations should be appropriate to the patient's needs. It is probably wise to err on the side of conservatism so that the patient rapidly regains the ability to protect his own respiratory tract from soiling by blood or debris. A number of ENT procedures are done as day-case surgery and heavy premedication is inappropriate.

It is sometimes said that topical analgesia should not be applied to the larynx during ENT anaesthesia in case the patient inhales material from the pharynx at the end of the operation. Even so, it is obviously impossible to adhere strictly to this rule because anaesthesia in some cases depends to a greater or lesser degree on topical analgesia. Fortunately, once they have recovered from the general anaesthesia most patients seem to have a protective cough reflex arising from areas lower in the respiratory tract than those reached by the topical analgesia. For example, after thorough application of topical analgesia for bronchoscopy, the problem when the patient is wakening is to stop rather than start them coughing. However, there seems no point in routinely spraying the larynx with local analgesic solution for every nose and throat operation (e.g. for tonsillectomy), as satisfactory anaesthesia does not depend on it.

Patients who have undergone tracheal anaesthesia should have regained their protective reflexes before extubation and it is important after throat and nose operations that all patients should recover in the lateral or semi-prone position.

Many ENT operations are performed with reduced theatre lighting, the patient's face usually being partly or completely hidden by surgical drapes. This makes careful observation of the patient's colour and vital signs more difficult than in many other anaesthetics and the anaesthetist must be particularly vigilant. Monitoring (Chapter 20) should be as comprehensive as possible.

Induction and maintenance of anaesthesia should be smooth and rapid, avoiding straining and hypercarbia. The head and neck is a very vascular region, and any engorgement produced by coughing or a rise in $P\text{CO}_2$ may take several minutes to subside, with a prolonged deterioration of operating conditions. A wide choice of spontaneous or controlled respiration techniques is satisfactory for most ENT surgery but the surgeon may request hypotensive anaesthesia for some middle-ear or laryngeal operations.

● INDIVIDUAL OPERATIONS

Tonsillectomy and Adenoidectomy

The (at times) near-barbaric guillotine tonsillectomy performed on the unsuspecting and often unpremedicated child has to most anaesthetists' relief largely given way to dissection tonsillectomy. For this the patient should come to the anaesthetic room adequately premedicated and anaesthesia be induced by the intravenous (or less commonly, the inhalation) route. Suxamethonium is usually used to provide muscle relaxation to perform intubation. Orotracheal tubes of the preformed RAE type (Chapter 18) are ideal because the tubes fit in the slit of the Doughty blade used with the Boyle–Davis gag without kinking and give the surgeon adequate access. Maintenance is commonly with nitrous oxide, oxygen and a volatile agent with spontaneous respiration, but controlled respiration is also satisfactory. It is common practice to provide analgesia with injection of local anaesthetic, for example, 0.5% bupivacaine into the tonsillar fossa at the end of the procedure. The patient is usually extubated on the side, deeply anaesthetised and recovered in the 'tonsil position'. This is a semi-prone position where the patient is prevented rolling onto his face by placing a pillow under the chest and by flexing the knees and hips.

Bleeding Tonsil

Even after the careful technique of dissection tonsillectomy, a small proportion of the patients bleed a few hours after the operation. These patients present one of the most frightening emergencies to face the anaesthetist and must be approached with the utmost care.

The child has usually lost a significant proportion of his blood volume, and much of this may be present in the stomach. An intravenous drip must always be set up, blood cross-matched and, if necessary, a blood transfusion started preoperatively. The operation should not start until the child is first adequately resuscitated. Anaesthesia should be induced on the operating table with the child carefully held on his left side and the table about 15° head-down.

An inhalation induction with nitrous oxide, oxygen and halothane is probably safest and usually very easy, the weak and exhausted child making little protest. Efficient pharyngeal suction must be instantly available and cricoid pressure applied to prevent regurgitation. Orotracheal intubation is carried out under the nitrous oxide, oxygen and halothane when anaesthesia is deep enough.

Some anaesthetists prefer a more typical 'crash induction' with thiopentone and suxamethonium after pre-oxygenation. The problem with this technique is that when the mouth is open there is often a confusing 'curtain' of blood and mucus and anxious moments may pass before the anaesthetist can see to pass the tracheal tube.

Operations on the Nose

The most common operations confined to the nose are the removal of nasal polyps and submucous resection (SMR) of the nasal septum or septoplasty.

These operations are now usually carried out under general anaesthesia using a tracheal tube and pharyngeal pack. Some anaesthetists prefer to use a reinforced laryngeal mask in the spontaneously breathing patient for these operations. In addition, it is usual to improve surgical access and reduce bleeding by the topical application of cocaine solution 5%, always taking care to stay within the safe dose of that drug. It is usual also to inject a small amount of local analgesic with vasoconstrictor deep to the mucous membrane of the septum to aid the dissection and reduce bleeding.

Operations on the Paranasal Sinuses

The same general anaesthetic technique as employed for nasal operations is used. The commonest sinus operation was the Caldwell–Luc operation on the maxillary antrum, for which a drainage hole (antrostomy) was made between the sinus and nasal cavity. These operations have largely been replaced by fibre-endoscopic sinus surgery (FESS) procedures, where the surgeon can operate through a small hole under direct fibreoptic vision. The principles of anaesthesia remain the same.

Ear Operations

Most of these operations are now carried out with an operating microscope. The surgeon requires an uncongested operating field. A smooth, spontaneous respiration anaesthetic with the patient a few degrees head-up will often provide these conditions, in most cases, but it is probably more reliable to avoid hypercarbia by controlled respiration in long and extensive middle-ear operations when the surgeon may require hypotensive anaesthesia. In middle-ear operations, for example, tympanoplasty, it is probably safer not to use nitrous oxide at all, or to stop it a few minutes before the graft is applied, because the nitrous oxide may put the graft under tension and ruin the operation (see Chapter 6).

Microsurgery of the Larynx

Microsurgery of the larynx involves the use of the operating microscope and the surgeon may want to visualise the movements of the vocal cords in some cases. Additionally lasers are being increasingly used for some of these operations (see below). Anaesthesia can be achieved by a variety of techniques, two of which, insufflation anaesthesia through a small tube such as a suction catheter, or intermittent inflation using the Sander's injector, have already been mentioned. A third more popular method involves the use of a special type of cuffed tracheal tube, for example, a microlaryngeal tube (Fig. 25.1). This polyvinyl chloride (PVC) tube has a small diameter of 5 mm allowing the surgeon enough access and a high-volume, low-pressure cuff which prevents blood or debris entering the lungs.

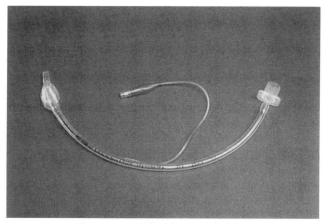

Figure 25.1 Microlaryngeal tube.

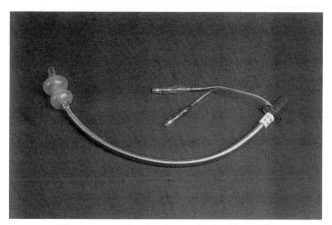

Figure 25.2 Steel tube with double cuff.

Laser Surgery

Laser (light amplification by stimulated emission of radiation) is used to excise lesions of the larynx in both adults and children. The advantage of laser surgery over conventional surgery is that the laser beam can be made to pinpoint the lesion precisely and thus reduce bleeding and postoperative oedema. The two main problems with laser surgery are the possible risk of eye damage to the personnel, which is prevented by wearing protective glasses to absorb the laser beam; and that the laser beam produces intense heat and may cause ignition of plastic, rubber or silicone tubes if it comes into contact with them. To prevent this, tubes were (and still are) wrapped in aluminium foil to protect them from igniting. Steel tubes are available with double cuffs (Fig. 25.2), so that in the event of one cuff bursting, the second can be inflated and the airway protected. It is also recommended that these cuffs be filled with saline rather than air (which is more combustible) to prevent them from igniting.

Some anaesthetists avoid using tracheal tubes altogether by using techniques of insufflation or jet ventilation through a Sander's injector mentioned above. An important consideration is to use a non-explosive gas mixture such as 30% oxygen in nitrogen or helium. Anaesthesia is then usually maintained using total intravenous techniques. Whatever precautions are used a vital component is good understanding between the surgeon and anaesthetist.

Laryngectomy

The anaesthetic management of these cases depends on whether the patient has already had a tracheostomy performed. If so, the anaesthetist must replace the silver tube with a cuffed tracheostomy tube and then administer the anaesthetic by that means. If the patient has not already had a tracheostomy, and has no stridor, then anaesthesia is induced and intubation performed in the same way as described in the previous section. When a patient presents with stridor, it is vital to ascertain the nature and degree of obstruction at the larynx by performing an indirect laryngoscopy or a flexible fibreoptic endoscopy while the patient is awake to determine whether there is enough space to introduce a tracheal tube. Where intubation is judged to be impossible, the surgeon performs a tracheostomy under local anaesthesia and general anaesthesia is only induced once the airway is secure. In cases where intubation is judged to be feasible, the choice is to intubate the trachea under deep halothane and oxygen anaesthesia or perform a fibreoptic intubation while the patient is awake (see Chapter 18). Careful planning is essential with involvement of senior anaesthetists and surgeons. Whatever technique is used, the surgeon must always be scrubbed and ready to perform a tracheostomy should this be required.

During surgery, a problem may arise when the larynx is divided from the trachea and the anaesthetic system has to be transferred from the tracheal tube to the newly inserted cuffed tracheostomy tube at the permanent tracheostomy site. It is vital that a choice of sterile tracheostomy tubes and catheter mounts for connection to the anaesthetic machine be available and tested before the incision is made in the larynx. As the patient has usually been given a muscle relaxant, there may be some anxious moments when the tracheal tube is partially withdrawn from the larynx until the surgeon succeeds in replacing it with the cuffed tracheostomy tube.

It should also be borne in mind that the blood loss at these operations may be quite heavy, especially if there are lymph glands to be dissected out. Some of the patients may be very frail and careful monitoring is essential.

26

Anaesthesia for Eye Surgery

•Intraocular pressure •Oculocardiac reflex •Other special features •Local analgesia •General anaesthesia •Common operations

Although the most localised of all branches of surgery, there are nevertheless certain features of anaesthesia for eye surgery that merit special consideration.

● INTRAOCULAR PRESSURE

The sclera and cornea together form the globe of the eye (Fig. 26.1), the contents of which are referred to as being 'intraocular'. The intraocular space is divided unequally into a smaller anterior part containing aqueous humour and a larger vitreous body containing vitreous humour. There

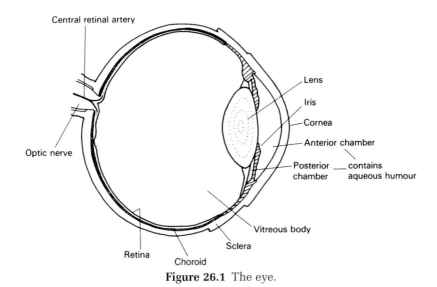

Figure 26.1 The eye.

is a constant production and removal of aqueous humour and in the important disease glaucoma, where the drainage of aqueous humour is obstructed, there is a pathological rise in intraocular pressure. Normal values of intraocular pressure are in the region of 10–20 mmHg.

Factors Raising Intraocular Pressure

Two drugs whose mydriatic (pupil-dilating) action causes obstruction to free drainage of aqueous humour from the angle of the anterior chamber, thereby increasing intraocular pressure, are atropine and cocaine. These agents should therefore not be applied locally to the eye in glaucoma. Parentally administered atropine is not considered to cause a significant increase in intraocular pressure.

The other anaesthetic agent in common use which causes a rise in intraocular pressure is suxamethonium. The rise in pressure in this case is caused by the extraocular muscles of the orbit squeezing the globe during suxamethonium-induced fasciculation.

Other anaesthetic factors increasing intraocular pressure are venous engorgement due to coughing, vomiting, straining or a head-down tilt, hypoxia and hypercarbia. Extraocular causes are a periorbital haematoma produced when performing a retro-ocular block, and the pressure on the eye produced by large volumes of local anaesthetic or even pressure from an anaesthetic mask.

Factors Decreasing Intraocular Pressure

Falls in intraocular pressure tend to be less dramatic and are caused by most intravenous induction agents (except ketamine), volatile agents and opioid analgesics. Hypotension, hypocarbia and a head-up tilt are other factors that decrease the intraocular tension.

● OCULOCARDIAC REFLEX

Traction on the extraocular eye muscles (as inevitably occurs in squint operations) may cause cardiac arrhythmias, especially bradycardia or even cardiac asystole. These reflex effects may be abolished by administering intravenous atropine in a dose of about 1 mg for an adult with a proportionately smaller dose for children (20 µg/kg) or glycopyrrolate in a dose of 0.5 mg for adults and 10 µg/kg for children. In practice, much smaller doses are usually effective. Subcutaneous or intramuscular atropine or glycopyrrolate given as premedication does not reach a high enough blood level to give protection against these adverse effects.

● OTHER SPECIAL FEATURES

During eye surgery, although the anaesthetist is not vying with the surgeon for the same area, the airway is somewhat inaccessible and the head and neck largely obscured. Particular vigilance is therefore required in monitoring the patient. Another feature of eye anaesthesia is that on no other operating list is the anaesthetist so likely to meet the extremes of age in one session. It is not unusual on one list to have patients ranging from small babies to the frail and elderly, the latter usually having cataract operations.

Many drugs which may have anaesthetic implications are administered before or during eye surgery. Examples include Cyclopantilate 1% drops to dilate the pupil and paralyse the ciliary muscle. Excessive absorption of this drug causes symptoms and signs similar to atropine poisoning. Phenylephrine drops are used to dilate the pupil. If systemically absorbed the α-agonist action of this drug may cause hypertension and cardiac arrhythmias. Timolol and other β-blocking drugs are used for treatment of glaucoma and may precipitate asthma. Mannitol is used as a diuretic and caution is required when performing intravenous induction in these patients as profound hypotension may occur. Acetazolamide is a carbonic anhydrase inhibitor and is used in congenital glaucoma. It may cause metabolic acidosis.

● LOCAL ANALGESIA

Surface Analgesia

This is useful for operations on the conjunctiva and cornea and is easily produced by local analgesic eye drops. Probably the most popular of these are the rather short-acting proxymetacaine (Ophthaine) 0.5%, amethocaine 0.5%, and lignocaine 4%, none of which dilates the pupil. Cocaine 2%, although it causes transient cloudiness of the cornea and dilatation of the pupil, is still used at times because its powerful vasocontrictor action is useful for reducing oozing during operations on hyperaemic eyes.

Local infiltration with 0.5% lignocaine in 1 : 200 000 adrenaline gives excellent analgesia for operations on the eyelids.

Peribulbar and Retrobulbar Blocks

For intraocular operations, such as cataract surgery, good analgesia is readily obtained by topical analgesia of the conjunctival sac associated with one of the above blocks. The principle of the technique is to deposit the local anaesthetic in the vicinity of the short and long ciliary nerves. These are contained in the conus formed by the extraocular muscles (lateral, medial, superior and inferior recti).

Peribulbar block is injection of local anaesthetic into the fatty tissues surrounding the cone and therefore includes injecting large volumes of solutions which then diffuse through; it therefore requires more time to work.

In a retrobulbar block technique, the local anaesthetic solution is injected behind the eyeball and into the conus. Small volumes of local anaesthetic are required and the onset is quick. Retrobulbar block carries the risk of retrobulbar haematoma and optic nerve damage and has been largely replaced by peribulbar block and sub-Tenon's injection.

Sub-Tenon's Injection

This technique where the local anaesthetic is deposited by a special needle underneath the Tenon's capsule has recently become popular.

Local blocks provide excellent analgesia, and are easy to perform and very cost effective because patients can be sent home on the day of surgery. Additionally the nausea, vomiting and confusion that follow general anaesthesia are avoided.

If possible, patients for eye surgery under local analgesia should be well sedated. Nevertheless, it must be remembered that many of these patients are frail and elderly and great care must be taken when prescribing drugs that may depress the cardiovascular or respiratory systems.

Current recommendations require that the sedation and monitoring of the patient be carried out by an anaesthetist even if the block has been performed by the surgeon. It is becoming increasingly common for the local analgesia also to be performed by the anaesthetist.

● GENERAL ANAESTHESIA

As one of the most important factors in general anaesthesia for eye surgery is the avoidance of postoperative nausea and vomiting, many anaesthetists routinely include an anti-emetic in the premedication.

Provided that the considerations mentioned are taken into account various spontaneous and controlled ventilation anaesthetic techniques give excellent operating conditions for eye surgery. It is good practice to spray the vocal cords with topical local analgesic to minimise coughing at extubation or the possibility of straining on the tracheal tube if anaesthesia is too light. With spontaneous respiration techniques, the depth of anaesthesia must be sufficient for the eye to remain stationary.

● COMMON OPERATIONS

Squint

These operations are nearly always carried out on small children, who should be well premedicated. Some anaesthetists would intubate after a thiopentone or propofol and suxamethonium induction, and maintain anaesthesia with nitrous oxide, oxygen and volatile agent, but most would prefer using a laryngeal mask airway in the spontaneously breathing patient. There are no other special features about these cases apart from taking precautions to suppress the oculocardiac reflex, as already discussed (see above) and to prevent nausea and vomiting.

Cataract Extraction and Lens Implant

The procedure of cataract extraction is now frequently accompanied by the implantation of a plastic replacement lens at the same operation. These patients are invariably elderly and surgery can be safely carried out under local analgesia.

Peribulbar Anaesthesia

As stated this is the injection of local anaesthetic into the tissues surrounding the conus and its effect is due to the diffusion of the local anaesthetic through the tissues. Lignocaine 2% or prilocaine 3% is a satisfactory local anaesthetic agent which may be mixed with hyaluronidase (5 IU/ml) to improve its efficacy. Adrenaline 1:400 000 may also be mixed with the local anaesthetic solution to improve its duration and reduce the chances of haemorrhage. A facial nerve block is not usually required because the spread of the solution usually involves the superficial fibres of the facial nerve. Usually two injections of about 5 ml each are required and these are performed with a fine 25 G needle and never deeper than 3 cm. An intraocular pressure reducing device should be applied to the eye for about 10 min.

Retrobulbar Block

This is injection of the solution into the conus and behind the eyeball. Most anaesthetists prefer to block the facial nerve to weaken the orbicularis oculi muscle so that the injection can be performed without a squeezing action. This block is not commonly performed because of the risk of retrobulbar haematoma and damage to the optic nerve.

Sub-Tenon's Injection

This involves injection of local anaesthetic underneath the middle of the Tenon's capsule. A small incision is made in the conjunctiva usually in the infero-medial aspect of the globe after it has been made numb with the local anaesthetic amethocaine. A special cannula is then guided along the sclera underneath the Tenon's capsule where a small amount of local anaesthetic solution, usually 7 ml, is deposited.

Very few patients having cataract surgery will require general anaesthesia. When required, this is given along the principles mentioned below.

Retinovitreous Surgery

An example is repair of a detached retina. The patients are often young and surgery can take a long time so general anaesthesia is usually required. Induction of general anaesthesia is with an appropriate dose of intravenous induction agent and short-acting opioid. Maintenance is by a volatile agent administered through a laryngeal mask airway of the reinforced variety or a tracheal tube. A total intravenous technique using propofol with or without an opioid is another option. Apart from spraying the larynx with local analgesic solution at intubation to prevent coughing when the tracheal tube is removed at the end of the operation, it is also wise to keep anaesthesia deep enough at the end of the operation for extubation to be performed without inducing coughing. While good anaesthetic technique and the use of anti-emetics postoperatively should minimise the extent of coughing, nausea and vomiting, fortunately, with modern improvements in surgical instruments and especially in suture materials, the danger of causing damage to the surgical work is much reduced.

Perforating Eye Injuries

These cases combine the danger of extrusion of the intraocular contents, should intraocular pressure rise, with the risks of vomiting and regurgitation inherent in any emergency anaesthetic (see Chapter 24). Where possible surgery should be delayed and pharmacological prophylaxis for acid aspiration should be instituted. When airway difficulties are not predicted, some anaesthetists would give generous doses of intravenous induction agent, usually propofol, and a large dose of a non-depolarising muscle relaxant (usually rocuronium) while cricoid pressure is applied by an assistant, and then intubate the trachea. With this 'modified' rapid sequence induction technique, the use of suxamethonium and the risks of increased intraocular pressure are reduced. The downside is the danger of aspiration and hypoxia if airway difficulties are encountered. If there is any doubt about the intubation, then probably most anaesthetists would feel that the safest compromise would be to intubate using suxamethonium and applying cricoid pressure. Padding on the eye and giving a small dose of nondepolarising muscle relaxant prior to suxamethonium to reduce the rise in intraocular pressure are used but are of doubtful value.

27

Anaesthesia for Dental and Maxillofacial Surgery

•Anaesthesia for out-patient dentistry •Anaesthesia for in-patient dentistry •Maxillofacial surgery

● ANAESTHESIA FOR OUT-PATIENT DENTISTRY

The number of anaesthetics given in the dentist's surgery has declined because it is no longer considered safe for a single operator to give the anaesthetic and perform the surgery. Current recommendations require the presence of two qualified staff, one operating and the other giving the anaesthetic, and stricter guidelines for monitoring patients and the training of staff in resuscitation skills. Out-patient dental surgery is now only performed in well-established units with dedicated anaesthetic staff. Despite these tight regulations there is still concern about the safety of these procedures and indeed in future all dental treatment requiring general anaesthesia will have to be carried out in a hospital setting.

Successful and safe dental anaesthesia depends on adequate preoperative preparation and using essentially simple techniques. Problems pertinent to this type of surgery include the fact that the majority of these patients are children, who are anxious and frightened, and the surgery is short. The anaesthetist is challenged with providing adequate anaesthesia with quick recovery, as most of these patients go home after surgery.

General Anaesthesia

Patients are now usually anaesthetised supine instead of in the dental chair, thus avoiding a vasovagal attack under anaesthesia, the consequences of which may be serious, if not fatal, when an acute fall in blood pressure goes unrecognised. It is essential to ensure that the patient can open the mouth sufficiently and has an unobstructed airway. Dental abscess with swelling leading to inadequate mouth opening may prove an extremely difficult problem when the patient is anaesthetised and relatively relaxed. If induction of anaesthesia is achieved intravenously, propofol is commonly used, because its effects wear off quickly enough to allow the patient to leave the surgery shortly afterwards. Many children receive a gaseous induction, often with nitrous oxide, oxygen and sevoflurane. The use of nasal anaesthetic masks leaving the mouth free for operation is usual and a pharyngeal pack of either gauze or absorbent sponge should be used to prevent inhalation of blood or tooth fragments. It is vital to ensure that the pack is removed at the end of the procedure before the patient wakes up. Nasotracheal or orotracheal intubation in out-patient dental practice is uncommon but a laryngeal mask airway is a suitable alternative.

Invariably, patients are allowed to recover lying on their side and are then usually returned to a recovery room. The patients are often allowed home shortly after the anaesthetic, and for this reason must be accompanied by a responsible adult and encouraged to rest at home. They should not be allowed to go on public transport, drive a car or do anything which might be dangerous as a result of relatively impaired judgement.

Local Anaesthesia with Sedation

Some dentists employ either continuous or intermittent administration of methohexitone, diazepam or midazolam for either anaesthesia or sedation during prolonged periods of conservative dental treatment. It is sensible, however, to use a single agent which should be titrated so that the patient is comfortable but can be aroused verbally. Although dentists are often very skilled in these procedures, fatalities have occurred, largely before it was accepted that two experienced people are needed to be present, one to carry out the dental treatment and the other to administer the sedative agents, maintain the airway and monitor the patient.

Relative Analgesia

Many dentists employ relative analgesia for sedation during dental treatment, particularly in children. Entonox (50% nitrous oxide, 50% oxygen) is administered through a nasal mask, providing sedation and analgesia for extractions and conservation work. This is often augmented by local anaesthetic techniques. The dentists take considerable trouble to train children to tolerate relative analgesia, emphasising that with this technique they will not go to sleep. If the child is then subjected to a general anaesthetic involving gas induction, which to them is identical to relative analgesia, the fact that this technique has then been used to put them to sleep may well make them intolerant of relative analgesia in future. For this reason, intravenous induction is more appropriate.

● ANAESTHESIA FOR IN-PATIENT DENTISTRY

As already indicated, in-patient dental treatment is often necessary in patients who either are unfit for out-patient anaesthesia or require extensive treatment. The commonest cases are multiple extractions, dental clearances, surgical removal of particularly difficult teeth, for example, wisdom teeth (8s), and apicectomies or conservative dental treatment. Some short cases on otherwise fit, young patients are increasingly performed on a day-case basis (Chapter 31).

Anaesthetic Technique

Intravenous induction with propofol or thiopentone is usually followed by a muscle relaxant to facilitate nasotracheal intubation. Although suxamethonium can be used, it is best avoided to prevent muscle pains and a short-acting non-depolarising agent – atracurium, vecuronium or mivacurium – is preferable. Most anaesthetists prefer to use a plain uncuffed nasal tube for dental treatment, resorting to the cuff only when major oral or maxillofacial work is required. Bleeding can be a real problem during nasal intubation. This may be prevented by instilling zylometazoline drops (Otrivine®) to produce vasoconstriction of the nasal mucosa. A tracheal tube previously softened in warm sterile water or saline may also reduce the bleeding. A good pharyngeal pack is essential and must be removed prior to extubation. The patients are commonly allowed to breathe nitrous oxide/oxygen and a volatile adjuvant and ventilated for the duration of the operation.

Intravenous infusion is not usually employed although an indwelling cannula is essential. Extubation is carried out with the patient lying on his side, the nasotracheal tube being withdrawn into the oropharynx to provide an adequate airway until the patient is fully recovered. When the intubation has been difficult, it is safer to leave the nasotracheal tube in the trachea and only remove it when the patient is fully conscious.

Several problems may occur in the immediate postoperative period. Patients often feel nauseated and may vomit, so anti-emetics are widely used. After extractions (particularly of the molar teeth), which are often traumatic, soft tissue swelling and inability to open the mouth are common. It is therefore routine practise to administer intravenous steroids, usually dexamethasone, to reduce this swelling. Postoperative pain is often considerable and the patients require adequate analgesia. Some surgeons infiltrate the empty sockets with 0.5% bupivacaine to provide prolonged analgesia after surgical extraction, to good effect.

Some patients presenting for in-patient dental treatment do so because they suffer from medical conditions that make them unfit for out-patient dentistry. Dental clearance is a common procedure in patients with congenital or acquired heart disease before operative correction under cardiopulmonary bypass (CPB), and anaesthesia in these cases may require specialised techniques. Pre-oxygenation and very small doses of intravenous induction agents are essential if hypoxia and hypotension are to be prevented.

Mentally retarded patients or those with learning disabilities are often referred for in-patient hospital treatment and, apart from the problems in communicating with these patients and in getting them to accept dental anaesthesia, it is important to consider their mental condition and consequently the drug therapy that they may be receiving. Many may be epileptic or may be on several psychiatric drugs, for example, tricyclic antidepressants or monoamine oxidase inhibitors. Children with Down's syndrome or other congenital abnormalities may also have heart disease and it is important to have adequate documentation of such patients before anaesthesia. Patients with other congenital conditions, such as blood coagulation defects and blood disorders such as sickle cell disease, also present for in-patient dental anaesthesia, and again adequate preoperative screening and preparation are essential to prevent serious complications.

● MAXILLOFACIAL SURGERY

The type and complexity of procedures which are performed by maxillofacial surgeons depend on their expertise. Some examples of operations performed include mandibular and maxillary osteotomy, excision of salivary glands, surgery for fixation of fractures of the bones of face, and excision of tumour in the oral cavity which may include major microvascular free flap (see Chapter 29). Although most maxillofacial operations are carried out on an elective basis, some may be done after acute trauma, when it is important to try to ensure that the patient has an empty stomach. If the operative technique involves wiring together the upper and lower jaws to stabilise fractures, then postoperative vomiting could be disastrous. For this reason, a preoperative anti-emetic is frequently prescribed. Some anaesthetists also use metoclopramide to promote gastric emptying (Chapter 38) immediately before anaesthesia. In patients whose postoperative airway may be in doubt, elective intra-operative tracheostomy will be considered, and in patients in whom severe facial swelling, bleeding and oedema are present, preoperative tracheostomy may be necessary. In such cases, premedication is avoided to guard against the dangers of respiratory depression, but most other patients benefit from preoperative sedation.

As in plastic surgery, it is essential to achieve a smooth induction and maintenance of anaesthesia, avoiding carbon dioxide retention and venous congestion. A longer-acting intravenous induction agent (e.g. thiopentone) is usually most satisfactory, although in patients whose airway is in doubt, and hence where the transient apnoea caused by thiopentone may be dangerous, gaseous induction of anaesthesia is usually safer. Muscle relaxation using suxamethonium before intubation is again used only when there is doubt about the ability to ventilate the patient with a mask and airway should intubation prove impossible. A safer alternative is to perform tracheal intubation using a flexible fibreoptic laryngoscope (Chapter 18). This is best performed on the 'awake' patient after topical anaesthesia of the nasal cavity and pharynx with local anaesthetic. The patient is given a general anaesthetic only when the position of the tracheal tube is confirmed in the trachea (see Chapter 18).

As it is usually important that the patient be awake at the end of the operation immediately before extubation, particularly when the jaws have been wired together, most anaesthetists favour a relaxant and fentanyl technique using intermittent positive pressure ventilation (IPPV). This technique not only allows the patient to be awake in the immediate postoperative period, but also prevents excessive rises in CO_2 and reduces the possibility of venous congestion. The patient is placed on the table in the head-up position, which again helps to reduce venous pressure in the operative field. A streamlined cuffed nasal tube, for example, a preformed RAE (Chapter 18), is usually used, allowing good surgical access in and around the mouth. The cuffed tube not only allows artificial ventilation (which is relatively difficult through an uncuffed nasal tube with the correspondingly large leak), but also seals the airway and, together with a good pharyngeal pack, prevents aspiration of blood and other debris.

As considerable blood loss may occur during maxillofacial surgery, despite the use of hypotensive techniques in conjunction with an impeccable anaesthetic, a wide-bore intravenous cannula should be inserted in case blood transfusion becomes necessary. As with any operation where hypotension may be used (and may be prolonged), direct arterial blood pressure monitoring is essential.

Postoperatively, the patients should be looked after in a recovery room or intensive care unit for several hours, as the not uncommon postanaesthetic complications of nausea and vomiting, restlessness and hypotension may all be much more difficult to deal with in a patient in whom the jaws have been wired together. It is important that the nurses be made aware of which wires link the upper and lower jaw and are supplied with a pair of wirecutters with which to separate these jaws in an emergency.

28

Hypotensive Anaesthesia

•Hypotensive anaesthesia •Controlling vascular tone •Reduction of cardiac output •Background anaesthetic technique for elective hypotension •Ganglion-blocking drugs •α-Adrenergic-blocking drugs •β-Adrenergic-blocking drugs •Direct-acting peripheral vasodilator drugs •Extradural and spinal anaesthesia

● HYPOTENSIVE ANAESTHESIA

With the advances in surgical techniques and the use of the operating microscope, the need for profound hypotension (e.g. systolic blood pressure, 60 mmHg) during surgery has declined, but a chapter on hypotensive anaesthesia underlying the basic principles and drugs involved is still useful.

Operative blood loss occurs as a result of either arterial bleeding, venous bleeding or capillary oozing, and the control of these three forms of blood loss is achieved in different ways. A reduction in systemic arterial blood pressure by using hypotensive drugs will reduce but not abolish arterial bleeding, because cut vessels will always bleed. Venous bleeding is worsened by venous congestion and a high venous tone and therefore techniques such as intermittent positive pressure ventilation (IPPV) and posture will help to reduce venous congestion, while regional anaesthetic techniques (e.g. epidurals) abolish venous tone. Capillary ooze depends on arterial blood pressure and venous congestion, but can also be abolished by localised vasoconstriction using dilute solutions of a vasoconstrictor (e.g. adrenaline).

The reduction of systemic arterial blood pressure by a hypotensive anaesthetic technique is used in two distinct situations. First, to make possible operations that would otherwise be impossible (e.g. neurosurgery and cardiac surgery) and, secondly, to reduce operative blood loss and make surgery easier (e.g. plastic, maxillofacial, orthopaedic, ear, nose and throat (ENT) and eye surgery). Hypotensive anaesthetic techniques vary widely, the main distinction being between drugs that can produce an extremely rapid reduction in blood pressure (e.g. sodium nitroprusside (SNP)) and those that produce a relatively gradual fall in blood pressure (e.g. ganglion-blocking drugs and epidurals). As mentioned, hypotensive anaesthesia should be employed as an extension of the concept of balanced anaesthesia, using specific drugs to produce arteriolar vasodilatation. The supplementation of hypotensive techniques with a good anaesthetic, together with IPPV and posture, is also essential.

CONTROLLING VASCULAR TONE

The pharmacology behind hypotensive anaesthesia lies in controlling vascular smooth muscle tone, because vasodilatation without expansion of the fluid volume results in hypotension. Blood vessel size is controlled by sympathetic nervous system activity (Chapter 2) and increase in sympathetic activity produces vasoconstriction, while abolition of sympathetic activity produces vasodilatation. With the exception of those drugs which act directly on the smooth muscle of the blood vessel walls, hypotensive techniques interrupt the sympathetic outflow at various sites.

The preganglionic sympathetic nerves leave the spinal cord to synapse within the sympathetic ganglia. Acetylcholine is the transmitter substance at these synaptic sites, this being a nicotinic action. Remember that acetylcholine is also the transmitter at the parasympathetic ganglia. Noradrenaline, however, is the transmitter substance between the postganglionic sympathetic neuron and the smooth muscle of the blood vessels. Sympathetic outflow may therefore be interrupted in the following ways:

1. Central sedation produced by general anaesthesia causing a degree of vasodilatation.
2. Ganglion blockade and competitive inhibition of acetylcholine (e.g. pentolinium, trimetaphan).
3. Direct competition with the effects of noradrenaline (α-adrenergic-blocking drugs, e.g. phentolamine).

In addition, hypotensive anaesthesia may also be achieved by direct-acting smooth muscle vasodilators (SNP, glyceryl trinitrate (GTN)) and by reducing the cardiac output, thus inevitably reducing blood pressure.

REDUCTION OF CARDIAC OUTPUT

Cardiac output depends on venous return to the heart, which itself depends on both a negative intrathoracic pressure and on the pumping action of muscles surrounding blood vessels. Muscular relaxation together with IPPV (instead of the negative pressure created during spontaneous ventilation) will tend to reduce venous return to the heart and hence reduce cardiac output. Isoflurane or halothane, usually in combination with IPPV, also produces vasodilatation and therefore hypotension. Halothane also directly reduces cardiac output. This it does by:

1. direct myocardial depression
2. slowing the heart rate as a result of vagal stimulation
3. decreasing the rate of conduction of impulses through the heart, and
4. inhibiting the baroceptor reflex, thereby preventing the reflex rise in heart rate resulting from hypotension.

The cardiovascular effects of enflurane are similar to those of halothane. Isoflurane, however, does not produce significant myocardial depression, making it now the best volatile agent for producing moderate hypotensive anaesthesia.

● BACKGROUND ANAESTHETIC TECHNIQUE FOR ELECTIVE HYPOTENSION

A small dose of isoflurane combined with IPPV provides a good background anaesthetic for elective hypotension. This is best augmented by muscle relaxation using curare, as this drug also possesses ganglion-blocking effects which tend to interrupt sympathetic activity.

This combines with both the effects of isoflurane and the mechanical effects of ventilation to produce a moderate fall in blood pressure which can be enhanced with various pharmacological agents.

● GANGLION-BLOCKING DRUGS

These drugs (pentolinium, trimetaphan) block preganglionic to postganglionic neuronal transmission by competitive inhibition of acetylcholine, the transmitting substance released in all autonomic ganglia, both sympathetic and parasympathetic. As these drugs act on both parts of the autonomic nervous system, they produce effects resulting from both sympathetic and parasympathetic blockade.

Main Actions of Sympathetic Blockade

Sympathetic nervous activity maintains peripheral vascular tone and interruption of this by sympathetic blockade will produce vasodilatation and therefore hypotension. This fall in blood pressure will be posturally sensitive, being made worse if the patient is in the foot-down position. Hypotension resulting from sympathetic blockade is augmented by the effects of (a) gravity, (b) venous pooling, and (c) a decreased cardiac output, resulting from the decreased venous return, as more blood is retained in the periphery.

Main Actions of Parasympathetic Blockade

Although the desirable effects of ganglion blockade are essentially to produce hypotension as a result of vasodilatation, the effects of these drugs are also seen at the parasympathetic ganglia. Interruption of parasympathetic activity produces:

1. mydriasis (due to blockade of the ciliary ganglion)
2. decreased intraocular pressure
3. decreased gastric secretion
4. decreased intestinal tone
5. difficulty in micturition, and
6. tachycardia.

This tachycardia may be due either to parasympathetic blockade or possibly to a baroceptor reflex resulting from the hypotension produced. In clinical practice the increased heart rate produced by ganglion-blocking drugs presents the greatest problem, the effects being most marked with trimetaphan, and least with pentolinium. Trimetaphan also exhibits tachyphylaxis, i.e. increasing doses of the drug are required to maintain the same effect. This tachycardia is often adequately controlled with a β-adrenergic-blocking drug (e.g. propranolol).

The ganglion-blocking agents are generally used to produce a relatively slow fall and rise in blood pressure most suited to plastic surgery and similar procedures. The duration of the hypotensive effect varies from one agent to another, being about 15–20 min with trimetaphan and 45 min with pentolinium.

● α-ADRENERGIC-BLOCKING DRUGS

The transmitting substance released from the postganglionic sympathetic nerve (see Fig. 2.5) is noradrenaline, the site of action being an α-adrenergic one. α-Adrenergic-blocking agents all produce vasodilatation by competitive inhibition at the α-site. The drugs used may conveniently be divided into those producing a relatively permanent effect lasting for several days which is irreversible (phenoxybenzamine), and those producing acute α-blockade lasting for 10–30 min (phentolamine). α-Adrenergic blockade not only produces peripheral vasodilatation which may result in compensatory tachycardia, but also produces congestion of mucous membranes and constriction of the pupil. These drugs do not block the positive chronotropic or positive inotropic effects of adrenaline on the heart. Details about the pharmacology of phenoxybenzamine and phentolamine are given in Chapter 13. Several other drugs (e.g. droperidol and some phenothiazines such as chlorpromazine) also possess mild α-adrenergic-blocking activity. The ergot alkaloids, with the exception of ergometrine, also produce peripheral vasodilatation and are used for treating migraine.

The combined α- and β-blocking effects of labetalol are particularly useful in the production of elective hypotension. The vasodilatation resulting from α-blockade wears off considerably more quickly than the β-blocking effect.

● β-ADRENERGIC-BLOCKING DRUGS

The main contribution of these agents to hypotensive anaesthesia results from the bradycardia and the consequent reduction in cardiac output. There is no doubt that a tachycardia greatly increases intra-operative blood loss and that, conversely, a dry and satisfactory operating field is often achieved with normal blood pressure but a slow heart rate. For this reason many anaesthetists use intravenous propranolol in fit patients to reduce the heart rate and therefore reduce bleeding. The individual β-blocking agents are discussed in more detail in Chapter 13.

● DIRECT-ACTING PERIPHERAL VASODILATOR DRUGS

Although some direct-acting vasodilators (e.g. hydralazine and diazoxide) are used in the long-term control of hypertension, the prolonged action of these agents makes them unsuitable for the acute intra-operative control of blood pressure. GTN and SNP are the most commonly used vasodilator drugs.

Sodium Nitroprusside

This drug, which is administered as an intravenous infusion, produces an extremely rapid fall in arterial blood pressure which is dose dependent and which is brought about by peripheral vasodilatation. SNP dilates arteries and veins equally and, for this reason, maintains blood flow to vital organs at lower blood pressures than most other hypotensive techniques. It is widely used for elective hypotension in operations where fine and rapid control of blood pressure is essential (e.g. neurosurgery, cardiac surgery and vascular surgery). It is also used as a vasodilating agent in intensive care and to treat acute hypertensive emergencies. The action of nitroprusside is short lived, wearing off within 2 min of discontinuation. The normal dose used should not exceed 1.5 mg/kg as a total dose or 10 μg/kg/min.

Glyceryl Trinitrate

Available as an intravenous infusion for intra-operative hypotension, this drug produces a slower fall and rise in blood pressure than nitroprusside, but this may sometimes be beneficial. GTN is also used in intensive care in similar situations to SNP. The drug provides accurate and fine control of blood pressure by peripheral vasodilatation.

● EXTRADURAL AND SPINAL ANAESTHESIA

These are discussed in detail in Chapter 41.

29

Anaesthesia for Plastic, Microvascular and Burn Surgery

•Plastic surgery •Microvascular reconstructive surgery •Craniofacial reconstruction •The burned patient

● PLASTIC SURGERY

Procedures performed by plastic surgeons include operations to correct congenital deformities, for example, cleft lip and palate, hypospadias, syndactyly; operations on the skin and muscle, for example, skin graft and pedicle flaps; operations for cosmetic purposes, for example, rhinoplasy, face lifts, breast augmentation and reduction, liposuction; and operations for microvascular and craniofacial reconstruction.

Although general anaesthetic techniques for plastic surgery do not differ greatly from those commonly used, additional drugs and manoeuvres are often employed specifically to reduce blood loss. While plastic surgery on the limbs is often carried out under tourniquet, a small amount of bleeding in an operation on a highly vascular area (e.g. the face) can be extremely troublesome. Elective drug-induced hypotension during anaesthesia may be used, but certain additional techniques are often employed. These are mainly designed to reduce the possibility of venous congestion in the operation site, and also to a certain extent to reduce systemic blood pressure. A smooth anaesthetic technique, which avoids coughing, straining or other manoeuvres likely to raise venous pressure during induction, is essential. Where possible, the operative site is placed at a higher level than the heart, for example, in facial surgery the patient is positioned with a 10–15° head-up tilt. Carbon dioxide, being a potent vasodilator, must not be allowed to accumulate and for this reason the patients are often either ventilated or allowed to breathe spontaneously round a circle system containing soda-lime to absorb the carbon dioxide produced (Chapter 8).

The drugs used are preferably those which produce a slow fall and rise in systemic blood pressure, since rapid alterations may well produce reactionary haemorrhage and bleeding under the skin flaps towards the end of the operation. The surgical technique includes local infiltration of solutions containing adrenaline to produce localised vasoconstriction and therefore reduction in bleeding, and it is important to monitor the patients for possible arrhythmias which may result from inadvertent intravenous injection of adrenaline.

The techniques of intubation for plastic surgery operations may require considerable skill, particularly in patients with tumours, scarring and facial deformity which may make conventional direct laryngoscopy difficult or impossible. Many anaesthetists now routinely use the flexible fibreoptic laryngoscope, which has superseded blind techniques, to intubate patients with a difficult airway (Chapter 18). The intubation may be performed under topical anaesthesia of the upper airway and sedation. Intra-oral or intranasal haemorrhage will require control by oropharyngeal packs, which are inserted at induction and which must be checked for removal before the patient is extubated. These may be of either absorbent gauze or sponge and are used in conjunction with both cuffed and uncuffed nasal intubation.

Control of postoperative pain, nausea and vomiting is important and intravenous fluids must be given until patients are able to take adequate amounts of oral fluids.

● MICROVASCULAR RECONSTRUCTIVE SURGERY

Recent advances in surgical techniques using the operating microscope have made possible many operations in which free musculocutaneous flaps are grafted, together with anastomosis of their blood supply, to cover defects created when tissue is removed following trauma, or after excision of tumours. An example is a transverse rectus abdominis muscle ('TRAM') flap operation for breast reconstruction in which the transverse abdominis muscle and its blood vessels are grafted to the area where the breast tissue has been removed.

The general principles of anaesthesia for plastic surgery (see above) apply to these cases. These procedures are generally lengthy and may last for up to 6–12 h. The anaesthetist is challenged to provide conditions on which depend the viability of the flap and the success of the operation. During the initial part of the surgery, when the lesion is excised and the donor site is harvested, blood loss is minimised by using a technique providing moderate hypotension (systolic blood pressure 80 mmHg), usually achieved with intermittent positive pressure ventilation (IPPV) using muscle relaxant, morphine and isoflurane. Isoflurane is an ideal volatile agent as very little is metabolised (0.2%) and it produces vasodilatation in normovolaemic patients. Additionally drugs such as phentolamine (α-blockers) or labetolol (α- and β-blockers) may be used to produce hypotension (Chapter 28).

During anastomosis of the vessels, maximal vasodilatation and a normal blood pressure aid surgery. It is vital therefore to keep the patient's temperature normal (by keeping the theatre warm, administering warmed intravenous fluids, humidifying gases with heat and moisture exchangers in the breathing circuit and using warming mattresses), avoid hypocapnia and infusing fluids to maintain a state of relative hypervolaemia. The surgeon may inject papaverine in the vessels to produce local vasodilatation. Where appropriate, regional blockade with local anaesthetic should be combined with general anaesthesia to produce sympathetic blockade and vasodilatation.

After the vessels have been anastomosed, an unobstructed blood flow can be achieved by continuing vasodilatation and adjusting the viscosity of the blood to avoid haemoconcentration by infusing appropriate fluids and by repeated measurement of blood haematocrit. Some anaesthetists use dextran 70 in saline after the vessels have been grafted to prevent the adherence (rouleaux formation) of the red blood cells. Dextran also prevents thromboembolism.

It is therefore not surprising that additional monitoring in these cases should include direct arterial blood pressure and central venous pressure monitoring, urinary output, and measurement of core and skin temperature and serial analysis of blood gases, haematocrit and clotting factors.

Postoperatively, these patients should be kept warm and well perfused and analgesia provided with patient-controlled analgesia (PCA) morphine or epidural local anaesthesia (Chapter 42). Patients in whom free microvascular reconstructions have been carried out in the head and neck are best looked after in the intensive therapy unit (ITU). An additional risk in this group is of airway difficulties, should a haematoma occur in the neck. Some surgeons routinely perform a tracheostomy to avoid this but a period of stabilisation in ITU with extubation when the swelling has reduced will avoid tracheostomy in many patients.

● CRANIOFACIAL RECONSTRUCTION

Craniofacial reconstruction for the treatment of severe anatomical abnormalities, usually congenital in origin, is now becoming a more widely used technique, although only in specialised centres. It combines all the problems of maxillofacial surgery and neurosurgery, together with those related to prolonged anaesthesia for microvascular surgery. The patients are frequently children, often with other congenital abnormalities and cardiac defects, and may be technically extremely difficult to anaesthetise and intubate. The surgical techniques involved are unique and the requirements of each operation related particularly to airway management must be discussed with the surgeon on an individual basis.

● THE BURNED PATIENT

The initial assessment and resuscitation of every burned patient should be the same as for any patient with trauma (Chapter 24), but the size and the depth of the burn should also be assessed. Examination and resuscitation should be done simultaneously. It is vital to look for respiratory injury caused by dry heat or smoke inhalation. Early intubation is preferred before complete airway obstruction sets in. Carbon monoxide and cyanides may also be inhaled and their levels and blood gas measurement should be performed. Special co-oximeters to measure carboxyhaemoglobin may also be required.

Many formulae are used to estimate the size of the burn, but the one most commonly used is the 'rule of 9s', where various regions of the body surface represent a 9% area or multiples thereof, for example, one upper limb is 9% of body surface and one lower limb is 18%, front and back of trunk are 18% each, head and neck 9%, and genitalia 1% and so on. It is generally agreed that a child with 10% burns or an adult with 20% should be resuscitated with intravenous fluids. A patient with more than 30% burns requires care in a special burns unit. The type of fluid used (crystalloid or colloid) and the rate at which these are infused vary from unit to unit.

Analgesia can be provided with entonox or intravenous opioids. Burned patients may present for anaesthesia during the acute resuscitative phase where airway, fluid management and ventilatory support may be required. The definitive treatment is surgical, with skin grafting of the burned tissue. Some partial thickness burns may be treated conservatively. The burned patient is likely to require multiple procedures, including debridement, skin grafting and reconstructive procedures. Special problems include the airway, which may be affected by direct injury in the acute phase, or by scarring later on. Sites for peripheral venous cannulation may be exhausted or be inaccessible. There may be difficulty in placing monitors and because of the large area of exposed burned tissue, heat loss can be extreme and body temperature should be maintained with warmed fluids, humidifiers, warming mattresses and a warm theatre. Fluid and blood loss can be substantial and should be replaced, urine output and central venous pressure monitoring usually being employed to guide this.

The same techniques of anaesthesia are suitable for the burned patient as are used for other surgical procedures, but suxamethonium should be avoided in the burned patient (for as long as 6 months after the burn) to avoid hyperkalaemia and cardiac arrhythmias. In addition, these patients are resistant to non-depolarising muscle relaxants. Intravenous or even intramuscular ketamine is useful for short procedures, for example, repeated burn dressing. EMLA cream applied topically is useful to harvest skin for grafting.

30

Anaesthesia for Abdominal and Gynaecological Surgery

•Anatomy •Techniques of anaesthesia •Postoperative nausea and vomiting •Position of the patient •Gynaecological surgery •Laparoscopy and endoscopic surgery

A chapter devoted mainly to anaesthesia for abdominal surgery is justified because it embraces a high proportion of elective and emergency anaesthesia; some of the special features of emergency anaesthesia are discussed in Chapter 24. The triad of anaesthesia – narcosis, analgesia and muscular relaxation – is referred to in Chapter 1 and it is during anaesthesia for abdominal surgery that provision of good muscular relaxation is of paramount importance to aid surgical access. The methods of achieving this are described below.

● ANATOMY

The skin and muscles of the abdominal wall are supplied mainly by the lower intercostal nerves. However, it is more important to have some knowledge of the segmental levels of the spinal cord which supply the various almost horizontal strips of skin, called 'dermatomes', at the various levels. Figure 30.1 shows that the skin in the region of the xiphisternum is supplied from the sixth thoracic segment, the umbilical level is innervated from T10 and it is not until the suprapubic region that the first lumbar segment is involved. The reasons for this perhaps surprising innervation of the anterior abdominal wall by thoracic nerves is that these intercostal nerves follow the ribs until the latter swing upwards in the form of their costal cartilages or, in the case of the lower ribs, end floating freely. The intercostal nerves continue forwards in the line of their earlier pathway in company with the posterior part of the ribs, and this leads them round onto the front of the abdomen where they supply almost horizontal dermatomes. The innervation of the abdominal wall by thoracic and the first lumbar segments of the spinal cord means that for any spinal or epidural block

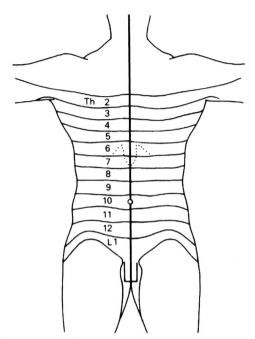

Figure 30.1 Segmental innervation of abdominal wall dermatomes.

to be effective for surgery on the abdomen, some sympathetic nerve fibres must also be blocked with vasodilatation and a tendency to hypotension.

The peritoneum is a serous membrane consisting of two layers resembling a deflated plastic bag. The anterior layer (the parietal peritoneum) lines the inner aspect of the anterior abdominal wall, while the posterior layer (the visceral peritoneum) closely invests the viscera which protrude into it from behind. If they protrude far enough into the peritoneum, it meets again behind them to form a mesentery. The parietal and visceral layers of peritoneum are usually closely applied to each other, being separated only by a little serous fluid. The potential space between the two layers is readily converted into a real one by the entry of air at operation, or by the injection of carbon dioxide or other gas through a needle into the closed abdomen – as occurs during laparoscopy.

The parietal peritoneum is supplied by nerve fibres from the same segments that supply the overlying skin. Like the underlying viscera, the visceral peritoneum is normally insensitive to cutting or burning, but the nerve endings in the viscera and mesenteries do register pain in response to inflammation and stretching.

Sensory Innervation of the Viscera

Sensory nerve fibres from the abdominal viscera are carried along two pathways – the sympathetic and the parasympathetic. The sensory nerves which run with the sympathetic nerves pass through the coeliac plexus and then in the greater, lesser and least splanchnic nerves to the sympathetic chain and thence to the spinal cord at the T5–12 segments (Fig. 30.2).

The parasympathetic component travels in two parts – a larger vagal part carrying sensation from most of the abdominal viscera, including the alimentary canal down to the transverse colon, and a smaller pelvic part carrying sensation from the rest of the bowel and the pelvic organs via the pelvic splanchnic nerves to the second, third and fourth sacral segments of the spinal cord. The vagal component (like the sympathetic) passes through the coeliac plexus, but then passes through the thoracic cavity and neck to the brain without ever joining the spinal cord. Thus, while spinal or epidural analgesia to the level of the fifth thoracic segment will produce complete block of the sympathetic component of intra-abdominal sensation, it has no effect on the vagal component, which can be blocked only by infiltration of local analgesic into the coeliac plexus, or into the vagal trunks higher in the abdomen or in the neck.

In summary, the nature and distribution of sensory nerves within the abdominal cavity allows gentle handling, cutting and suturing of

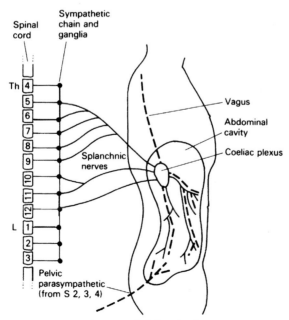

Figure 30.2 Pathways of abdominal sensory nerves.

uninflamed viscera, provided that no tension is put on mesenteries, without either sympathetic or parasympathetic blockade. Rougher handling, or surgery on inflamed viscera, requires full blockade of both sympathetic and parasympathetic pathways.

● TECHNIQUES OF ANAESTHESIA

Most abdominal surgery is made easier by (indeed, some operations are impossible without) good muscular relaxation. The only common exceptions are elective operations for inguinal or femoral hernia repairs. For these, the mild degree of relaxation associated with a spontaneous respiration anaesthetic using nitrous oxide, oxygen and volatile agent should be sufficient and is preferred by some anaesthetists.

Like all striated muscle, that of the abdominal wall musculature tends to be in a state of less than full relaxation: this is called muscle tone. This tone in the muscles may be raised to much stronger levels of contraction in response to noxious stimuli sending large numbers of impulses up the sensory nerves to the spinal cord. There, the information is transmitted to the motor side of the spinal cord, whence impulses are carried down the motor nerves and across the neuromuscular junctions to the muscle fibres. This sensory-to-motor reflex arc has to be broken to produce muscular relaxation and this can be done on the sensory side, the motor side or both of them or, nowadays, most effectively at the neuromuscular junction. Some of the techniques of anaesthesia producing relaxation are discussed below.

Spontaneous Respiration Anaesthesia

Spontaneous respiration anaesthesia with single agents (e.g. chloroform, ether or cyclopropane) was the classical method of providing anaesthesia for abdominal surgery. Unfortunately, good muscular relaxation with these agents is produced only in the deepest planes of anaesthesia – indeed, only when the patient is near respiratory arrest. For prolonged upper abdominal surgery such as a gastrectomy, so great was the necessary 'soaking' with these powerful agents that the patients tended to be drowsy and sick for hours afterwards, with a high incidence of respiratory and venous embolic phenomena. As a result, and as anaesthetic techniques improved, this type of anaesthesia for abdominal surgery has largely disappeared from the medically advanced parts of the world. However, in less well-endowed areas, it may still be acceptable to use one of these agents (diethyl ether) because it is so safe. Even then, it may often be possible to administer it from an accurate and temperature-compensated vaporiser like the Epstein-Macintosh-Oxford (EMO) (Chapter 9).

Muscle-relaxant Anaesthesia

Muscle relaxants transformed anaesthesia for abdominal surgery, great depths of anaesthesia no longer being necessary. Excellent operating conditions may be obtained with the lightest of general anaesthesia from which the patient quickly recovers. With the possible exception of hernia operations, as mentioned above, it is customary to perform tracheal intubation for most abdominal operations and this may be done by producing muscle relaxation with either suxamethonium or one of the non-depolarising relaxants. Relaxation is usually maintained by using one of the latter group. The question is, how light should the general anaesthesia be? If only nitrous oxide and oxygen are used for maintaining anaesthesia, the patient may have awareness or recall at some stage during the operation. There is no doubt, therefore, that the nitrous oxide should be supplemented with additional anaesthetic in the form of a trace of a volatile agent and a parenteral analgesic like fentanyl or morphine. Another alternative is to avoid volatile agents altogether and maintain anaesthesia with an infusion of propofol.

Regional Techniques

As methods of producing muscular relaxation for abdominal surgery, spinal and epidural analgesia have been much less used since the advent of muscle relaxants. Both techniques tend to produce relaxation by blocking the sensory side of the reflex arc. The local analgesic agents for producing spinal block are usually powerful enough to produce motor block, so that side of the reflex arc is also broken. The drugs used for epidural analgesia, however, do not usually produce such intense motor block so that more muscle tone may remain, especially in response to painful impulses being carried up the unblocked vagal pathways.

Combined Regional and General Anaesthetic Techniques

Excellent operating conditions may be provided by combining regional and general anaesthesia especially for operations requiring muscle relaxation combined with some degree of hypotension, for example, abdomino-perineal resection of the rectum and pelvic exenteration operations. An additional advantage of this technique is the excellent postoperative pain relief that can be provided by epidural infusion of local anaesthetic and or opioids (see Chapter 12).

● POSTOPERATIVE NAUSEA AND VOMITING

Inclusion of this subject in this chapter does not imply that the problem is confined to abdominal and gynaecological surgery. But the incidence is higher in this group of patients and measures to prevent and treat postoperative nausea and vomiting as described in Chapter 12 should be followed.

● POSITION OF THE PATIENT

The lithotomy and Lloyd–Davis position are used for some major abdomino-perineal and some gynaecological procedures. Care should be taken to protect the patient's back, peripheral nerves, eyes and pressure points. A steep head-down position may also be requested by the surgeon producing diaphragmatic splinting, necessitating muscle relaxation. The venous return is increased and adequate fluids should be given to prevent hypotension when the patient is placed supine.

● GYNAECOLOGICAL SURGERY

This consists essentially of lower abdominal and vaginal surgery. Many of these operations, for example, laparoscopy, and dilatation and curettage (D&C), are suitable for day surgery (Chapter 31). The anaesthetic techniques required for abdominal gynaecological surgery do not differ from those for other abdominal procedures. The possible exception is pelvic exenteration and radical vulvectomy for malignancy where the haemorrhage associated with the extensive dissection of pelvic lymph glands may be reduced by a hypotensive technique. Of the various methods available, the best method is a combined technique of light general anaesthesia with muscle relaxation and epidural local anaesthetic.

For vaginal surgery, a wide choice of techniques using spontaneous or controlled ventilation are acceptable. Some anaesthetists prefer to use a combined technique of regional anaesthesia (spinal or epidural) with light sedation or general anaesthesia.

Also included in the vaginal operations are the various operations associated with abortions, both spontaneous or therapeutic. In these cases it must be remembered that bleeding from the cavity of the uterus may occur for the same reasons as mentioned in Chapter 38 on obstetric anaesthesia, and it must be remembered that volatile agents in high concentrations may cause uterine relaxation. An injection of an oxytoxic such as syntocinon is usually given, and this may produce transient hypotension.

One real gynaecological emergency is a ruptured ectopic pregnancy. The bleeding varies in extent, but at its most severe may be one of the most frightening emergencies with which an anaesthetist has to deal. Attempts must always be made to resuscitate the patient, but in the most severe cases proper restoration of the blood pressure cannot be achieved until laparotomy is performed and salpingectomy carried out on the side from which the bleeding is occurring. Recently it has become popular in cases where there is doubt about the diagnosis to perform a preliminary laparoscopy.

● LAPAROSCOPY AND ENDOSCOPIC SURGERY

Laparoscopy has been used for many years in general surgery and gynae-cology, for both diagnostic and limited therapeutic purposes, for example, tubal sterilisation. Recent advances in fibreoptic and video technology and the availability of surgical instruments designed to pass through these 'endoscopes' has opened up a new era of surgery which is often called 'minimally invasive' (keyhole) surgery. By this is meant that complex surgical operations, for example, cholecystectomy, hernia repair and even hysterectomies which require large incisions in the abdominal wall can now be performed through tiny holes, large enough only to pass the oper-ating endoscopes and instruments. Advantages of these techniques include less tissue damage, bleeding, postoperative pain, nausea and vomiting. This allows early postoperative mobilisation, fewer complications and frequently the ability to perform these procedures as day cases (Chapter 31).

These techniques have also added to the diagnostic accuracy of what were once blind procedures, for example, diagnostic hysteroscopy instead of D&C.

The basis of every laparoscopic technique is to introduce gas into the peritoneal cavity with a needle, so that the abdominal or pelvic viscera fall away from the anterior abdominal wall. The laparoscope can then be more safely passed and the abdominal contents visualised. Some of the complications, for example, damage to a blood vessel or viscera by the needle, are directly related to the technique, but there are others which are related more to the anaesthetic.

The gas generally used is carbon dioxide, or less commonly nitrous oxide. The reason for choosing one of these gases is that they are highly diffusible and so are rapidly absorbed into the circulation and excreted by the lungs. Unfortunately, carbon dioxide in large quantities in the blood-stream can cause hypotension or cardiac arrhythmias, especially if volatile agents are used. Nitrous oxide, while safer when absorbed into the blood-stream, can at least theoretically support combustion and most surgeons are not happy to use it when employing diathermy within the peritoneal cavity.

In gynaecological laparoscopy, the patient is usually placed steeply head-down so that the pelvic contents may be seen more easily. Diaphragmatic descent, already hindered by the weight of the abdominal contents in this position, is made even more difficult by the intra-abdominal pressure exerted by the gas. For this reason, controlled ventilation is usually required to maintain adequate ventilation and especially elimination of carbon dioxide. However, if high intrathoracic pressures have to be applied, a point may come where blood is prevented from entering the chest and heart, so that cardiac output and blood pressure fall. This condition may be worsened by a vena-caval occlusion effect similar to that seen in obstetrics as the high intra-abdominal pressure compresses the inferior vena cava. It is therefore important that the anaesthetist monitors the patient's blood pressure, especially as abdominal distension becomes pronounced.

Postoperatively, the patient's cardiovascular system must be monitored carefully for arrhythmias and for hypotension. She should probably be kept in the recovery room for at least 30 min after the release of the gas from the peritoneal cavity. By no means all the gas is released in this way, and blood gas measurements have shown that the P_{CO_2} sometimes does not reach its maximum level until 30 min after gas release.

A perhaps surprising postoperative symptom after laparoscopy is the occurrence of shoulder tip pain. This is believed to be caused either by gas under the diaphragm, or more likely by blood or other fluid running up to the lower surface of the diaphragm in the head-down position. Lower abdominal pain also occurs, especially after gynaecological procedures such as sterilisation, and probably results from fallopian tubal spasm.

Modern gynaecological surgery may also involve the use of lasers and hysterectomy is being replaced by endometrial ablation by laser or diathermy. All the precautions such as the wearing of protective glasses should be followed. The risk of explosion and fire is less than that when lasers are used in ear, nose and throat (ENT) surgery (see Chapter 25). Large quantities of irrigation fluids such as glycine are used during endometrial ablation and this may cause a few problems. If large amounts of glycine are absorbed in the circulation, hyponatraemia, low osmolality of the plasma and haemolysis of the red cells may result. Accurate count of fluids in and out of the patient should therefore be kept and patients should be watched for signs and symptoms: nausea, vomiting, headache, hypoxia and convulsions if large quantities are absorbed in the bloodstream.

31

Anaesthesia for Day Surgery

*•Preoperative assessment •Premedication •Anaesthetic techniques
•Recovery and discharge*

Day surgery means that the patient is admitted, operated on and discharged home on the same day. There are several reasons why day surgery has become popular in recent years. First, there are obvious savings in terms of hospital beds and staff, because the patients do not stay overnight and in the face of increasing health costs this makes day surgery a desirable option; secondly, patients have less disruption of their personal life; and thirdly, they are at less risk of hospital infection and possibly fewer post-operative complications. Advances in surgical and anaesthetic techniques have now made it possible to perform >50% of cases on a day-stay basis.

Although gynaecological procedures, for example, dilatation and curettage (D&C) and laparoscopy, are the most common operations performed, others such as dental, general surgical, for example, varicose vein operations, herniorrhaphy, and urological and plastic surgical procedures can also be safely performed on this basis. Any operation of a reasonable length, not associated with major bleeding or sepsis and after which the patient's pain can be controlled with simple oral analgesics, can be done as a day case. Many operations on children are also performed as day cases (Chapter 37).

For a successful outcome it is important to pay meticulous attention to all aspects of anaesthesia, i.e. preoperative assessment, anaesthetic techniques and discharge procedures.

● PREOPERATIVE ASSESSMENT

Either day surgery is performed in purpose-built day units, or patients are admitted as day patients to normal wards on a normal operating list. To avoid delay and cancellation, patients should be selected when they are first seen in the out-patient clinic. This is done according to criteria agreed and understood by surgeons, anaesthetists, and ward and clinic nurses.

Some important considerations about patient selection are as follows, but local policies vary greatly.

Age

It is generally recommended that patients <6 months and >70 years are unsuitable for day-case surgery. With experience many units are modifying this rule.

General Condition

Only patients with physical status ASAI or II (Chapter 14) should be considered for day surgery. This will exclude patients who are grossly obese, and with systemic diseases which cause limitation of activity, for example, chronic bronchitis, severe asthma, poorly controlled diabetes or hypertension.

Anaesthetic History

Patients with previous anaesthetic complications, for example, airway problems, or with a history of one of the serious hereditary conditions, for example, malignant hyperpyrexia, are unsuitable.

Domestic Circumstances

Patients who cannot be escorted and looked after at home by a responsible adult are not suitable for day surgery.

Surgical Procedures

Criteria for appropriate surgical procedures are mentioned above.

It is common practice in most units to ask patients to fill in a preoperative questionnaire when first seen in the out-patient clinic to determine suitability for admission. This questionnaire follows the lines of the pre-anaesthetic assessment interview (Chapter 14). It enables the surgeon to tell at a glance if the patient is fit for day surgery and also speeds the anaesthetist's assessment of the patient when admitted for surgery. When the patient is booked for surgery they are given a set of standard instructions about preoperative fasting and postoperative care at home. Routine blood tests are only carried out where necessary.

PREMEDICATION

The aims of premedication are discussed in Chapter 14. Day surgery patients are likely to be apprehensive and anxious, and explanation by staff can do much to allay this anxiety. Worry that anxiolytics may delay recovery is unfounded and short-acting benzodiazepines, for example, temazepam, can safely be used if required but not on a routine basis. Opioids are generally avoided because of their side-effects. Emphasis is, however, placed on other aims of premedication, especially prevention of nausea and vomiting and of acid aspiration syndrome. Some anaesthetists routinely prescribe metoclopramide and ranitidine to adult day surgical patients. EMLA cream is useful in children and obviates the need for systemic drugs.

● ANAESTHETIC TECHNIQUES

Anaesthetic techniques for day surgery should be simple, produce rapid induction, adequate intra-operative analgesia and amnesia and most importantly provide rapid recovery. The basic principles of providing general anaesthesia are the same as for in-patient surgery, but some anaesthetic drugs are better suited for day surgery than others.

General Anaesthesia

Induction

Induction of anaesthesia is usually intravenous. Any agent can be used but propofol has the distinct advantages that it induces sleep quickly, anaesthesia can easily and safely be maintained with an infusion and emergence is rapid (Chapter 4). Other advantages are that the incidence of post-operative nausea and vomiting is low and it is easier to insert a laryngeal mask after induction with propofol than it is after thiopentone. Inhalation induction is indicated in small children, although with the advent of EMLA this has declined. For inhalation induction, halothane was the most popular agent used but sevoflurane is currently preferred in both adults and children (Chapter 10). Isoflurane and the newer agent desflurane irritate the upper respiratory tract and may make induction difficult.

Maintenance

Maintenance of anaesthesia is with a volatile agent with 60–70% nitrous oxide in oxygen. As regards emergence from anaesthesia, there is not much to choose between isoflurane, halothane or enflurane, but this is significantly quicker with the newer agent desflurane. Total intravenous anaesthesia using propofol infusion is a popular alternative and is now increasingly used (Chapter 4).

Anaesthesia is maintained with a laryngeal mask airway (LMA) or a tracheal tube. The LMA can be used for spontaneous or controlled ventilation, frees the anaesthetist's hands and results in a lower incidence of sore throat. Suxamethonium is not required to insert an LMA and hence side-effects of this muscle relaxant are avoided.

Analgesia during the procedure is provided by the short-acting opioid analgesics, for example, fentanyl or alfentanil, but non-steroidal anti-inflammatory drugs given intravenously (e.g. ketorolac) or rectally (e.g. diclofenac) are extensively used and provide excellent analgesia without side-effects. Wherever possible, local anaesthetic blocks or infiltration in the wound are used to supplement analgesia and reduce the necessity for systemically administered analgesics.

The introduction of short-acting non-depolarising muscle relaxants, for example, atracurium and vecuronium, has made it possible to administer light general anaesthesia. Mivacurium has an even shorter duration of action. If judiciously used, these agents may not even require reversal at the end of the operation. Suxamethonium should be avoided wherever possible because of its side-effects (Chapter 11).

Regional and Local Anaesthesia

Central neural blockade in the form of single-shot spinal anaesthesia may be suitable for a variety of procedures including urology (e.g. cystoscopies), herniorrhaphy and varicose vein operations. Advantages include the avoidance of nausea, vomiting, drowsiness and acid aspiration, and the provision of excellent analgesia. Disadvantages include the time required and the risk of post-dural puncture headache (PDPH), although this is less with the use of finer pencil-point needles for spinal anaesthesia. If used, patients should have regained full sensory function and motor power before discharge. Nerve blocks, for example, axillary block for hand surgery are frequently used with excellent results. Eye blocks are an excellent choice for cataract surgery (Chapter 26). Some minor operations can be safely performed under local infiltration anaesthesia by the surgeon.

Sedation may be required for some of these procedures and when used the patients should be adequately monitored.

● RECOVERY AND DISCHARGE

Patients are recovered after day-case anaesthesia in a similar manner to any other anaesthetic. Criteria used to discharge patients vary in different units but the following are a general guideline.

The patient should be awake and oriented, should have had stable vital signs for 30 min, should be able to tolerate oral fluids and be able to pass urine. Finally they should be able to stand and walk unaided. If the patient is not in pain and is not nauseous or sick and the wound is satisfactory, then they are ready for discharge. It is usual to give the patient written instructions not to drive or operate machinery for 24 h and they should be discharged only in the company of a responsible adult who should be able to look after the patient for 24 h. Instructions are given about wound care, and analgesia and anti-emetics are prescribed. The patient is given a contact number to ring if there are any problems.

Using carefully chosen routines and techniques, day-case surgery not only is safe but may be preferable to the patient and is proving exceptionally economical as a means of dealing with surgical waiting lists.

32

Anaesthesia for Patients with Systemic Disease – Renal, Hepatic and Ischaemic

•Renal disease •Renal failure and renal transplantation •Hepatic and renal function related to anaesthesia •Patients with hepatic failure •Ischaemic disease

● RENAL DISEASE

Routine urological surgery does not normally require specialist anaesthetic techniques, but many patients presenting for prostatectomy and other urological procedures are elderly and suffer from other diseases, particularly of the cardiovascular and respiratory systems. Careful preoperative assessment is important to ensure their fitness for anaesthesia and particularly their ability to tolerate mildly hypotensive techniques which are commonly used for prostatic surgery. Lumbar extradural or spinal anaesthesia is often used to decrease intra-operative blood loss and induce mild hypotension. Patients with a history of cardiovascular or cerebrovascular disease are unsuitable for such procedures. Papillary carcinoma of the bladder is usually treated by repeat cystoscopy and cystodiathermy, and as these patients have a high incidence of repeat anaesthesia, the possibility of hepatotoxicity from multiple exposures to volatile agents or the development of hypersensitivity to intravenous agents (Chapter 4) must be borne in mind. The introduction of flexible cystoscopy, which can be satisfactorily performed under topical anaesthesia, will substantially reduce the need for general anaesthesia in these patients. Operations on the upper urinary tract and kidney involve careful positioning of the patient in the lateral position, and breaking the table to permit maximum exposure of the loin. Other problems of urological anaesthesia relate to specific features of renal disease. These may be summarised as impaired or absent excretion of water, electrolytes, urea and many drugs. Renal disease and failure may be accompanied by reduced production of erythropoietin, which controls the formation of red blood cells, and excess production of renin, which through the renin–angiotensin mechanism controls arterial blood pressure (Chapter 2). Excess renin production produces hypertension, renin release being stimulated by a fall in renal perfusion, the reflex being designed to maintain kidney blood flow. Abnormal renin production may occur as a result of renal artery stenosis.

● RENAL FAILURE AND RENAL TRANSPLANTATION

Impaired or absent renal function produces not only disorders of fluid and electrolyte balance but also alteration in the levels of renally produced hormones. Such patients are therefore anaemic, acidotic and often hypertensive and may present considerable problems during anaesthesia.

Preoperative Considerations

The patients are often extremely nervous and used to hospitals because they have had many previous admissions. In addition, the excitement of a possible transplant after many years on dialysis leaves them far from calm.

Cardiovascular problems may include hypertension – often treated by β-adrenoceptor blockade and methyldopa or angiotensin-converting enzyme (ACE) inhibitors, for example, captopril (Chapter 13) – mild congestive cardiac failure and sometimes even pulmonary oedema. It is important to control potential cardiovascular problems by preoperative dialysis to remove excessive fluid.

Metabolically, the problems of uraemia, acidosis and hyperkalaemia must be controlled preoperatively by dialysis if anaesthesia is to be uneventful. As postoperative dialysis includes locally heparinising the patient, this is best avoided until the second or third postoperative day to prevent possible haemorrhage at the operative site resulting from systemic absorption of the heparin. Immediate preoperative dialysis treatment is therefore essential. Increased calcium excretion and secondary hyperparathyroidism may also result from renal disease.

Routine drug therapy in patients with renal disease may include antihypertensives, diuretics and in some cases steroids, which must be maintained intra-operatively in the normal way (Chapter 14). The anaemia which results from renal disease is chronic, resulting from a decreased production of erythropoietin. These patients can compensate for their chronic anaemia in several ways, and the combination of anaemia and acidosis, in particular, maintains tissue oxygen delivery. For this reason, it is essential for patients to retain their mild acidosis during operation, since correction to normal values will impair tissue oxygenation.

Preoperative Information

Although many patients in renal failure will be starved and preoperatively prepared in the usual way, certain information is important. Details of the time when the patients last ate or drank, the time of their last dialysis and their current drug therapy are all essential. It is important also to have measurements of their current urea, electrolytes and haemoglobin after their last dialysis treatment, together with their age, post-dialysis weight and blood pressure. Patients are often given a resonium enema preoperatively to reduce their serum potassium concentration, as hyperkalaemia is probably the most serious intra-operative complication. If major surgery is planned, preoperative cross-matching, usually involving red cells specially prepared for the patient, must be carried out well in advance and the site of the patient's arteriovenous dialysis fistula must be known so that blood flow through it can be protected.

Anaesthetic Technique

Oral premedication is usual in these patients, since intramuscular injections may produce haematomata following systemic absorption of the heparin used during dialysis. Intra-operative steroid cover may also be necessary in certain cases. Intravenous induction is carried out using an intravenous infusion of normal saline placed under local anaesthetic in the back of the hand, saline being preferred to 5% dextrose. It is important to avoid using forearm or anticubital veins because these may be needed later for dialysis treatment. Pre-oxygenation is followed by a propofol, fentanyl, relaxant sequence, usually with atracurium. This non-depolarising neuromuscular blocking drug, which is uniquely metabolised in plasma and the duration of action of which is therefore independent of renal function, has contributed considerably to the anaesthetic technique in these patients. Suxamethonium is usually avoided since it produces a rise in serum potassium following muscle fasciculation, although it may be specifically indicated in certain circumstances where the patient is inadequately prepared or starved.

Intermittent positive pressure ventilation (IPPV) maintaining the Pa_{CO_2} at the patient's normal level is used to avoid alterations in the chronic metabolic acidosis which facilitates oxygen delivery to the tissues.

Routinely, 66% nitrous oxide in oxygen is used, although some anaesthetists may supplement this with a small dose of isoflurane, and indeed may ventilate the patient with a volatile agent without using relaxants. Non-depolarising neuromuscular blocking drugs tend to be partly metabolised in the liver and partly excreted unchanged in the kidneys; for this reason their action may be excessively prolonged in patients with renal failure. However, the patients are usually reasonably fit and require an adequate dose of relaxant to achieve muscle relaxation. It is important therefore to administer relaxants only at the beginning of the operation, since it is usually incremental administration during the procedure which results in inadequate reversal at the end unless atracurium is used. Central venous pressure monitoring may also be used, particularly in anephric patients, unable to excrete fluid load, because postoperative fluid balance may be critical for maintaining an adequate blood flow through the fistula.

The arteriovenous fistula is the patient's lifeline to dialysis: flow must therefore be maintained to avoid clotting. Avoiding hypotension due to hypovolaemia or cardiac depression is essential. Local techniques include wrapping the arm in warm gamgee or a stellate ganglion block to increase local blood flow.

Intra-operative monitoring should include electrocardiography (ECG) – particularly to detect hyperkalaemia (peaked T waves) – and measurement of arterial blood pressure. This should always be by an indirect method as the use of arterial lines, particularly in the arm, may damage an artery potentially suitable for fistula formation.

● HEPATIC AND RENAL FUNCTION RELATED TO ANAESTHESIA

Many drugs administered as part of routine anaesthesia undergo some metabolism in the liver before being excreted by the kidneys. The link between adequate hepatic and renal function is therefore important when considering the doses of drugs to be given and their normal duration of action. Non-depolarising muscle relaxants, in particular, demonstrate this balance between metabolism and excretion, and if one or other organ's function is impaired then the other will compensate. This means that additional hepatic metabolism will occur in renal failure and vice versa, although both processes may take considerably longer.

The liver is involved not only with metabolising drugs, but also in generating and maintaining adequate concentrations of plasma proteins, these having many functions including the binding of certain drugs (Chapter 3). The degree of protein binding influences the potency and duration of the action of various drugs, and inadequate hepatic function may produce hypoproteinaemia and thus impaired protein binding.

The liver also synthesises some clotting factors including prothrombin, and hepatic failure may be complicated by disorders of coagulation.

Inadequate renal function inevitably produces problems of fluid and electrolyte excretion, as well as influencing the duration of action of various drugs that depend on renal excretion in the unchanged form. It is particularly important during anaesthesia to prevent renal insufficiency occurring as a result of hypovolaemia, since this may exacerbate pre-existing renal failure.

● PATIENTS WITH HEPATIC FAILURE

The importance of the liver in drug metabolism, plasma protein synthesis and blood coagulation has already been discussed. Nevertheless, as the liver is normally capable of regeneration and therefore ultimately of regaining normal function, it is essential that any anaesthetic technique should not produce more hepatic damage. Careful use of drugs, particularly induction agents, analgesics and muscle relaxants – all of which are metabolised to a greater or less degree in the liver – is essential. However, the most important factor is to maintain an adequate hepatic blood flow and therefore oxygen supply.

The liver receives two-thirds of its blood supply from the portal vein arising from the splanchnic circulation, and one-third from the normal arterial supply. Normal portal blood flow and oxygenation is therefore an important factor in avoiding further hepatic damage during operation. Catecholamine release, which is produced by several anaesthetic agents, will produce splanchnic vasoconstriction and a reduction in portal venous blood flow, whereas other agents which produce splanchnic vasodilatation (e.g. halothane, enflurane and isoflurane) are more likely to maintain normal oxygenation of the liver. This is in strange contrast to the normally held view that halothane is toxic to the liver and emphasises that hepatotoxicity is an extremely rare phenomenon, and that, in normal circumstances, volatile agents like halothane or isoflurane are good maintainers of hepatic blood flow.

Hepatic failure sometimes results in renal failure, thought to be caused by the need to excrete high levels of bilirubin. Hepatorenal failure may occur in jaundiced patients and for this reason diuretics, particularly mannitol, are often given together with a fluid load immediately preoperatively to produce an osmotic diuresis which can protect against the development of this syndrome.

● ISCHAEMIC DISEASE

Although ischaemic disease can occur in many different organs or places in the arterial tree, the occurrence of problems in one area, for example, aorta or heart, should imply a more widespread, though perhaps, at present, symptomless incidence of disease. The problems of patients with ischaemic heart disease are dealt with in Chapter 15 and those of patients with vascular disease in Chapter 33. In general, the symptoms of ischaemic disease relate to relative hypoxia of an organ which may ultimately produce vascular occlusion and infarction. The main organs affected by ischaemia are the brain, heart and kidneys, together with the peripheral circulation, usually of the lower limbs.

Patients who have suffered cerebral ischaemia are usually affected in the form of a stroke, the severity of which ranges from mild speech impairment or forgetfulness to complete hemiplegia. The symptoms may also be either transient or permanent. Such patients should be assumed also to have myocardial disease, at least until a normal ECG is obtained. Renal ischaemia will produce organ malfunction, presenting as renal impairment frequently associated with hypertension, while widespread atherosclerosis can present with numerous symptoms, for example, leg pain from claudication or transient ischaemic attacks from carotid artery stenosis.

33

Anaesthesia for Vascular Surgery

General considerations •*Preoperative assessment* •*Preparation for anaesthesia* •*Extracranial vascular surgery* •*Vascular radiology*

● GENERAL CONSIDERATIONS

Improvements in surgical techniques and equipment (especially suture materials and operating microscopes), in methods of diagnosis (especially vascular radiology) and in anaesthesia have led to the steady expansion of vascular surgery as a surgical subspeciality.

While a small proportion of treatable arterial disease is caused by congenital abnormalities or by syphilis (once an important cause of arterial disease), the major cause of occlusive vascular disease is now atherosclerosis. This generalised disease affects all the arteries in the body, including the coronary, cerebral and renal arteries. Vascular surgery has now progressed to the stage where not only the arteries to the vital organs may be operated on, but also those in the peripheral vascular tree (e.g. of the limbs). It is important to remember that the widespread nature of the disease indicates that the blood supply to the vital organs is imperfect and that anaesthesia must be carefully planned and carried out to reduce complications.

Patients presenting for vascular surgery are often elderly and have other serious conditions associated with atherosclerosis, for example, hypertension, diabetes, and chronic obstructive lung and renal diseases.

Most drugs used for treating hypertension produce some degree of sympathetic blockade leaving a vagal (parasympathetic) preponderance, so that many patients show some degree of bradycardia. These patients, like patients with sympathetic blockade produced by spinal and epidural analgesia, have difficulty compensating for factors that may produce hypotension, for example, sudden blood loss or a head-up tilt. For this reason it was formerly thought that therapy (e.g. β-adrenoceptor blockade) should be stopped preoperatively, but it is now believed that these risks are less than those of myocardial or cerebral damage during anaesthesia and surgery when anti-hypertensive drugs have been withdrawn.

Cigarette smoking is closely correlated with the incidence and severity of vascular disease. While patients coming for elective vascular surgery will have stopped or greatly reduced their consumption, some patients coming for emergency surgery may be heavy smokers.

It is common for surgeons to induce regional heparinisation in the vascular distribution of an artery being operated on to reduce the incidence of thrombosis during arterial clamping. This is achieved by intravenous injection of 5000–10 000 IU heparin, which does not usually produce complete systemic anticoagulation. If it does, however, the problems produced are more likely to be surgical than anaesthetic, although they would certainly deter most anaesthetists from using, for example, continuous epidural analgesia as a method of postoperative pain relief.

● PREOPERATIVE ASSESSMENT

In some vascular surgical cases haste may be so imperative that thorough preoperative assessment may have to be curtailed to save the patient's life. Given time, however, the generalised nature of the atherosclerosis necessitates thorough preoperative evaluation. The history-taking, for instance, should enquire particularly about chest pain indicating angina or previous myocardial infarction, the presence of intermittent claudication, blackouts indicating severe cerebrovascular disease, breathlessness due to cardiac or respiratory disease or ankle oedema, which may be due to right-sided cardiac failure. Most patients will be on some type of long-term medication, for example, anti-hypertensive drugs, digoxin, anti-arrhythmics, diuretics, anticoagulants or insulin or oral hypoglycaemics. Continuation of these drugs over the operative period will have to be decided upon.

Laboratory investigations should include a full blood count, a full biochemical profile, including renal and liver function tests, 12-lead electrocardiogram (ECG), a chest X-ray examination and sometimes blood gas analysis or other lung function tests. Since preoperative myocardial ischaemia is an important determinant of morbidity and mortality in these patients, specific tests designed to detect this may also be performed. These include ambulatory ECG monitoring, radionuclear thallium scanning and, in selected cases, coronary angiography.

● PREPARATION FOR ANAESTHESIA

As already mentioned, most patients undergoing vascular surgery are suffering from generalised degenerative arterial disease. Younger, healthier patients may be suffering from acute hypovolaemia (as from a stab wound) or from the effects of multiple injuries (as after a road traffic accident). In addition, most vascular operations are lengthy and sudden rapid blood loss may occur. Consequently, for all major vascular surgery the following are required:

1. At least one large-bore (14G or 12G) venous cannula. This venous line must also be provided with a warming coil and thermostatically controlled water bath and some means of speeding the blood transfusion.
2. A central venous and/or pulmonary artery catheter.
3. An arterial pressure line.
4. An ECG to include lead II to monitor dysrhythmias and lead CM5 to monitor myocardial ischaemia.
5. A means of measuring core and skin temperature.
6. A thermostatically controlled water or warm air (Bair hugger) blanket for use during the operation.
7. A urinary bladder catheter.
8. A nasogastric tube, since many of these patients suffer from some degree of postoperative ileus.

Other standard anaesthetic monitoring, for example, pulse oximetry and end-tidal CO_2 monitoring must also be included.

Elective Aorto-iliac Surgery

This is commonly for elective repair of an aortic aneurysm or for the relief of occlusive aorto-iliac disease, the latter usually by grafting or by endarterectomy. This is major surgery but there is less urgency and, as a result, time for preoperative investigation and preparation of the patient.

During surgery, the aorta is clamped above the lesion as a consequence of which afterload to the heart increases resulting in hypertension, tachycardia and myocardial strain. The kidneys, spinal cord and the intestines will receive less blood supply and acid metabolites will accumulate below the clamp. These changes will to some extent be determined by the site of the clamp (above or below the renal vessels), myocardial function, duration of clamping and the presence of collaterals. In slowly progressive occlusive disease there is time for a collateral circulation to develop so that clamping and unclamping of the aorta tend to produce less dramatic fluctuations in blood pressure.

Unclamping results in restoration of blood flow to the pelvis and legs with resultant hypoperfusion to the brain and heart. This is prevented by optimising the preload to fill the circulation during clamping and by adequate cardiovascular monitoring.

Techniques suitable for anaesthesia include an oxygen–nitrous oxide muscle-relaxant technique with opiate and/or inhalational adjuvants.

Regional anaesthesia using epidural local anaesthetics and/or opiates combined with light general anaesthesia has the advantages of vasodilatation and superior pain control, but many anaesthetists fear the risks of performing epidural anaesthesia in patients who are anticoagulated.

Ruptured Abdominal Aortic Aneurysm

The rupture of an abdominal aneurysm, whether into the peritoneal cavity, retroperitoneally or into the bowel, is potentially lethal and carries a high mortality. Death occurs either from massive blood loss or from the associated hypotension which is poorly tolerated by patients with arteriosclerosis. These may be extreme surgical emergencies where resuscitation is not possible until the abdomen has been opened and the aorta clamped.

It has been suggested that the muscular fasciculations associated with suxamethonium may cause further bleeding from the aneurysm. These may be reduced or avoided by preliminary administration of a small dose of a non-depolarising relaxant or by intubation with one of this group of relaxants, for example, vecuronium or atracurium. Unfortunately the reduction in intra-abdominal pressure resulting from muscular relaxation can also cause renewed bleeding by removing pressure 'tamponade' and it is wise to anaesthetise the patient on the operating table with the surgeon ready to start. These patients are all at risk from inhalation of gastric contents and a 'crash induction' (Chapter 24) technique should be performed.

Maintenance of anaesthesia is as for elective cases (see above). The patient's cardiovascular status is carefully monitored and blood or other intravenous fluids are given as appropriate, as blood loss is significantly higher than in elective cases.

Impaired coagulation may be seen either due to depletion of clotting factors caused by the massive blood transfusion, or occasionally due to disseminated intravascular coagulation.

These patients should almost always be electively ventilated for several hours postoperatively.

Dissecting Aneurysm of the Aorta

This is not a true aneurysm, but a break occurring in the intima (inner lining) that allows blood to escape from the lumen of the aorta and to track longitudinally between the layers of the aortic wall, sometimes for a considerable distance. If rupture occurs through the outer coats of the aorta, the outcome is quickly fatal. If this does not occur, various complications may result from occlusion of various branches of the aorta which may occur if the dissection spreads as far as their points of origin from the aorta. Thus, renal or spinal cord ischaemia may result from occlusion of the renal or lumbar arteries.

Treatment is usually conservative with attempts to relieve the severe pain associated with the condition and induced hypotension to try to contain the dissection. Thoracic epidural analgesia is one method of achieving both these aims. Surgery is sometimes performed to provide a re-entry ostium to relieve the pressure occluding the important renal or lumbar arteries. Dissection usually starts in the thoracic aorta, and to prevent the marked rise in blood pressure which occurs on clamping the aorta, it is sometimes necessary to induce hypotension, for example, with sodium nitroprusside.

Femoropopliteal Surgery

Surgery on arteries distal to the inguinal ligament is still on relatively large-bore arteries in patients with generalised cardiovascular disease, but the problems of surgery itself are considerably less. Should haemorrhage occur it is more easily controlled than in the abdomen and clamping and unclamping problems are minimal, not only because these arteries are smaller but because they have usually been occluded, or relatively occluded, for some time. Furthermore, surgery is only taking place on one limb. The commonest operations are femoropopliteal bypass using synthetic grafts or a strip of the patient's own long saphenous vein, or endarterectomy.

Peripheral Vascular Emergencies

These may be caused by trauma, embolism or sudden extension of a thrombus. Trauma usually occurs in younger patients who are basically fit, unless they are suffering from multiple injuries. In these cases anaesthesia has the usual potentially dangerous implications of any emergency, but otherwise is largely concerned with the appropriate correction of blood loss. Emboli usually arise either from a fibrillating atrium, from a mural thrombus associated with myocardial infarction, or less commonly as a detached vegetation from a heart valve in subacute bacterial endocarditis. In all these conditions the patient may be seriously ill from the underlying disease, but fortunately the operations can often be easily carried out under local infiltration analgesia. Rapid occlusion of an artery may also occur with thrombus formation, although this is not usually as dramatic as in the case of trauma or embolism.

Whatever the cause, the sudden nature of the arterial obstruction tends to produce vasospasm in the surrounding small vessels. This reduces the adequacy of any collateral circulation past the obstruction. Sympathetic nerve block (e.g. lumbar sympathetic chain block) may improve the peripheral circulation by relieving the spasm.

Microvascular Surgery

See Chapter 29.

● EXTRACRANIAL VASCULAR SURGERY

This type of surgery is designed to restore the blood supply in the arteries carrying the oxygen supply to the brain and to prevent thrombi from the atheromatous plaques in these vessels causing further strokes. The commonest operations are bypass grafting or endarterectomy. As the arterial disease is generalised, clamping of the vessel to be operated on may result in acute cerebral ischaemia. For this reason, many surgeons insert a temporary arterial bypass from the common carotid artery proximally to the internal carotid beyond the occlusion. Many patients are treated hypertensives and, as a sudden rise in blood pressure may lead to cerebral haemorrhage and a fall in blood pressure to a reduction in cerebral blood flow, it is important during anaesthesia to maintain the blood pressure as near their treated level as possible.

Many of the requirements of neurosurgical anaesthesia (Chapter 36) apply also to anaesthesia for surgery on the arteries supplying the brain. For example, anything but very mild degrees of hypercarbia or hypocarbia should be avoided. On emergence from anaesthesia, about one-third of patients develop severe hypertension, with the threat of cerebral haemorrhage. An infusion of labetalol (Trandate) or the slow injection of propranolol, sometimes with hydralazine, has been suggested as a means of controlling blood pressure at this time.

In many centres these procedures are now performed with the patient awake to facilitate neurological assessment. Regional anaesthesia is then performed with superficial and deep cervical plexus blocks (C2–4 nerve roots).

● VASCULAR RADIOLOGY

Most vascular radiological investigations can be carried out under local analgesia except in children and uncooperative adults. Injection of the radio-opaque dye is not exactly painful, but produces a somewhat unpleasant burning sensation which may cause the patient to move and spoil the quality of the films. For this reason, in less cooperative patients, better results are likely to be obtained under general anaesthesia.

The investigation in this branch of radiology, which is most commonly carried out under general anaesthesia, is translumbar aortography. For this the patient lies prone on the X-ray table and a long needle is inserted through the lumbar region into the aorta. Dye is then injected forcibly into the aorta and the table moves so that the X-ray camera can take sequential pictures of the dye as it passes down the lower limbs. Once again, anaesthesia is being carried out in patients with less than perfect cardiovascular systems – this time in the prone position. In this position, even with supports under the patient's hips and chest, carbon dioxide is likely to be retained if respiration is allowed to be spontaneous, and for this reason controlled ventilation is preferred. Almost all vascular radiology is now performed via an arterial catheter inserted under local anaesthesia in the groin. This has minimised the use of general anaesthesia in the radiology department, except in children and uncooperative adults.

34

Anaesthesia for Thoracic Surgery

•Endobronchial and one-lung anaesthesia •Pneumonectomy or lobectomy •Bronchopleural fistula •Oesophagectomy •General anaesthesia for bronchoscopy •Local anaesthesia for bronchoscopy •Tracheostomy •Chest drains •Postoperative thoracic care

The thorax contains both the lungs and pleura, the trachea and bronchi, the oesophagus, the heart and the great vessels. This chapter deals with anaesthesia for surgery of the lungs, trachea, bronchi and oesophagus, cardiac surgery being dealt with in Chapter 35.

The lungs are each surrounded by two layers of pleura – the parietal pleura attached to the chest wall, and the visceral pleura which surrounds the lung itself. The negative pressure existing within the pleural space is responsible for maintaining the lung in the expanded position, even in expiration. An increase in negative intrapleural pressure brought about by thoracic wall expansion during inspiration, together with the two layers of pleura remaining adherent due to surface tension, is responsible for lung expansion. If the pleural space is exposed to atmospheric pressure caused either by air entering it from inside via the bronchi (bronchopleural fistula) or externally due to chest wall injury, the resulting pneumothorax allows the lung to collapse. This collapse is further enhanced by the negative pressure created during inspiration, but can be prevented by positive pressure inspiration – in other words, artificial ventilation. Intermittent positive pressure ventilation (IPPV) is therefore an essential part of thoracic anaesthesia, maintaining the lungs in an expanded state during the operation with the chest open. This equal expansion of both lungs also prevents 'mediastinal flap', which results from uneven inflation of the lungs during normal breathing in the presence of a pneumothorax and may result in severely impaired venous return.

Thoracic anaesthesia in the presence of an open chest is comparatively straightforward provided that artificial ventilation is employed; an identical anaesthetic technique to that employed for abdominal laparotomy is perfectly suitable for thoracotomy provided that the surgeon is able to work with both of the patient's lungs expanded and ventilated. Many of the complications of thoracic anaesthesia result from the need to collapse one of the lungs in order to provide surgical access for lung or oesophageal resection. Most anaesthetists therefore employ a nitrous oxide/oxygen, relaxant, analgesic anaesthetic technique, using IPPV, supplemented by thoracic epidural anaesthesia, the latter also providing optimal postoperative analgesia. Although in the past a considerable amount of thoracic anaesthesia, particularly in patients with tuberculosis, was carried out under local or regional anaesthesia alone, this has now been largely superseded by general anaesthetic techniques.

● ENDOBRONCHIAL AND ONE-LUNG ANAESTHESIA

If the surgeon is happy to operate on a moving lung, thoracic anaesthesia is possible with an endotracheal tube, but many surgeons prefer to operate on a still lung or to be able to retract the lung away from the operative field in, for example, oesophagectomy. Selective intubation of either the right or left main bronchus (Fig. 34.1) allows independent ventilation of either right or left lung while the other lung is allowed to collapse.

Double-lumen endobronchial tubes are widely used for this purpose and consist of two separate tubes lying side by side, either in the anterior–posterior or lateral plane, one of which is long, cuffed and designed to fit

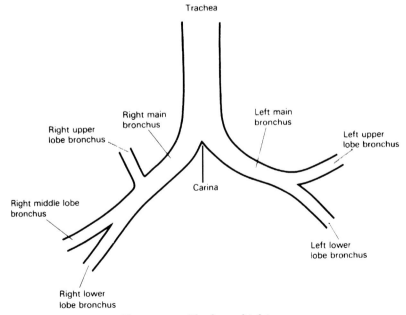

Figure 34.1 The bronchial tree.

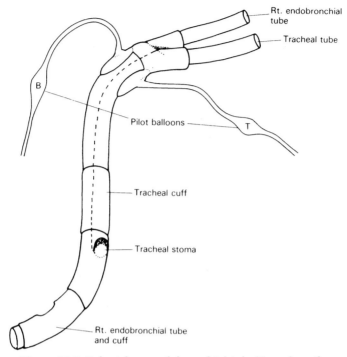

Figure 34.2 Robertshaw endobronchial tube/Bronchocath.

in either the right or left main bronchus while the other terminates in the trachea (Fig. 34.2). Such tubes allow independent ventilation of either the right or left lung and for this reason it is usual to use a left-sided tube where possible, thereby avoiding placing a bronchial cuff in the upper part of the right main bronchus and possibly occluding the right upper lobe. Occasionally the right upper lobe bronchus arises from the trachea rather than the right main bronchus and in both these situations right upper lobe collapse may occur, although an abnormal right upper lobe bronchus should have been detected by bronchoscopy before intubation. In addition to allowing independent ventilation of the right and left lung, endobronchial anaesthesia isolates an infected lung from its 'clean' partner. In cases of chronic lung infection – such as bronchiectasis or bronchopleural fistula with an empyema – inadvertent spillage of pus from the bad to the good lung may result in severe postoperative complications. Before the advent of double-lumen tubes, a bronchus blocker was often inserted under direct vision through a bronchoscope into the main bronchus of the infected lung, thereby preventing spillage and allowing the good lung to be intubated with an endobronchial tube.

● PNEUMONECTOMY OR LOBECTOMY

Resection of all or part of one lung is usually performed for either neoplastic disease or bronchiectasis, a chronic inflammatory condition of the lung which usually affects the bases and produces severe destruction of lung tissue. Many of the patients presenting for lung resection are severely incapacitated by breathlessness but nevertheless tolerate operations reasonably well. By the nature of the disease they are often heavy smokers and may already have a limited exercise tolerance. Diagnosis has usually been made by preoperative bronchoscopy but, if there is any doubt, anaesthetic induction should allow for a further bronchoscopy before intubation. An intravenous infusion is set up under local anaesthesia, the patient is pre-oxygenated for a full 5 min and anaesthesia is then induced with intravenous analgesia, propofol and a muscle relaxant, either suxamethonium, later to be followed by atracurium or vecuronium, or a non-depolarising relaxant in the first instance. A range of endobronchial tubes should always be available, a large and medium Robertshaw for a man and a medium and small Robertshaw for a woman. Some anaesthetists prefer the disposable Bronchocath as an alternative and other varieties are available. The position of the tube is checked by first inflating the tracheal cuff and confirming ventilation of both lungs. The endobronchial cuff is then inflated until there is no leak back past it when positive pressure is applied solely down that half of the double-lumen tube, auscultation confirming that only that lung is being inflated (with special attention to the right upper lobe with right-sided tubes). Some anaesthetists insist on using a fibreoptic bronchoscope inside the endobronchial tube, to confirm correct positioning. The correct functioning of the tube should be rechecked when the patient has been positioned on the operating table. This check should be repeated when the patient has been positioned in the full lateral position for the operation, because the tube may slip during turning.

Anaesthesia may then proceed in the usual way until the chest is opened and it is necessary to collapse the upper lung. It is important to realise at this point that in normal circumstances in an erect subject, while blood flows predominantly to the dependent part of the lung, some gas flows to the top of the lung. With the patient on their side, this variation in blood and gas flow still occurs, with a relatively higher proportion of blood flowing to the dependent lung. If the upper lung is then collapsed, but still perfused, a further imbalance will develop between gas and blood supply to the dependent lung. This is known as a ventilation/perfusion imbalance and may result in relative hypoxia. It is therefore essential to increase the inspired oxygen concentration during one-lung anaesthesia. This may be achieved by using either 50% oxygen in nitrous oxide together with supplementary analgesia, or 100% oxygen and a volatile agent, for example, isoflurane, or total intravenous anaesthesia (TIVA) with an air/oxygen

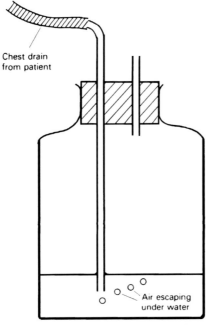

Chest drain
from patient

Air escaping
under water

Figure 34.3 Underwater seal bottle.

mixture. The two former techniques have the advantage that the patient wakes easily at the end of operation and is able to sit up and breathe deeply in the early postoperative period.

One-lung anaesthesia should not be undertaken if, when the lung is collapsed, the patient is unable to maintain adequate oxygenation even with supplementary oxygen during anaesthesia, as they will never be able to lead a normal life when breathing air. Other indices of inadequate oxygenation during one-lung anaesthesia are a rising pulse rate or blood pressure occurring soon after the lung has been collapsed. In any of these events the anaesthetist and surgeon should consult before proceeding with the operation.

If the lung has not been totally resected, it is important at the end of the operation to ensure its complete re-expansion, which requires considerable pressure on the reservoir bag of the anaesthetic circuit. The thoracic cavity must be drained after all operations to avoid accumulation of either air or blood which may impede lung expansion. Air is drained through an apical thoracic drain and blood through a basal one, both linked to underwater seal bottles (Fig. 34.3).

These allow air and blood to leave the chest but prevent air being sucked into the chest during the negative inspiratory phase. When satisfactory lung expansion has been achieved and the chest wall is closed, neuromuscular blockade is reversed and the patient sat upright in bed and given supplementary oxygen. An early postoperative chest X-ray is essential to ensure adequate expansion of the remaining lung and also the correct placement of chest drains. During transfer of the patient, if the drains are raised from the floor their tubing should be clamped to prevent the water being siphoned back into the chest.

Postoperative analgesia is often a problem after thoracotomy, and intercostal blocks at the time of operation may considerably help to relieve pain. Since systemic analgesics are often relatively ineffective, continuous thoracic epidural anaesthesia (Chapter 42) is now used in almost all cases. This allows painless deep breathing and coughing in the postoperative period when infection or collapse of the remaining lung tissue may produce severe complications. Other techniques such as paravertebral or intrapleural blocks are also useful and relatively free from some of the side-effects of epidural, such as hypotension, but are by no means 100% effective.

● BRONCHOPLEURAL FISTULA

A fistula between the lung and the pleural cavity allows free flow of air in and out of the pleural space. Provided that a valvular system does not exist, the affected lung will collapse and external chest drainage will only permit re-expansion so long as the chest drain remains in position. If the pleural contents, usually fluid, become infected and form an empyema, surgical treatment is usually indicated; however, a normal induction and endobronchial intubation would result in severe complications. In the presence of a bronchopleural fistula, IPPV results in increased intrapleural pressure and therefore the creation of a tension pneumothorax; for this reason patients with bronchopleural fistulae must be allowed to breathe spontaneously until endobronchial intubation has been accomplished. In addition, if infection is present either as an empyema or as chronic bronchiectasis, the patient should be positioned prior to induction so that spill of the infected material into the opposite lung does not occur. Induction of anaesthesia should ensure that the patient does not stop breathing, and for this reason an inhalational induction in the sitting position is usually thought to be ideal. Once intubation of the opposite lung has been achieved, a normal one-lung thoracic anaesthetic technique may be used and pus from the offending lung can be aspirated up the opposite endobronchial tube lumen.

● OESOPHAGECTOMY

In oesophagectomy, endobronchial and one-lung anaesthesia are employed simply to facilitate operative dissection and anastomosis of the oesophagus in the chest. For the lower third of the oesophagus a left thoracotomy is usual, though for higher lesions a right-sided approach is more convenient. In either situation the overlying lung is usually collapsed during the operative procedure, although as lung resection is not involved, straightforward re-expansion of the lung without subsequent problems is generally achieved. Postoperative pain seems to be greater than sometimes occurs with pneumonectomy, and considerable care is necessary to avoid postoperative chest infections.

● GENERAL ANAESTHESIA FOR BRONCHOSCOPY

Bronchoscopy is used for either diagnostic or therapeutic purposes, and with the advent of the fibreoptic bronchoscope many procedures do not now require full general anaesthesia. Rigid bronchoscopy, however, is still carried out in many centres, particularly before thoracic work, as it is often easier directly to visualise and biopsy tumours with this technique. The anaesthetic requirements are that the patient should be relatively lightly anaesthetised, oxygenated and able to wake quickly postoperatively, to maintain their own airway and to cough up any blood and other secretions which have accumulated during the procedure. An indwelling needle is essential and pre-oxygenation is followed by a technique using incremental propofol and suxamethonium, supplemented by artificial ventilation with a Venturi system using oxygen attached to a side limb of the bronchoscope. High-pressure Entonox is sometimes used in place of oxygen to provide a greater depth of anaesthesia and possibly reduce the risk of awareness during this procedure. It is important to ensure adequate oxygenation at all times as many patients have considerable cardiovascular or other problems exacerbated by the hypoxia which may result from a severe coughing spasm.

If a 'Stortz' bronchoscope is used, the closed system with a viewing window over the end of the bronchoscope allows direct connection to a coaxial circuit via the special side port and a conventional anaesthetic using spontaneous ventilation with nitrous oxide, oxygen and halothane or isoflurane.

High-frequency oscillation and high-frequency jet ventilation are two newer ventilatory techniques which are particularly suitable for use during rigid bronchoscopy. They rely upon very rapid small volume oscillations of gas flow in and out of the lungs with minimal changes in airway pressure. As such, they provide adequate alveolar ventilation, arterial oxygenation and carbon dioxide extraction without significant lung movement, making them ideally suited to this procedure. They have also been used in patients with bronchopleural fistulae and severely reduced pulmonary compliance, such as shock lung and pulmonary contusion, to prevent the development of high airway pressures. They are not widely available at present and are still considerably more expensive than conventional ventilators.

Fibreoptic bronchoscopy seldom requires general anaesthesia, although if required a propofol/nitrous oxide/oxygen and isoflurane technique using a small endotracheal tube, which allows the fibreoptic instrument to be passed alongside, or a larger tube through which the bronchoscope can be introduced, is usually found to be sufficient.

● LOCAL ANAESTHESIA FOR BRONCHOSCOPY

Bronchoscopy is a relatively unpleasant procedure, particularly when a rigid instrument is used, but some patients are only suitable for a local anaesthetic technique. In this event premedication is often used and the patient's mouth and pharynx are then anaesthetised by encouraging them to suck an amethocaine lozenge. The overall amount of local anaesthetic to be used is then poured out, thus avoiding the easy error of inadvertently administering an overdose of lignocaine. Progressive anaesthesia of the posterior pharyngeal wall, the fauces, the pyriform fossae and the larynx are then carried out, usually with the patient in the semi-recumbent position, and finally a small dose of midazolam is usually administered intravenously before the bronchoscopic procedure. Local anaesthesia of the larynx is contraindicated in patients in whom biopsies are being taken, because this prevents adequate postoperative coughing and expectoration of blood and other secretions.

● TRACHEOSTOMY

Although tracheostomy may be performed as an emergency or life-saving procedure, it is usually limited nowadays to patients requiring prolonged artificial ventilation or those undergoing laryngectomy as a result of neoplastic disease or trauma. Soft-cuffed, non-irritant endotracheal tubes have considerably reduced the incidence of tracheostomy in intensive care. The procedure, usually carried out under general anaesthesia except in severely ill or unconscious patients, involves making an aperture in the trachea, usually at the region of the second and third tracheal rings, with the creation of an anterior (Björk) flap attached to the skin to provide a ledge over which the tracheostomy tube is inserted.

Anaesthetic complications which may arise from tracheostomy are largely limited to those concerned with the initial intubation of the patient – which will have been done already if they are receiving artificial ventilation. In patients with carcinoma or other obstructive lesions, extreme difficulty may initially be experienced in inserting an endotracheal tube, and this may require considerable preoperative manipulation using extremely small uncuffed endotracheal tubes, introducers, etc. Tracheostomy may also occasionally be required before thyroidectomy in patients with a large retrosternal thyroid producing tracheal compression. This may result in a soft trachea (tracheomalacia) postoperatively, which some surgeons prefer to protect with a temporary tracheostomy.

Intra-operative anaesthetic management varies between a spontaneous respiration technique and IPPV. The former has the advantage that the patient breathes during the changeover period between endotracheal and tracheostomy tubes, which may help if the tracheostome is difficult to cannulate. It is essential before tracheostomy that the size of the tube required be available together with all the relevant connections, to allow reconnection to the anaesthetic equipment under the towels. If this is not done a vital part is invariably found to be missing. It is important also to have a range of tracheostomy tubes available, as in some cases a small internal diameter trachea is extremely difficult to predict. Once inserted, and before attachment to the ventilator, the tracheostomy tube should be sucked out to remove secretions and to allow the free passage of a suction catheter, thereby ensuring that it has not been misplaced into the anterior mediastinum, since only a few litres of air in the mediastinum may cause considerable cardiovascular embarrassment. Usually a cuffed tracheostomy tube is inserted and left in position for a few days before being replaced by a longer-term silver tube.

Percutaneous Tracheostomy

This is now frequently used in intensive care patients undergoing long-term ventilation for respiratory failure. The technique utilises the Seldinger principle whereby a guidewire is introduced into the trachea over which a series of dilators are railroaded. Finally a conventional cuffed tracheostomy tube is introduced into the tracheostome. This technique, which can be safely performed in the intensive care unit, is particularly useful in very sick patients who are unsuitable for transfer to theatre, but normally requires administration of a general anaesthetic. Since most patients are already sedated and ventilated, this does not usually present a problem, although a specialist must be present to administer anaesthesia and look after the endotracheal tube and airway during the changeover period to the tracheostomy.

● CHEST DRAINS

As already mentioned, chest drains placed either at the apex of the lung to drain air or at the base of the lung to drain blood are always connected to an underwater seal drainage bottle (see Fig. 34.3). The tubing from the patient is attached via a rigid, transparent tube, which passes under the surface of the water, the depth to which the tube is inserted in the water presenting a small resistance to expiration, usually of 3–4 cm. The initial level of water in the bottle must be accurately recorded to allow the additional volume of blood collecting to be measured. It is important also to ensure that the surface area of the water in the chest drainage bottle is large by comparison with the diameter of the chest tube, because considerable turbulence may occur as gas bubbles violently out of the chest during coughing or maximal expiration. In addition, if the drainage bottle is narrow, a small amount of fluid or blood draining from the chest will considerably raise the fluid level and therefore the depth to which the chest tube is submerged and the resistance to expiration. If the tube is submerged to an inadequate depth, a large inspiration will draw up water, and then, when this is exhausted, air will be sucked up the tube.

● POSTOPERATIVE THORACIC CARE

In most thoracic units, postoperative artificial ventilation is relatively rare, and patients are nursed in a high-dependency area on the normal thoracic ward. Experienced nursing care, together with oxygen, suction and the necessary equipment for emergency intubation and ventilation, should be readily available. Postoperative respiratory failure may develop for several reasons, but should not be due to the patient being unable to manage on one lung, as this should have been detected at the time of operation (see above).

Pulmonary oedema, infection and, more commonly, postoperative pain leading to collapse and consolidation are the usual causes of respiratory failure in the immediate postoperative period, and of these the control of pain is probably the most important. Accurate volume replacement is also essential, particularly as many of the patients have concomitant cardio-vascular disease. The development of atrial fibrillation, particularly where a lung tumour has involved the pericardium in the older age group of patients, is common, and intra-operative digitalisation is recommended in all thoracotomy patients over the age of 60, to prevent the development of fast postoperative atrial fibrillation, which may precipitate cardiac failure. Chest drains are usually left in position for several days until both air and fluid have stopped leaking. They are then clamped but left in place for a further 24 h when the patient is examined by X-ray. If there has been no accumulation of air or blood, they may then be removed safely.

35

Anaesthesia for Open Heart Surgery

•Technique of cardiopulmonary bypass •Preoperative patient assessment •Anaesthetic technique •Anaesthetic management during surgery •Postoperative management

The development of cardiopulmonary bypass (CPB), and its recent refinement into a relatively safe and routine technique, has permitted a significant broadening of the scope of cardiac surgery. Whereas previously operations were limited to comparatively simple procedures such as repairs of minor congenital defects, the ability to operate on a still, non-beating heart which is not in circuit with the vascular system has enabled complex intracardiac procedures such as valve replacements, septal defect repairs, aorto-coronary bypass grafting and even cardiac transplants to be performed.

Heart operations can be divided into 'closed heart' procedures, such as pericardectomy, closed mitral valvotomy and ligation of persistent ductus arteriosus, in which the heart and lungs function normally, and 'open heart' procedures, in which blood to the heart and lungs is diverted – 'bypassed' – to an extracorporeal circuit (ECC) comprising a pump and gas exchanger, allowing arrest of lung ventilation and heart beat. Most cardiac surgical operations are now performed on an arrested heart during CPB, and as such procedures become more common so the incidence of reoperations has increased: re-entering a chest poses special risks and technical difficulties. This chapter describes the anaesthetic management of adult patients undergoing open heart surgery.

Although there are aspects to patient assessment and anaesthetic technique which are unique to cardiac surgery, it should be stressed that all the general considerations for good, safe anaesthetic management apply equally in anaesthesia for cardiac procedures.

● TECHNIQUE OF CARDIOPULMONARY BYPASS

Extracorporeal Circulation

If the patient's heart and lungs are to be arrested and bypassed, a device to pump and oxygenate the blood must be utilised, to substitute for the heart and lungs, respectively. The essential components of the CPB circuit therefore include: (a) a filter, (b) a reservoir, (c) a pump, (d) a heat exchanger, (e) an oxygenator, and (f) tubing.

Pump

Mechanically driven roller pumps are most commonly used. Blood flow is usually constant ('non-pulsatile') and is produced by rotating rollers compressing flexible tubing against a rigid semicircular track; this can be modified to produce a pulsatile waveform, which may improve tissue perfusion and organ preservation.

Oxygenator

The gas exchange unit mimics the lung, and must therefore expose a large surface area of blood for oxygen uptake and carbon dioxide elimination. There are two main types of oxygenator:

1. direct blood-gas contact oxygenator
   (a) rotating disc oxygenator
   (b) bubble oxygenator
2. membrane oxygenator
   (a) flat sheet
   (b) hollow fibre.

Direct contact oxygenators are cheap and efficient but tend to damage blood components; their use is declining. The membrane oxygenator is more anatomically and physiologically similar to the lung, having a micro-porous membrane which separates gas and blood phases and allows gas exchange to occur. There is less damage to blood cells, efficiency is good and cost has decreased relatively such that these are now the oxygenator type of choice.

Bypass Circuit

This is illustrated in Figure 35.1. Venous blood bypasses the patient's heart via a cannula placed in the right atrium; if the right atrium is to be opened during surgery two cannulae are inserted, in the superior and inferior venae cavae, which are then snared. The venous blood drains under gravity

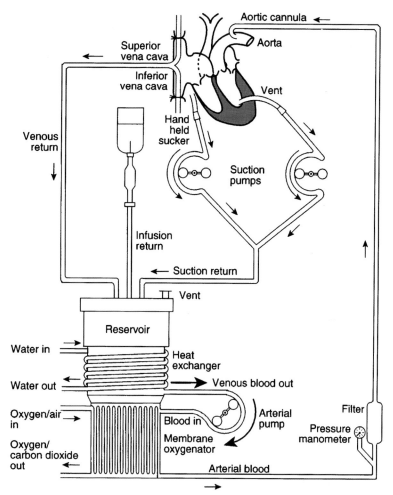

Figure 35.1 Cardiopulmonary bypass circuit.

by a siphon effect through a filter and into the reservoir, from where it is pumped through the heat exchanger and oxygenator into a cannula placed in the ascending aorta (or less frequently, the femoral artery). Bubble oxygenators also require a defoaming unit. If bypass is partial, with some pulmonary blood flow, or if the aortic valve is regurgitant, the left ventricle may fill with blood and distend, in which case a separate venting cannula inserted through the apex of the heart is used. Hand-held suckers powered by additional pumps are routinely employed ('soft' or 'pump' suction), and blood scavenged from the wound by these devices is returned to the bypass reservoir for reinfusion.

Circuit Priming

The bypass circuit is primed with fluid before being connected to the patient. Originally this prime comprised anticoagulated whole blood; however, it is now recognised that this is expensive and potentially dangerous, and a bloodless prime consisting of a clear crystalloid solution (e.g. Ringer's lactate, Hartmann's solution, 1.5–2.0 l) is therefore used. Some centres supplement this with additives according to individual recipes, for example, heparin (100 IU/kg body weight), mannitol (0.25 g/kg) or sodium bicarbonate (1 mmol/kg). The clear prime will dilute the patient's blood which reduces haematocrit, decreasing oxygen carriage (detrimental), but this is outweighed by the decreased blood viscosity which increases tissue perfusion (beneficial). In the case of paediatric heart operations, the dilution of the patient's blood may be excessive and red cells may be added to maintain the haematocrit at an acceptable level.

● PREOPERATIVE PATIENT ASSESSMENT

The patient is visited by surgical, anaesthetic, physiotherapy and postoperative care teams and the operation and postoperative period are explained. This is crucial to decrease patient anxiety and hence cardiovascular stress. A general anaesthetic assessment is performed, as before any operation, but some additional factors are addressed. Coronary artery disease has a strong association with diabetes mellitus, hypertension and smoking; smokers, and patients in heart failure, may have compromised pulmonary function. Patients with valvar heart disease are at risk of infective endocarditis and require a dental check, and treatment if necessary. The nature and severity of the cardiac lesion is evaluated using routine investigations (electrocardiography (ECG), chest X-ray) and more specialised tests (exercise ECG, echocardiography, cardiac catheterisation and angiography, radionuclide imaging) (Table 35.1). Besides yielding information on the anatomical (surgical) nature of the lesion, they permit an assessment of ventricular function.

Preoperative Drug Therapy

Most patients will be receiving cardiac drugs preoperatively. Many of these, including β-adrenergic-blocking drugs (e.g. atenolol), calcium-channel-blocking drugs (e.g. nifedipine) and nitrates are continued up to the time of surgery. Increasingly, patients are presenting on angiotensin-converting enzyme (ACE) inhibitors (e.g. lisinopril); when or whether to discontinue them is controversial as they cause significant vasodilatation postoperatively. Diuretics are continued until the day before operation,

Table 35.1 Laboratory investigations

Haematology	Full blood count	(Haemoglobin > 11 g/dl)
	Sickle cell test	(Where appropriate)
	Clotting screen	(Normal prothrombin time)
	Blood cross-match	(Usually 4 units)
Biochemistry	Urea/creatinine and electrolytes	(NB: Danger of hypokalaemia in patients receiving long-term diuretics; renal impairment in diabetics)
	Blood glucose	(Diabetics at risk of coronary artery disease)
	Liver function tests	(May be abnormal in right ventricular failure)
	Cardiac enzymes	(In emergency patients undergoing coronary artery grafting)
	Blood gases	(Assessment of pulmonary function/gas exchange)
Microbiology	Midstream urine and urinalysis	
	Swabbing of nose, throat and perineum	
	Hepatitis status	(Where appropriate)
	Human immunodeficiency virus (HIV)	(Where appropriate)
Radiology/others	ECG	($\pm$ Exercise stress test)
	Chest radiograph	(Cardiomegaly, pulmonary oedema)
	Pulmonary function tests	(Where appropriate)
	Echocardiography	(Cardiac anatomy and function)
	Cardiac catheterisation and angiography	(Ejection fraction, coronary anatomy)

while digoxin is usually stopped 36–48 h preoperatively (to decrease hypokalaemia-associated dysrhythmias per- and postoperatively). Anticoagulants (e.g. warfarin) are stopped 2–3 days before surgery to normalise prothrombin time; if this renders the risk of thromboembolisation unacceptably high, the patient may be switched from warfarin to an intravenous heparin infusion (discontinued 6 h preoperatively), or warfarin may be continued and the coagulation defect corrected per-operatively by infusion of fresh frozen plasma. Aspirin is discontinued 2 weeks before operation to permit recovery of platelet function.

Patients presenting for emergency coronary surgery are commonly receiving glyceryl trinitrate (GTN) and/or heparin infusions; the former may be continued throughout the procedure, while the latter is stopped 6 h preoperatively if time and patient condition permit.

● ANAESTHETIC TECHNIQUE

Premedication

A careful explanation, with sympathetic rapport, is the most important preoperative preparation. Traditionally, a heavy opiate-based premedication is used (e.g. morphine, 10–15 mg) combined with hyoscine (0.2–0.4 mg). Atropine is generally avoided to prevent excessive tachycardia. Doses may be decreased in patients with a low cardiac output. Alternatively, an oral dose of benzodiazepine (e.g. diazepam, 5–10 mg; temazepam, 10–20 mg) may be used, especially if the patient is unduly anxious. GTN may also be administered (e.g. as a skin patch), and oxygen is given through a face mask. Since the induction sequence in cardiac anaesthesia is relatively long, there is a case for inclusion of metoclopramide and an H_2 antagonist (e.g. ranitidine) or a proton pump inhibitor (omeprazole) with the premedication to decrease the risk of acid aspiration.

Induction

The aims of induction of anaesthesia for cardiac surgery are to produce unconsciousness while maintaining a stable cardiovascular system in which myocardial oxygen demand is minimised and myocardial oxygen supply is maximised. The main determinants involved are (systemic arterial) blood pressure and heart rate; coronary blood flow occurs during diastole and a slow pulse (long diastole) and high diastolic pressure therefore optimise oxygen supply, while oxygen demand is related to ventricular wall tension (high systolic pressure, itself related to contractility and systemic vascular resistance). Hence during induction of anaesthesia:

1. Systolic hypertension and tachycardia should be avoided by producing a smooth loss of consciousness without coughing or straining. Intubation should not be attempted until sufficient depth of anaesthesia and relaxation are achieved.
2. Myocardial depression with decreased cardiac output and diastolic hypotension should be avoided.
3. Tachycardia and excessive bradycardia should be avoided.

Induction of anaesthesia is a critical time for many of these patients and drug dosages may need to be modified. Patients with poor ventricular function may require greatly decreased amounts of anaesthetic drugs, which must therefore be titrated in against patient response. Resuscitative drugs and a defibrillator must be available in the anaesthetic room.

Before induction of anaesthesia, a peripheral intravenous cannula and an arterial cannula (usually radial) are placed under local analgesia, and a pulse oximeter and ECG leads are connected (Fig. 35.2). The patient is pre-oxygenated. Fentanyl (5–20 μg/kg) supplemented by a small dose of

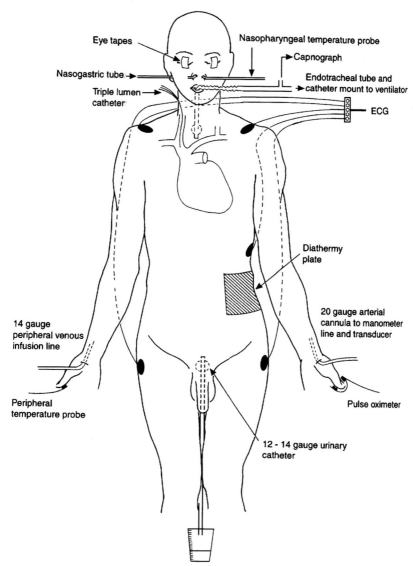

Figure 35.2 Cannulation and monitoring before open heart surgery.

thiopentone (1–2 mg/kg) or etomidate (0.1–0.2 mg/kg) will usually achieve unconsciousness while maintaining haemodynamic stability; pancuronium bromide (0.1–0.2 mg/kg) or vecuronium (0.1–0.2 mg/kg) is used for muscle paralysis prior to tracheal intubation with a low-pressure cuff oral endotracheal tube. Intermittent positive pressure ventilation (IPPV) is mandatory since the chest will be opened. A triple-lumen central venous catheter is placed in the right internal jugular vein – one lumen is used for measuring central venous (right atrial) pressure and administration of drugs, another lumen is used for infusing cardiostimulant drugs (e.g. inotropes), while the third lumen is used for infusing vasodilators (e.g. GTN). If cardiovascular status is critically compromised prior to anaesthesia, the central venous catheter may be inserted before induction of anaesthesia under local analgesia, to permit rapid administration of cardioactive drugs during induction; occasionally a Swan-Ganz pulmonary artery catheter is passed preoperatively to monitor cardiac function more closely.

A urinary catheter is inserted, and nasopharyngeal and peripheral temperature probes are applied.

● ANAESTHETIC MANAGEMENT DURING SURGERY

The operation comprises three periods:

1. Pre-bypass period, involving patient positioning and preparation, skin incision, sternotomy, systemic heparinisation and cannulation of the aorta and right atrium/venae cavae.
2. CPB period, involving establishment of extracorporeal circulation, myocardial preservation and definitive cardiac surgery.
3. Post-bypass period, during which the patient must re-establish normal circulation, aortic and venous cannulae are removed and the chest is closed.

Pre-bypass

As with induction of anaesthesia, the aim is to achieve anaesthesia while retaining cardiovascular control, and to optimise myocardial oxygen supply versus demand. Anaesthesia is usually maintained with nitrous oxide and oxygen, supplemented with inhalational agents (e.g. halothane, isoflurane) and increments of narcotic opioids (e.g. fentanyl); alternatively total intravenous anaesthesia may be employed. Systemic arterial and central venous pressures and heart rate are kept within predetermined parameters (typically, their preoperation values); syringe pumps are used to infuse vaso- and cardioactive drugs through the dedicated central venous catheter ports. If required, atropine (0.6 mg) or isoprenaline (10 μg) is given to increase heart rate; less commonly esmolol (50 µg/kg/min), or deepening of anaesthesia, to decrease heart rate. Intravenous fluids or occasionally inotropes are used to increase arterial blood pressure, while volatile anaesthetics, GTN (0.5–5 µg/kg/min) or sodium nitroprusside (SNP; 1–5 µg/kg/min) are used to decrease blood pressure. Prophylactic antibiotics are administered, to decrease the risk of wound infection and infective endocarditis. Sternotomy is very stimulating and commonly associated with a marked increase in arterial pressure and heart rate which must be countered. Sternotomy is particularly hazardous in reoperations where the right ventricle may be adherent to the sternum and at risk of damage during sternal sawing; external defibrillator paddles should be attached and blood should be available in theatre for immediate transfusion. Arterial blood gases, plasma potassium concentration, haematocrit and activated clotting time (ACT) are measured. Aprotinin may be infused to decrease postoperative bleeding although it may increase the risk of vein graft occlusion. Before aortic cannulation, heparin (300 µg/kg) is given through the central venous catheter, with aspiration to guarantee intravascular delivery and the ACT is rechecked before commencing CPB to ensure anticoagulation is adequate (ACT >400 s). Typically the arterial pressure is lowered moderately (80–90 mmHg) prior to aortic cannulation to decrease the risk of aortic dissection/rupture.

During Cardiopulmonary Bypass

Anaesthesia

Ventilation is discontinued once CPB is established, with a low (2 l/min) flow of oxygen or air to keep the lungs slightly inflated. Maintenance of anaesthesia during CPB is complicated by dilution of drugs by the pump prime, by adsorption of certain drugs onto ECC components and by the inability to use the lungs for delivery of inhalational anaesthetics. This is partly offset by decreased drug metabolism during induced hypothermia, an effect not to be relied upon to avoid awareness and respiratory movements. Volatile anaesthetic agents can be administered through the gas flow of the oxygenator, but this creates problems with gas scavenging. Therefore, anaesthesia on bypass is usually maintained by supplemental intravenous doses of opioids (fentanyl, 2–10 µg/kg; morphine, 10–60 mg) and/or benzodiazepines (diazepam, 5–10 mg; midazolam, 5–10 mg) or more recently by an infusion of propofol (7 mg/kg/h).

Cardiopulmonary Bypass

A blood flow from the pump of 2.4 l/min/m^2 body surface area is required at 37°C, with a 30% decrease for each 10°C drop in temperature. The optimum perfusion pressure during CPB is controversial but is usually maintained at 50–80 mmHg by use of vasoconstrictor (α_1-agonist, e.g. metaraminol 1 mg) or vasodilator (α_1-antagonist, e.g. phentolamine 1 mg) drugs to modify the systemic vascular resistance.

Tissue perfusion is difficult to assess clinically while on bypass, but urine output is a useful index. A diuresis is common during and following bypass due to the crystalloid fluid load used in the pump prime and the cardioplegia solution.

Coagulation Control

As soon as CPB is established with complete mixing of patient's blood and pump prime, the ACT is again measured, and rechecked every 30 min, being maintained at >400 s by incremental doses of heparin to the ECC.

Myocardial Preservation

During bypass, oxygenated blood from the aortic cannula flows in an anterograde direction to perfuse the body, but also flows retrogradely down the ascending aorta, causing the aortic valve to shut and perfusing the myocardium through the coronary arteries (Fig. 35.3). The heart beats, although since the venous return does not fill the heart, it does not eject any blood. Surgery is performed on a non-beating heart with empty chambers – to stop the heart beating, ventricular asystole or fibrillation must be induced. The commonest method of achieving an immobile heart while preserving the myocardium from ischaemic damage is to cross-clamp the aorta immediately proximal to the aortic cannula and infuse cold (4°C) cardioplegic solution (containing potassium and procaine in Ringer's solution) under pressure into the aortic root. The cardioplegia closes the aortic valve and perfuses the myocardium through the coronary arteries, causing asystolic cardiac arrest in diastole; hypothermic cardiac preservation is supplemented by pouring ice-cold saline into the pericardium ('surface-cooling'). An initial volume of cardioplegia of 1000 ml is used, with further infusions (500 ml) every 30 min or if myocardial activity returns. This local cooling of the heart achieves a cardiac temperature of about 15°C, sufficient to prevent ischaemic damage for about 1 h, and may be assisted by more modest whole-body hypothermia (28–30°C) generated by the heat exchange unit of the ECC. Occasionally the whole body is cooled to 15–18°C on CPB and the entire circulation then stopped ('deep hypothermic circulatory arrest'), allowing surgery to be performed on the aortic root and arch.

An alternative method of achieving a relatively still heart is to induce (warm) myocardial ischaemia by cross-clamping the aorta as above,

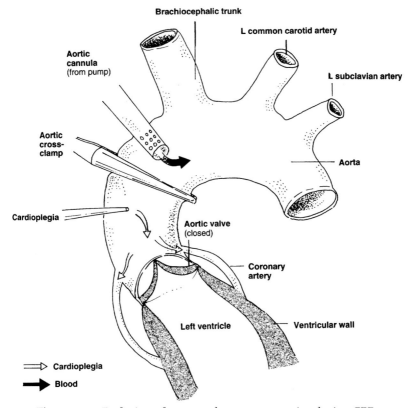

Figure 35.3 Perfusion of aorta and coronary arteries during CPB.

but then to make the heart fibrillate with an electrical 'fibrillator'. This technique does not offer myocardial protection, and therefore any procedure must be performed within the 10 min available at 37°C before ischaemic damage occurs. In practice, this is sufficient time to anastomose the bottom (coronary) end of one aorto-coronary vein graft.

In both cases myocardial reperfusion is reinstated by removing the aortic cross-clamp, permitting renewed perfusion of the coronary arteries with warm oxygenated blood from the aortic cannula. Reperfusion and rewarming are usually sufficient to induce spontaneous heart beating, but occasionally persistent ventricular asystole requires electrical (epicardial) pacing or adrenaline bolus, while ventricular fibrillation requires internal defibrillation (10–30 J) applied directly across the ventricles. Failure to defibrillate the heart may be due to potassium imbalance, hypothermia or overfilled ventricles.

Blood-gas Analysis

Arterial blood gases are monitored and checked frequently, and oxygen/air flow to the oxygenator is adjusted to produce normal values. Occasionally a metabolic acidosis develops, suggesting inadequate tissue perfusion requiring an increased pump now with peripheral vasodilatation, and possibly sodium bicarbonate (1 mmol/kg). Haematocrit is adjusted to 0.25–0.3 by adding red blood cells, diuretics or haemofiltration, if necessary.

Potassium Balance

Plasma potassium concentration is important in cardiac surgery because of the risk of perioperative dysrhythmias. Total body potassium may be depleted because of long-term diuretic therapy, and the dilution and diuresis associated with the crystalloid pump prime further lower plasma potassium concentration; potassium may also migrate intracellularly during prolonged bypass. This is partly offset by the potassium load arising from incorporation of the potassium-rich cardioplegia into the circulating blood volume. Plasma potassium concentration should therefore be measured before, frequently during, and after CPB surgery, and plasma supplements administered as necessary.

Restoration of Circulation – Termination of Bypass

Before the heart can be expected to resume maintenance of the circulation, the patient must be warm (37°C), the blood gases and electrolytes must be within normal limits, and the heart must be in a stable, effective rhythm and rate. Therefore on completion of surgery the heart is reperfused with warm oxygenated blood from the CPB pump (by removal of the aortic cross-clamp; Fig. 35.3), usually causing it to beat spontaneously (though see above). Air is removed from the chambers of the heart if they have been opened during surgery. Lung ventilation is recommenced with 100% oxygen (nitrous oxide is avoided since the diffusion effect would expand any air bubbles remaining in the circulation). The venous line on the ECC is gradually constricted, causing an increasing proportion of the venous return to flow around the atrial cannula and into the heart itself, generating ventricular filling and hence increasing ventricular ejection. This is seen as 'blips' of increasing size on the otherwise flat arterial pressure trace. Eventually the venous line is clamped completely and all venous blood returns to the heart to be pumped physiologically; the pump is stopped and the patient is 'off bypass'.

Cardiac performance is now assessed visually and by examining systemic arterial and venous pressures. If arterial pressure is low, cardiac filling and ejection, and hence cardiac output, may be increased by transfusing blood remaining in the pump reservoir through the aortic cannula. If this procedure fails to increase arterial pressure but causes the central venous pressure to rise, the heart is failing and requires inotropic support. Available drugs include calcium chloride; β_1-adrenergic agonists such as dopamine, dobutamine, adrenaline, noradrenaline and isoprenaline; phosphodiesterase inhibitors such as milrinone; and occasionally glucagon or digoxin. Excessive arterial hypertension should, however, be avoided as this increases myocardial oxygen demand and places undue mechanical stress on aortic and cardiac suture lines. Increasing use of ACE inhibitors preoperatively has resulted in more patients being vasodilated, and hence hypotensive post-bypass; this may be treated with a vasoconstrictor (e.g. noradrenaline infusion). Dysrhythmias which compromise cardiac output/ blood pressure are treated with electrical cardioversion or pacing, or the appropriate antidysrhythmic drug. If cardiac function remains poor it may be necessary for the surgeon to insert a left atrial cannula to monitor left ventricular filling pressure and hence optimise circulating blood volume and ventricular filling; alternatively, a Swan-Ganz pulmonary artery catheter may be inserted which also permits measurement of cardiac output and systemic vascular resistance. The ECG is checked to exclude myocardial ischaemia, and a trans-oesophageal echocardiogram may be performed at this stage to check ventricular filling and performance, and valve competency. Left ventricular ejection may be further assisted by the use of vasodilator drugs (e.g. GTN or SNP) to decrease the afterload (systemic vascular resistance) – 'offloading' – and/or by insertion of an intra-aortic counter-pulsation balloon pump, which also augments coronary perfusion. In extreme cases it may be necessary to go back on bypass while the problem is re-evaluated. Recently, ventricular assist devices have been used to help support the circulation in the post-bypass period while the heart recovers or a transplant organ is sought. If the problem is due to pulmonary hypertension preventing blood flow from the right heart to the left heart through the lungs, nitric oxide may be administered in an attempt to induce pulmonary vasodilatation. Epicardial pacing may need to be instigated for bradydysrhythmias.

When the circulation is stable and effective, the heparin is reversed with protamine sulphate (3 mg/kg). This may cause peripheral vasodilatation and pulmonary vasoconstriction with resulting hypotension and is therefore given slowly through a peripheral venous cannula; in excess it is itself an anticoagulant. Once administration of protamine commences the pump suckers are switched off to prevent coagulable blood being introduced into the pump reservoir. The ACT is again checked to confirm adequate reversal of anticoagulation. If excessive bleeding persists, consumption of clotting factors and platelets during bypass may be responsible, and therefore a clotting screen and platelet count should be performed followed by administration of fresh frozen plasma and platelets if necessary.

Thromboelastography is increasingly being used in the theatre setting to check coagulation and direct therapy.

The cannulae are removed, haemostasis is achieved, and drains are placed in the pericardium, mediastinum and, if opened, the pleural cavities. Epicardial pacing wires are attached, and the chest is closed. The drains are put on suction and blood loss is measured in graduated collecting bottles.

● POSTOPERATIVE MANAGEMENT

Following completion of surgery, and while still anaesthetised and venti-lated, the patient is transferred to a postoperative care unit. This may be an intensive care unit, or increasingly a dedicated cardiac high-dependency unit. The patient is only moved out of the operating theatre once cardio-vascular stability is achieved, and arterial blood pressure, ECG and pulse oximetry are monitored during the transfer. The patient is initially venti-lated on the recovery unit while full monitoring is reinstigated. Blood pres-sure control is as important postoperatively as preoperatively – hypotension causes decreased aorto-coronary vein graft and myocardial perfusion, while hypertension increases myocardial oxygen demand and risks disruption of suture lines – and blood pressure monitoring (both arterial and venous) permits assessment of circulating blood volume and fluid balance. Vaso-active infusions are continued or commenced by infusion pumps as required. The muscle relaxant is reversed.

Patients tend to be peripherally cold and vasoconstricted postoperatively, therefore the use of vasodilators (e.g. GTN or SNP) is common to assist peripheral rewarming, decrease the afterload of the left ventricle and con-trol hypertension. As the patient vasodilates and warms peripherally, blood volume redistributes, with a decrease in effective circulating volume (decreased central venous pressure), and blood volume replacement is usually required; this is in addition to intravenous infusions required to replace measured blood loss in the postoperative period. The choice of fluid depends on the patient's haematocrit and coagulation status, but colloids such as albumin solution, gelatin, blood, fresh frozen plasma and platelets may each be indicated. Urine output is usually brisk (diuresis of pump prime and cardioplegia), again leading to relative hypovolaemia, but also to hypokalaemia; potassium supplements may again be required.

Dysrhythmias are common at this time and are treated promptly to prevent compromise of cardiac output and hence graft patency. Other com-mon problems include bleeding (with the attendant risk of cardiac tam-ponade), oliguria and poor gas exchange with hypoxia, all of which are dealt with appropriately.

Patients require postoperative analgesia and this is typically morphine or alfentanil infusions; once awake, this can be patient controlled.

Non-steroidal analgesics (e.g. diclofenac) are effective adjuncts. The need for sedation depends on the imminence of extubation; if this is delayed, a propofol or midazolam infusion may be commenced. If the patient shows cardiovascular stability, with satisfactory blood pressures and peripheral perfusion (peripheral skin temperature >30°C) and good urine output (>30 ml/h), is warm and is not bleeding excessively (measured loss <100 ml/h) and is conscious with satisfactory blood gases, an attempt is made at spontaneous ventilation, and then extubation. Postoperative ventilation is only indicated for the relatively brief period of gaining cardiovascular control and stability and allowing anaesthetic drugs to wear off – usually within 2 h of transfer from the operating theatre. Following most procedures, patients are easily weaned from the ventilator and extubated, difficulties most commonly being encountered in patients with pre-existing pulmonary disease. Following successful extubation, invasive monitoring continues until haemodynamic, respiratory and metabolic stability are assured, when lines are removed and the patient is transferred to the cardiac ward.

36

Anaesthesia for Neurosurgery and Neuroradiology

● APPLIED ANATOMY AND PHYSIOLOGY

The skull is a rigid closed box, except in neonates and infants before the various component bones have fused together. This box contains the brain, blood and cerebrospinal fluid (CSF), and it is an important feature of neurosurgery that an increase in the volume occupied by one of these components must be compensated for by a decrease in the volume of one of the others. Failure to do so leads to a rise in intracranial pressure. The brain itself is composed of grey and white matter, the grey matter being the cerebral cells themselves and the white matter consisting of the nerve fibres and their surrounding myelin sheaths. The brain is surrounded by three meningeal layers – the pia, the arachnoid and the dura mater. The first of these layers is closely applied to the brain and between it and the arachnoid is the subarachnoid space containing the circulating CSF. This space is enlarged in parts of the brain to form ventricles, which contain both CSF itself and areas for secretion of this fluid, the choroid plexuses. CSF circulates in the subarachnoid space, surrounding both the brain and the spinal cord, and is reabsorbed by the arachnoid villi which lie in the superior sagittal sinus over the surface of the brain. It is essential that circulation of CSF is unimpeded because obstruction to the canals leading to and from the ventricles causes local accumulation of CSF and hydrocephalus.

● CEREBROSPINAL FLUID

In normal man there is 120 ml of CSF, of which about 25 ml is in the spinal subarachnoid space. Its composition is similar to protein-free plasma. The functions of the CSF are both to buffer the brain against movements of the skull and to surround certain parts of the brain with a fluid capable of fluctuation in its concentration of ions, for example, sodium, potassium and bicarbonate. Changes in CSF bicarbonate concentration are responsible for alterations in respiratory rate and volume mediated by the chemoreceptors. Certain drugs can pass into CSF while others cannot, since its formation is one of selective secretion. The normal CSF pressure is about 120 mmH$_2$O in the recumbent position.

● CEREBRAL BLOOD FLOW

The brain is dependent for its blood supply on four main arteries: the two internal carotid arteries and the two vertebral arteries. These anastomose at the base of the brain, forming the circle of Willis (Fig. 36.1) which then gives off the anterior, middle and posterior cerebral arteries. Because of this anastomotic link, the brain can survive with occlusion of one or even two of its main arteries. Under normal conditions the brain receives about 15% of the cardiac output and the cerebral circulation is able to regulate its own blood flow. This means that between mean arterial blood pressures of 60 and 140 mmHg the cerebral blood flow is maintained at a constant level by local alteration in the diameter of blood vessels. This process is known as autoregulation.

● GENERAL PRINCIPLES OF NEUROSURGICAL ANAESTHESIA

Neurosurgical operations usually involve either the brain or spinal cord, operations on the brain requiring a craniotomy, i.e. removal of a flap of bone to gain access to the brain substance beneath. Operative treatment may range from the removal of either an intracerebral or extracerebral tumour to the clipping of an arterial aneurysm in the region of the circle of Willis, but anaesthesia for all these operations has many factors in common. Most important of these is the prevention of a rise in intracranial pressure (see below). This is achieved by a smooth, uncomplicated anaesthetic technique, avoiding increases in either venous blood pressure, carbon dioxide concentration or arterial blood pressure while at the same time maintaining cerebral oxygenation. It is also common to administer diuretics, either mannitol or frusemide, at induction of anaesthesia. Most anaesthetists tend to employ a technique using intra-operative analgesics such as fentanyl, alfentanil or remifentanil, muscle relaxation using either vecuronium or infusions of atracurium and intermittent positive pressure ventilation (IPPV) to produce moderate hypocapnia (Pco_2 3.5–4.0 kPa). Isoflurane in concentrations up to 1 MAC is the only volatile anaesthetic agent which does not cause cerebral vasodilatation and until recently was the most common agent used for maintenance of anaesthesia. This has now been replaced by infusions of intravenous agents, especially propofol. It is extremely important to ensure adequate fixation of endotracheal tubes and drips and to protect the eyes, all of which disappear under the drapes during the operation.

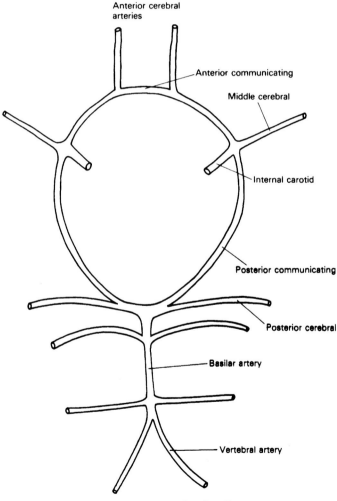

Figure 36.1 Circle of Willis.

● POSTERIOR FOSSA CRANIOTOMY

The posterior fossa approach is used for operations on the cerebellum and upper cervical spine. In the past, some surgeons preferred to have the patient sitting. This posture was also common for cervical laminectomy, but has largely been abandoned since it posed several severe anaesthetic problems. Patients in the sitting position are prone to hypotension, which will inevitably result in poor cerebral perfusion. Some surgeons also preferred to operate on a spontaneously breathing patient since many operations in the posterior fossa are in the region of the respiratory centre, and warning changes in respiratory pattern indicate to the surgeon that he is dangerously close to that centre. Air embolism may also be a problem since, when the skull is opened, many of the veins within the bone are held open and, if the venous pressure at this point is subatmospheric, air may enter the veins. Additional monitoring to detect air emboli, for example, Doppler, oesophageal stethoscope, must be used and if there is suspicion that air has entered the circulation, the anesthetist must warn the surgeon who then floods the wound with saline to prevent further emboli.

● INTRACRANIAL PRESSURE

The main factors tending to cause a rise in intracranial pressure together with the methods commonly employed to minimise them or to reduce intracranial pressure electively are summarised in Table 36.1. The use of diuretics such as mannitol or frusemide is designed to deplete the intravascular fluid volume and subsequently reduce CSF production. Actual drainage of CSF may be accomplished either by lumbar puncture or by direct puncture of the cisterna magna or lateral ventricles.

Table 36.1 Causes of raised intracranial pressure and their treatment

Cause	Treatment
$\uparrow CO_2$	IPPV hyperventilation
Volatile anaesthetics (e.g. halothane)	Avoid these drugs
Coughing, straining	Smooth induction, muscle paralysis
Obstructed airway	Armoured endotracheal tube
Hypertension	Elective hypotension
Head-down position	Raise head

● EMERGENCY NEUROSURGICAL ANAESTHESIA

This is often required in the treatment of intracranial bleeding – usually as a result of trauma. Collections of blood may arise either extradurally, subdurally or intracerebrally and may accumulate either rapidly or slowly. Many of the patients presenting for anaesthesia will already be unconscious or semi-conscious and irritable as a result of raised intracranial pressure and cerebral compression. It is important to avoid long-acting opiate analgesics because these may mask the eye signs and the level of consciousness, which are used to follow the progress of cerebral trauma. The anaesthetic technique employed is one of muscle relaxation and ventilation preceded by emergency intubation with suxamethonium to avoid regurgitation in the patient with raised intracranial pressure (Chapter 24). If the patient is unconscious the anaesthetic requirements initially may well be minimal and, indeed, decompression of intracranial haematoma through burr holes is often conducted under local anaesthesia. However, as the patient's brain is decompressed this may result in their level of consciousness lightening considerably and the anaesthetic may have to be deepened to prevent them waking up. Many patients with head injury require preoperative neuroradiology and are subsequently kept asleep and taken to theatre for surgery to decompress the brain, usually by burr holes or craniectomy.

● NEURORADIOLOGY

The introduction of the computed tomogram (CT) and magnetic resonance (MR) scanners into diagnosis has removed the need for much invasive neuroradiology under general anaesthesia. However, not only is anaesthesia still required sometimes for these diagnostic procedures, but also more commonly for therapeutic neuroradiological procedures, for example, embolisation of a cerebral aneurysm.

Carotid Angiography and Embolisation

This is generally performed to outline the vascular system of the brain and involves injecting dye into one or both internal carotid arteries and vertebral arteries. Diagnostic angiography is usually performed under local anaesthetic, but embolisation of a cerebral aneurysm, arteriovenous malformation or tumour involves inserting fine platinum wires in the affected area to occlude the feeding vessel and is a prolonged procedure. In some centres, the majority of cerebral aneurysms are treated by 'coiling' and a neurosurgical anaesthetic technique with full monitoring is required. This is best achieved by ventilating the patients with a short-acting opiate such as fentanyl (see earlier). Hyperventilation may improve the quality of the X-ray pictures by delaying the flow of dye through the cerebral vessels.

Anaesthesia for Computed Tomographic Scanning

Although most patients tolerate this procedure without anaesthesia, restless, semi-conscious patients and children often need sedating or even a full anaesthetic to remain still throughout the procedure. Like other radiological investigations where the anaesthetist is required to leave his patient for a considerable time while X-rays are taken, a semi-remote control form of anaesthesia is preferable. Again it is usually more satisfactory to ventilate the patient, although the procedure is often so short that while intermittent suxamethonium provides satisfactory muscle relaxation, the non-depolarising relaxants tend to last too long.

Anaesthesia for Magnetic Resonance Imaging Scanning

The demand for general anaesthesia for this procedure is again small, but poses considerable problems, related particularly to the anaesthetic equipment used. Since the radiological technique uses an extremely powerful electromagnetic field, normal equipment will malfunction and also cause the images to be degraded. The solution is either to keep all the equipment away from the magnetic field, or use all apparatus made from nonferrous metals (e.g. aluminium). This includes the anaesthetic machine, cylinders, all parts of the anaesthetic circuit and monitoring apparatus. Such equipment is now readily available. Meticulous attention to detail and familiarity of the anaesthetic staff with the technique and risks associated with anaesthesia in the MR scanner are vital if disasters are to be avoided. It is usually sufficient to utilise a spontaneous breathing technique, via a laryngeal mask airway (LMA), since most procedures only take between 20 and 30 min.

● SURGERY OF SPINE AND SPINAL CORD

Several neurosurgical procedures involve surgery in the region of the spinal cord, usually either for the decompression of nerves as a result of prolapsed intervertebral discs or for the decompression of the cord when the spinal canal is occupied by tumour. In most instances – except when the cervical region is involved – patients should lie prone and an anaesthetic technique employing ventilation is essential since these procedures often take a long time. However, because raised intracranial pressure is not a problem it is often sufficient to ventilate the patient with a volatile anaesthetic agent unless this causes a fall in systemic blood pressure. As the spine is an extremely vascular area, hypotensive anaesthesia is occasionally used to decrease the bleeding and particularly the venous ooze in the area of the operation. This is also considerably reduced if the operation site can be placed above the level of the heart, this being another advantage of the patient's being prone.

● POSTOPERATIVE NEUROSURGICAL CARE

Although many of the patients who have undergone spinal or cranial surgery are awake and conscious in the immediate postoperative period, some will still require active intensive treatment after their operation. This is particularly important in patients who still have raised intracranial pressure or when it is liable to rise, and in those who have undergone cerebral aneurysm surgery or coiling, when postoperative vasospasm is often a problem. Elective postoperative ventilation to control cerebral oxygenation and to produce a mild decrease in intracranial pressure is often employed, with continuous monitoring of both arterial and intracranial pressure. The latter is usually accomplished by placing a catheter within the ventricular system of the brain at operation. The patients are then treated with diuretics and possibly CSF drainage to control persistent rises in intracranial pressure. In the case of postoperative vasospasm, specific vasodilator therapy with calcium-channel blockers may be instituted to prevent local areas of cerebral ischaemia which may result in hemiplegia. In general, postoperative opiates are avoided in neurosurgical patients, codeine phosphate being used as an analgesic. They may also need an antiemetic, for example, metoclopramide or ondansetron, to treat the nausea which is not uncommon after intracranial operations.

37

General Anaesthesia in Neonates and Children

•Main differences between adults and children •Drugs in paediatric anaesthesia
•Monitoring •The management of anaesthesia •General comment

'Children are not small adults, although some adults can be large children'

● MAIN DIFFERENCES BETWEEN ADULTS AND CHILDREN

The most obvious difference is one of size, but the anatomy, physiology and pharmacology of the neonate differ from those of the adult in several important respects, and these modify the anaesthetic care that the patients are given.

General Metabolism

The oxygen consumption of a resting adult is about 3 ml/kg/min. After the first week of life this figure for a neonate is about 7 ml/kg/min, or approximately double that of the adult. This then slowly declines until around puberty when there is a brief increase. This high oxygen consumption has a number of important anaesthetic implications:

1. Since oxygen is converted into carbon dioxide (CO_2) in the body, the output of this gas per kg body weight is also double that of the adult and in order to excrete this volume of CO_2 the pulmonary ventilation of a neonate is correspondingly greater. This is achieved by doubling the respiratory rate, since the tidal volume is about the same (around 7 ml/kg). During anaesthesia the type of breathing circuit used, the gas flows into it and the amount of ventilation required must still enable the child to eliminate CO_2 efficiently.
2. If respiratory obstruction or arrest occurs during anaesthesia the oxygen reserves within the body are used up twice as quickly as in the adult – consequently a neonate will become seriously hypoxic in one-half of the time. There is thus much less margin for error.

3. Water and energy turnover are directly related to oxygen consumption, and are much higher in children. Children are therefore much more susceptible to lack of food and water and become dehydrated and hypoglycaemic more rapidly.
4. Neonates have a high resting cardiac output in order to supply enough oxygen, carbohydrate and other molecules to the active cells of the body and to remove metabolites.

Respiratory System

The main anatomical differences between neonates and adults occur in the upper airway. The head is disproportionately large compared to the rest of the body while the neck is shorter. The tongue is comparatively large and tends to obscure the anaesthetist's vision during laryngoscopy, while the lower jaw is on the small side. The epiglottis is folded upon itself and is floppy, tending to fall down in front of the opening to the larynx and to hinder successful intubation. It is common practice to try to catch the epiglottis under the blade of the laryngoscope and thus improve the view for intubation.

The adult larynx is essentially cylindrical, its narrowest part at the level of the vocal cords. The neonatal and paediatric larynx up to 8–10 years is circular or funnel-shaped; its narrowest portion is at the cricoid, a continuous ring of cartilage just below the thyroid cartilage (or 'Adam's apple'). During intubation it is important not to use a tube that is too tight, since prolonged and excessive pressure on the mucosa covering the inner surface of the cricoid may cause damage and oedema leading to the possibility of acute upper airways obstruction following extubation and long-term sub-glottic stenosis. The best fit is one which allows a slight leak when positive pressure is applied to the airway. The fact that the cricoid cartilage is narrower than the nasal passages means that an airtight fit can be obtained with both oral and nasal intubation without using cuffed tubes, and this is made use of during long-term intubation in the intensive care unit, where nasotracheal intubation is often employed.

It is not always possible to judge accurately the correct size of endotracheal tube needed before it has been passed and tested for leaks. Three sizes of tube should therefore be prepared – the estimated correct size, one size above and one below. The tube size refers to the internal diameter in mm. A rough estimate can be made from the following formula:

$$\text{Tube size (mm)} = \frac{\text{Age}}{4} + 4$$

Thus, for a 6-year-old child, the sizes that should be prepared are 5.5 (% + 4 = 5.5), 5.0 and 6.0 mm plain tubes. This formula may vary slightly for different types of endotracheal tube, and does not apply to children below 2 years for whom relatively large tube sizes are required. Nearly all neonates will accept a 3.0 mm tube without difficulty, though 2.5 and 3.5 mm tubes should also be available.

The length of the endotracheal tube is also crucial, since the neonatal trachea is only some 4 cm long, and there is therefore not much margin for error between a tube that is too short which may become displaced from the trachea, and one that is too long which will enter the right main bronchus. Nasal tubes need to be about 2 cm longer than oral tubes in the neonate. It is important not to cut the tube until you know what length the anaesthetist requires.

Intubation in the Neonate

Historically, intubation was often performed on the awake neonate before inducing anaesthesia. This was for safety reasons. Awake intubation could often be difficult and traumatic but now with better training in the skills of neonatal intubation this practice has all but been abandoned. Induction of anaesthesia, either intravenously or by inhalation, now precedes intubation which is usually carried out with the help of relaxant drugs. The anaesthetic assistant will usually be asked to help with obtaining venous access before induction and then to pre-oxygenate the patient before intravenous drugs are given. After that, help is required with intubation. The laryngoscope, which is normally straight bladed, is gently passed and the assistant uses the right hand to give the tube to the anaesthetist. During insertion of the tube it is helpful if the assistant applies gentle backward pressure on the larynx, thus helping to bring it into view. The correct anaesthetic circuit, plenty of adhesive tape and a small nasogastric tube should have been confirmed with the anaesthetist beforehand and be available for use immediately after successful intubation.

It is important that the whole process of induction and intubation is carried out in a warm environment, particularly with pre-term neonates. This is best achieved under an overhead radiant heater. Many neonates are nursed in the special care baby unit (SCBU) on a specially designed cot complete with a dedicated overhead grille. This also provides ideal conditions for anaesthetic induction.

Pulmonary Ventilation

In neonates, as in adults, pulmonary ventilation is mainly diaphragmatic. In the neonate, however, the thoracic component is not nearly so powerful. There are two reasons for this. First, the ribs are much more horizontal so that the possible lateral expansion of the chest is less. Secondly, and more importantly, the ribs are cartilaginous and therefore soft. In the event of respiratory obstruction (either partial or complete), or any other difficulty in respiration, instead of moving outwards to help respiration the rib cage is sucked inwards by the powerful action of the diaphragm, and this tends to decrease lung expansion, making the efforts of the diaphragm to suck air into the lungs less efficient. It is therefore especially important in this age group to use low-resistance apparatus and endotracheal tubes, and to ensure that the airway is maintained during anaesthesia so that there is as little resistance to breathing as possible.

As well as a low resistance, the other important point about neonatal anaesthetic apparatus is that it should have a low dead space. In the normal neonate the tidal volume is about 20 ml (7 ml/kg), of which about 30–40% (6–8 ml) is dead space, so that only 12–14 ml of the inspired gases actually take part in gas exchange at each breath (the alveolar ventilation). If a piece of apparatus with a large dead space of, for example, 10 ml is placed on the child's face, the total dead space (child + apparatus) will then amount to some 16–18 ml. Since the tidal volume is only 20 ml, the alveolar ventilation is therefore reduced to only 2–4 ml per breath.

Face masks are designed for closeness of fit and to minimise dead space. The Rendell-Baker face masks have now been superseded by clear plastic face masks with a cushion rim (Fig. 37.1). These are available in a circular or teardrop shape and can be flavoured to assist inhalational induction. Although dead space is slightly greater, they are better fitting and the transparent design allows for rapid detection of cyanosis or vomiting.

Oropharyngeal airways are available in a range of sizes from 000 to adult although they are often unhelpful in neonates. They should not be inserted upside down in the adult style because of the risk of damage to the palate.

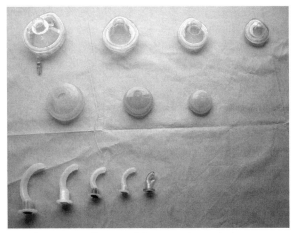

Figure 37.1 Range of face masks and airways.

Laryngoscopes are available with either a curved or straight blade and in a range of sizes from neonatal to adult. Because of the nature of the neonatal airway, particularly the anterior placed larynx, a straight blade is more useful for intubating babies up to 6 months; the blade is placed behind the epiglottis to facilitate intubation.

Breathing Circuits

The Ayre's T-piece (Fig. 37.2) is an ideal circuit for paediatric use. It is small and lightweight with a low resistance and there are no valves in the circuit. Fresh gas is provided through the side-arm and expired gas passes out down the wide-bore tubing to a small bag with an open tail and then into the atmosphere. Scavenging, however, is a problem. The addition of the open-ended bag was suggested by Jackson Rees, and enables artificial ventilation to be used. This is the Mapleson F system (Chapter 8). Inflation is accomplished simply by closing the tail and squeezing the bag, and expiration is allowed by releasing the bag and opening the tail. The bag also allows an assessment of tidal volume and respiratory rate. Continuous positive airways pressure (CPAP) can be applied by partial occlusion of the tail to assist spontaneous ventilation. Specially designed paediatric ventilators can be attached to the T-piece, replacing the bag. The apparatus dead space depends on the volume of the catheter mount and therefore during spontaneous ventilation this should be kept as small as possible. Disposable forms of the T-piece are available.

The Ayre's T-piece is applicable for children up to 20 kg. In larger children the dead space and resistance characteristics of adult circuits are more satisfactory. The circle system and the Humphrey ADE circuit are both suitable alternatives in paediatric practice.

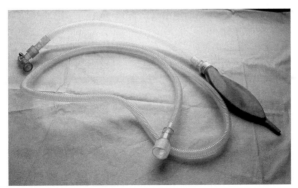

Figure 37.2 Jackson Rees modification of Ayre's T-piece.

Circulatory System

The resting cardiac output of the neonate is two to three times that of the adult. Cardiac output is dependent on heart rate rather than stroke volume since the ventricles are small and contract less efficiently than the adult heart. The resting pulse rate is variable, the normal ranging between about 110 and 160 beats/min. It may rise above 200 beats/min during crying. A heart rate below 100 is usually due to hypoxia and responds to treatment with oxygen rather than atropine. A bradycardia of below 60 represents an inadequate cardiac output and cardiac massage should be started immediately.

As the child grows older the variability becomes less and the average rate progressively declines (see Table 37.1).

The systolic blood pressure is 70–90 mmHg after birth, rising to 90–100 mmHg at 1 year of age, and then slowly up to adult values as a late teenager. Again, there is much variability in the very young. It can be conveniently estimated using the formula

$$\text{Systolic blood pressure (mmHg)} = 80 + (\text{age in years} \times 2)$$

Haematology

Neonatal haemoglobin consists mainly of fetal haemoglobin (HbF) which *in utero* has a stronger affinity for oxygen than maternal haemoglobin and therefore assists oxygen transport from mother to fetus. It progressively declines over 3 months to be replaced by adult haemoglobin.

The blood volume of the neonate is about 85 ml/kg, so a 3 kg baby contains approximately 250 ml blood. The haemoglobin is initially high, 18–20 g/100 ml but total haemoglobin falls rapidly after birth, reaching a low point of 12–14 g/100 ml at 2–3 months of age, then slowly rising again to reach adult values (14–15 g/100 ml) by early adolescence.

Table 37.1

Age	Pulse (beats/min)	Mean blood pressure (mmHg)
Term	95–145	40–60
3 months	110–175	45–75
6 months	110–175	50–90
1 year	105–170	50–100
3 years	80–140	50–100
7 years	70–120	60–90
10 years	60–110	60–90
12 years	60–100	65–95

The principles of blood transfusion during surgery are the same as in the adult, namely that blood should be given if the loss exceeds 15% of the blood volume, provided that the child is not anaemic. In a 3 kg neonate this amounts to a blood loss of about 35 ml. Measuring such small volumes is difficult; swabs should be weighed carefully and suction recorded. At best this produces a somewhat inaccurate assessment of the loss – normally an underestimate due to evaporation and undetected blood loss – and the volume measured must be supplemented by a visual estimate of blood loss, including that on the floor and on the drapes and gowns. It is advisable to be on the generous side when replacing operative blood loss. Clinical indices, especially tachycardia and hypotension, should also be taken into account.

All transfused blood should be warmed before being given. If rapid or major transfusion is necessary, neonates may be vulnerable to hypocalcaemia. Serum calcium levels should be checked and treated with calcium chloride or calcium gluconate if necessary. Small volumes of blood in special 40 ml 'baby packs' are available for neonatal transfusion. Blood can be administered via a burette but if rapid transfusion is required it is more convenient to use a syringe and three-way tap.

Heat Loss and Temperature Control

Up to about 3–6 months of age a baby is not able to control its temperature nearly as effectively as an adult. This is due to both impaired ability to conserve heat and a reduced capacity to increase its heat production. Both these factors are adversely affected by anaesthesia and surgery.

Sources of Heat Loss

A child has a greater surface area to volume ratio than an adult (2.5 times greater in the neonate) and therefore the potential for heat loss to the atmosphere is greater. Anaesthesia tends to produce skin vasodilatation and thus increase heat loss from the skin. In the premature neonate the layer of subcutaneous fat is deficient, so the baby is only poorly insulated. Heat loss occurs by radiation conduction and because of evaporation from wounds and from exposed bowel or other organs. The infusion of cold intravenous fluids tends to lower the baby's temperature even further.

Sources of Heat Production

1. *Shivering.* Unlike adults, who can raise their heat production by shivering, newborn babies are unable to shiver.
2. *Metabolism of brown fat.* Situated around the scapulae and the back of the neck and also lagging the major vessels of the thorax are deposits

of brownish fat whose metabolism produces a considerable amount of heat. Metabolism of brown fat is triggered by the sympathetic nervous system in response to a cold environment, and the sympathetic system is effectively blocked by many anaesthetic agents. Therefore the capacity to mobilise heat from brown fat is reduced by anaesthesia.

3. *Carbohydrate metabolism.* This is also increased in response to cold, and provides a ready source of heat production. Many neonates, however, have a tendency towards hypoglycaemia, because of reduced glycogen stores and the increased use of glucose and glycogen to produce heat may accentuate this. Although the neonate cannot shiver, the metabolism of both brown fat and carbohydrate can increase its heat production some three times, but this is reduced by anaesthesia.

The harmful effects of allowing a baby's temperature to fall include:

1. Decreased drug metabolism with prolonged action of muscle relaxants and opioids.
2. Changes in electrolyte, water and acid–base status leading to a worsening acidosis and hypoglycaemia.
3. Impaired clotting resulting in increased blood loss.
4. Failure of the baby to breathe at the end of surgery necessitating transfer to intensive care.
5. Reduced immune function leading to delayed wound healing and susceptibility to infection,
6. Scleroma, or neonatal cold injury. This is a condition which appears postoperatively, in which the metabolism of subcutaneous fat alters and it becomes hard to the touch. This change can first be detected in the calves and forearms, and may spread to cover the whole body. Mortality is high in severe cases, and there is no effective treatment, so prevention is imperative. The three main predisposing factors are prematurity, an ill child and hypothermia. Fortunately this is now an extremely rare condition.

Prevention of Hypothermia

In the unanaesthetised neonate the ambient temperature (e.g. in an incubator) should be kept at 32–34°C. During surgery the following precautions should be taken to prevent a fall in body temperature:

1. The theatre and anaesthetic room should be preheated to warm the walls and reduce radiant heat loss. An ambient temperature of 21°C is adequate for older children. Neonates may require an ambient temperature of 26°C but this results in uncomfortable working conditions. A sensible compromise is to warm the theatre to 21°C and concentrate on reducing heat loss in the immediate area around the anaesthetised child.

2. Exposure of the child should be kept to a minimum. This particularly applies in the anaesthetic room when intravenous cannulation may be difficult and prolonged. In theatre, careful draping should reduce the exposed area to a minimum. The child should be insulated with polythene or warm gamgee. The neonatal head represents a large surface area for potential heat loss and should always be covered.
3. Active warming methods should be employed. These include the electric warming mattress, or convector warm-air heating blanket (e.g. Bair Hugger) of which the latter is the most effective. An overhead grille can be used both in theatre and in the anaesthetic room.
4. All intravenous fluids and blood products should be warmed. Cleaning fluids to prepare the site of surgery should also be pre-warmed.
5. A heat and moisture exchanger (HME) should be incorporated in the anaesthetic circuit. In addition to humidifying anaesthetic gases they play an important role in reducing heat loss from the lungs. Heated water vapour humidifiers are available and are commonly used in the intensive care setting.
6. The doors should stay closed as far as possible to reduce draughts and convective heat loss.
7. Temperature monitoring is mandatory in all neonatal surgery. Core temperature should be measured using a nasopharyngeal, oesophageal or rectal probe.

Above the age of about 6 months precautions should be reduced or the child may easily become hyperthermic.

Water and Electrolyte Balance

The neonate consists of 80% water by weight and this falls to adult levels of 60% by 2 years. Water and electrolyte turnover in neonates is two to three times that of the adult, being closely related to the oxygen consumption. However, the ability of the neonate to deal with excesses or deficiencies in either is less than that of the adult, so more care has to be exercised in the amounts that are given or withheld. For instance, in adults it is customary to withhold all oral intake preoperatively to reduce the risk of inhalation of stomach contents. Stopping fluids in an adult for 12 h preoperatively (i.e. overnight) does no appreciable harm, but in a neonate it has the same effect as withholding water from an adult for two to three times as long (i.e. 24–36 h). Hence neonates and infants must not be starved for long periods. They should not be fasted for longer than 6 h. They can be given milk up to 4 h preoperatively and encouraged to take clear fluids up to 2 h before surgery. Similarly, feeds should be started as soon after the operation as is practicable.

During surgery a greater amount of fluid should be given (per kilogram) than to an adult. Provided that there is no fluid deficit before operation a suitable amount is 5–10 ml/kg/h plus some extra to account for evaporation and other losses. When losses are high, an amount nearer to 10 ml/kg/h should be given. Fluid loss ultimately must be assessed clinically. The maintenance fluid for neonates is 10% dextrose with added sodium and potassium. In infants and older children 4% dextrose with 0.18% sodium is usually adequate.

In a shocked infant fluid boluses of 10 ml/kg should be given and repeated if necessary. For resuscitation normal saline or Hartmann's solution can be administered in the first instance or alternatively a colloid solution can be given.

The normal response of adults to surgery is to retain fluid and sodium postoperatively, and neonates show much the same stress response. Some restriction of water and sodium intake is therefore desirable after surgery, as babies very readily become oedematous at this time. However, in assessing a reduced urine output, it is important to distinguish between stress response and inadequate replacement of fluid loss.

Hypoglycaemia

In the first few days of life babies may have a low blood sugar. Glycogen stores in the liver are low in the neonate and almost absent in the premature baby. This is because their stores are largely used up during delivery and take some days to be replenished, especially in ill babies who are not feeding properly. Severe hypoglycaemia (the signs of which are masked if the neonate is anaesthetised) may occur and cause brain damage. Regular blood glucose measurement is essential for all premature babies and neonates undergoing surgery. They should routinely receive 10% dextrose as maintenance fluid but the dextrose concentration can be increased or decreased to achieve normoglycaemia.

● DRUGS IN PAEDIATRIC ANAESTHESIA

Neonates are more sensitive to drugs in the first 2 weeks of life. Children require relatively larger doses than adults to achieve the same effect. Neonates have immature liver function with reduced capacity to break down drugs. The blood–brain barrier is also permeable, allowing centrally acting drugs to exert a greater effect. Babies are particularly sensitive to opioids and non-depolarising muscle relaxants, both of which should be given cautiously. They are, however, relatively resistant to suxamethonium, the dose required being approximately double that of the adult. Children are more resistant because of the relatively high cardiac output and metabolic rate. This allows drugs to be more rapidly removed from their site of action, metabolised and then excreted.

The doses of most drugs may be estimated from the adult dose (more easily remembered than children's doses) by using the formula:

$$\text{Child's dose (mg/kg)} = \frac{\text{Total adult dose}}{50}$$

For example, the normal intubating dose of suxamethonium in the adult is 100 mg. Therefore:

$$\text{Child's dose} = \frac{100}{50} = 2\,\text{mg/kg}$$

Alternatively it may be convenient to keep a record of the paediatric dosages of commonly used anaesthetic drugs in the anaesthetic room.

● MONITORING

It is essential to use a pulse oximeter for all paediatric and neonatal anaesthesia from before induction until they leave the recovery room to return to the ward. Oximeter probes that are suitable for infants and babies must be available in the anaesthetic room (Table 37.2).

Reliable blood pressure measurements can be made using automatic machines with a suitable sized cuff even in the smallest babies. A suitable selection of cuffs must be available. For some types of major surgery, direct arterial blood pressure measurements will be required and the radial or another artery will be cannulated in the anaesthetic room.

For older children, say over 1 year old, similar monitoring to that used for adults is usually suitable.

It is useful to be able to see a hand or some other part of the child during surgery. Monitoring may not always be reliable and in neonates especially should supplement rather than replace clinical observation.

Table 37.2 Recommended monitoring for a neonate

Always	Often	Occasional
Pulse oximeter	Oesophageal stethoscope	Direct arterial blood pressure
ECG	Blood glucose	Central venous pressure
Cuff blood pressure	Peripheral nerve stimulator	Blood gas estimation
Capnography		
Temperature probe		
Blood loss estimation		

● THE MANAGEMENT OF ANAESTHESIA

Premedication

The purpose of premedication is to reduce anxiety and improve conditions for induction of anaesthesia.

There has been a general trend towards using oral premedication for children (mainly benzodiazepines) so as to avoid an injection. Increasingly paediatric anaesthetists are not using premedication at all. This has become much more practical since the advent of topical anaesthetic cream (EMLA or Ametop) and the now widespread practice of allowing one parent to accompany the child into the anaesthetic room.

The use of anaesthetic cream has revolutionised intravenous induction in children. EMLA should be placed on the skin at the site of cannulation 60–90 min before anaesthesia when it will have reached its maximum effect. Ametop cream is a suitable alternative. It has the advantage of a faster onset of 30 min and can be used for infants as young as 1 month whereas EMLA can only be used over 1 year of age.

The most commonly prescribed premedicants are probably midazolam and temazepam but other benzodiazepines are also used. Some of the more established drugs including vallergan and chloral hydrate still have their advocates. There is a suggestion that midazolam given to the preschool age groups from 2 to 5 years of age may result in a reduction in postoperative psychological complications, including tantrums, nightmares and bed-wetting.

Intra-muscular premedication is unnecessarily painful and should be avoided if possible. Exceptions include suspected airway problems or children with excessive secretions when atropine should be given intramuscularly because of its variable absorption by the oral route.

Induction

It is now common practice for one parent to accompany their child into the anaesthetic room and be present while they are being anaesthetised. Generally this presence is felt to be advantageous to both child and parent. However, parents should realise that this attendance is not compulsory; in fact anxious and distressed parents may make conditions worse.

The anaesthetist should communicate with both parent and child throughout the induction period, explaining the various procedures involved. An informed child is usually much more composed and cooperative.

Intravenous and inhalational induction are both acceptable techniques and older children can be offered the choice. Intravenous induction is associated with fewer airway problems including coughing and laryngospasm. Propofol is most commonly used but it is not licensed below 1 month of age when thiopentone is the drug of choice.

Inhalational induction is indicated for the child with difficult venous access or a suspected airway problem. Sevoflurane provides conditions for a smooth rapid induction.

Neonates will require intubation for most types of surgery unless of short duration, because of the respiratory depressant effects of volatile anaesthetics. Once intubated, the work involved in breathing through a small tube increases dramatically and the child will require controlled ventilation.

Neonatal intubation has been described previously. The tube should be secured meticulously. Preformed north-facing paediatric endotracheal tubes are available which make tube fixation easier and reduce the incidence of endobronchial intubation and accidental extubation. Most intubated neonates also require a nasogastric tube.

Both the standard LMA and reinforced laryngeal mask airway (RLMA) are available in a range of sizes suitable for paediatric use (see Table 37.3). They are convenient for most day-case procedures and operations of short and intermediate duration where muscle relaxation is not required. Some anaesthetists will also paralyse and ventilate children using the LMA rather than an endotracheal tube. The insertion technique is similar to that in adults. An alternative method is to pass the LMA upside down behind the tongue before rotating it through 180°.

Intravenous access is critical and often difficult. It may be especially challenging in ex-premature infants and children between 3 months and 2 years, and veins in the feet may be a useful alternative.

Maintenance

It is important to reduce heat loss on transferring the neonate from the anaesthetic room to the operating theatre. Exposure should be minimised and warming devices activated. The infant is usually positioned supine with both hands raised at the level of the head. This allows examination of the hands for colour, temperature and pulse. The pulse oximeter is placed on the ear or same arm as the intravenous line allowing the blood pressure cuff to be placed on the other arm.

Table 37.3

Size of LMA	Weight of patient (kg)	Cuff volume (ml)
1	<5	2–5
1.5	5–10	4–7
2	10–20	5–10
2.5	20–30	10–15
3	>30	15–20

Intravenous access and tracheal tube placement should be checked and secured before the drapes cover the patient; an extension and three-way tap may be required for the drip. A minimum of two intravenous lines are necessary for major neonatal surgery.

Most anaesthetic techniques involve ventilation with oxygen, nitrous oxide and a volatile agent together with supplemental opioids.

Mechanical ventilators are specialised for paediatric use. They are not always adequate for very small infants and hand ventilation is sometimes necessary. Fluid loss is carefully observed from weighing swabs and noting suction loss. Fluid and blood can be given using a burette or more rapidly using a syringe and three-way tap.

At the end of surgery, nitrous oxide and the volatile agent are discontinued, the muscle relaxant is reversed with glycopyrrolate (or atropine) and neostigmine, and the baby is extubated awake in 100% oxgyen.

As children become older, the anaesthetic techniques resemble those used in adult practice. Indications for intubation or LMA insertion are similar although uncuffed tubes are used until approximately 8 years of age.

Postoperative Care

Ideally the postoperative child should be warm, awake and pain free. The neonate should be transferred back to the incubator as soon as possible. Monitoring should continue in the recovery area; a pulse oximeter is the minimum requirement. Ex-premature infants are susceptible to postoperative apnoeic episodes and should be monitored for 24 h with a pulse oximeter and apnoea alarm.

Postoperative Pain Relief

Local anaesthetic agents are used to provide conditions for a light general anaesthetic and postoperative pain relief. They are particularly useful in day-case procedures such as circumcision, herniotomy and orchidopexy, and the removal of various lumps and bumps. Caudal analgesia, peripheral nerve blockade and local infiltration are all commonly used techniques. In major surgery epidural analgesia is increasingly used. A catheter is inserted either using the lumbar route or alternatively via the caudal space in infants. Bupivacaine is routinely used although ropivacaine is gaining popular acceptance.

Mild to moderate pain can be treated by paracetamol, non-steroidal anti-inflammatory drugs (NSAIDs) or codeine phosphate used either individually or in combination. They should be given regularly in the immediate postoperative period.

Following major surgery morphine is given by either simple infusion or nurse-controlled analgesia (NCA). In older children patient-controlled analgesia (PCA) is well accepted but with encouragement and careful explanation, children can manage their own analgesia at a surprisingly young age.

Postoperative nausea and vomiting (PONV) is distressing. It is more common over the age of 2 years especially if morphine is being given. Routine anti-emetics should be prescribed, of which ondansetron is the drug of choice.

● GENERAL COMMENT

Neonatal anaesthesia is challenging. Consistent success requires good teamwork and meticulous preparation. There is very little room for error in these tiny patients.

38

Obstetric Anaesthesia and Analgesia

•Physiological changes in pregnancy •Special considerations •Caesarean section under general anaesthesia •Awake Caesarean section •Pain relief in obstetrics •The obstetric flying squads

The first part of this chapter is concerned with anaesthesia for obstetric patients. This branch of anaesthesia is unique in that even elective operations carry a high degree of risk. The reasons for this are included in the 'Special Considerations' section below. The second part of this chapter briefly discusses methods of pain relief in labour.

● PHYSIOLOGICAL CHANGES IN PREGNANCY

Changes due to the increased metabolic requirements of the growing fetus and placenta occur in most of the body systems. Some of the most important, from the anaesthetist's viewpoint, are outlined below.

Cardiovascular System

There is an increase in cardiac output from a non-pregnant level of about 4.5 l/min to 6.0 l/min. This is achieved by an increase both in heart rate (to about 85/min at term) and in stroke volume. Many organs have an increased blood flow, but the biggest increase is to the growing uterus and placenta. In the last trimester of pregnancy, occlusion of the inferior vena cava by the gravid uterus tends to occur in the supine position. This is discussed in more detail below.

Respiratory System

Minute ventilation is increased by an increase in tidal volume of about 40% over non-pregnant values without an increase in respiratory rate. This meets the increased oxygen requirements and disposes of the increased carbon dioxide production of the growing uterus, fetus and placenta. The P_{CO_2} at term is about 4.0 kPa (30 mmHg) compared with the normal 5.3 kPa (40 mmHg) in the pre-pregnant state. This has important implications for the anaesthetist who must ensure that in pregnant patients an anaesthetic technique is employed that is capable of achieving these lower than usual P_{CO_2} levels.

Blood Volume and Its Constituents

Both the plasma volume and the number of red cells increase in pregnancy. However, the increase in the red cells is proportionately less, so that there is a fall in the haemoglobin content of the blood to a level which should not be lower than 10 g/100 ml, provided that the woman takes supplementary iron and folic acid. This is the so-called 'physiological anaemia' of pregnancy.

The relevance of the physiological changes in the gastrointestinal and musculoskeletal systems is discussed below in the sections under vomiting and regurgitation and difficulties in intubation, respectively.

● SPECIAL CONSIDERATIONS

A number of factors affecting obstetric anaesthesia – some of them unique to obstetric patients – deserve special mention.

The 'Two Lives' Problem

The so-called placental 'barrier' is readily crossed by most pharmacological agents used in anaesthesia, including the thiobarbiturates and other induction agents, anaesthetic gases, volatile anaesthetic agents, opioids and benzodiazepines. The only frequently used drugs that do not cross the placenta in significant quantities are the muscle relaxants. While the fetus is *in utero*, it relies on the placenta for its supply of oxygen and its excretion of carbon dioxide. At birth this facility is abruptly removed, and the newborn, by redistributing its circulation and expanding its lungs, has to fend for itself in obtaining oxygen and excreting carbon dioxide. Thus it has to initiate and maintain regular respiration and it is its ability to do this which is so readily adversely affected by depressant anaesthetic agents.

Thus it is standard anaesthetic practice before obstetric anaesthesia not to give the mother any sedative premedication. Induction is then carried out by a sleep dose of intravenous agent (e.g. sodium thiopentone 4–6 mg/kg) and after intubation with suxamethonium; anaesthesia is maintained with 50% nitrous oxide and 50% oxygen and a volatile agent such as isoflurane (at least 1 MAC) until the baby is delivered. Thereafter, anaesthesia should be deepened by increasing the nitrous oxide concentration to 67% and administering opioids for pain relief.

Awareness in the Mother

The possibility that a patient is not deeply enough anaesthetised is always a danger with muscle-relaxant anaesthesia where the surgical operating conditions are achieved by the muscle relaxant rather than by depth of anaesthesia, as was the case when single agents, for example, chloroform or ether, were used. The risk of awareness can be particularly high in obstetric anaesthesia, where in the interests of the fetus anaesthesia is deliberately kept as light as possible.

The best that the anaesthetist can do is to choose a technique which is known to have a low incidence of awareness allied to minimal depression of the newborn and to perform it meticulously. The incidence is minimized to <1% by giving the mother a sleep dose of thiopentone rather than a fixed, small dose (200–250 mg) and at least 1 MAC volatile agent in 50% oxygen and 50% nitrous oxide until delivery of the baby.

Vomiting, Regurgitation and Aspiration

The difference between vomiting and regurgitation is discussed in Chapter 24. Vomiting occurs only at a very light level of anaesthesia. With modern intravenous induction agents (unless these are given very slowly) the patient is taken down rapidly to a depth of anaesthesia well below the level at which vomiting occurs, but may become deeply enough anaesthetised for regurgitation to occur. The induction agent is immediately followed by a muscle relaxant. This is usually suxamethonium, which may cause strong enough twitching of the abdominal muscles to increase the intragastric pressure and facilitate reflux. It then paralyses the patient so that regurgitation is again more likely. A tracheal tube is passed and once the cuff is inflated the patient's respiratory tract is secure against soiling by gastric contents until extubation at the end of the obstetric procedure.

There are several reasons why obstetric patients are likely to regurgitate. These factors are listed in Table 38.1, where they are considered in elective

Table 38.1 Factors facilitating reflux in obstetric patients

Danger factor	Elective obstetric procedures	Emergency obstetric procedures
'Big bump' problem	+	+
Heartburn problem	+	+
Full stomach problem	−	+

or emergency obstetric procedures. The commonest example of the former is elective Caesarean section, while the latter nearly always implies that the patient is in labour.

The 'big bump' refers to the gravid uterus, which in the second half of pregnancy occupies an increasingly large proportion of the abdominal cavity. It eventually occupies more space than any but the most enormous pathological tumours and in the recumbent position simply compresses the stomach against the diaphragm and tends to squeeze any gastric contents up into the oesophagus. This danger factor applies to both elective and emergency procedures, except possibly in women who are under 20 weeks pregnant, in whom the uterus is still relatively small, and in cases of retained placenta, where the uterus has already diminished in size.

Heartburn is a common symptom in pregnancy and implies reflux of acid gastric juice into the oesophagus due to incompetence of the lower oesophageal (gastro-oesophageal) sphincter. The reason for this incompetence is not known for certain, but is believed to be partly hormonal. A weak sphincter is more likely to give way before the increased intragastric pressure caused by the gravid uterus, especially in the recumbent position. About 80% of women complain of heartburn at term but it is wise to consider all patients in the second half of pregnancy to be at risk from oesophageal reflux. Once again, both elective and emergency patients are at risk.

On the whole, pregnant women digest food adequately – otherwise they would reach term in a uniformly cachectic state! In established labour, recent work has shown that digestion does slow down, but two factors tend to cause a further delay in gastric emptying. The first of these is prolongation of labour, a duration of over 12 h being likely to be associated with an increase in gastric contents. Secondly, the administration of opioids for pain relief by both the intramuscular and bolus epidural routes causes a marked delay in gastric emptying.

In summary, all pregnant patients are at risk from inhalation of gastric contents, but patients in prolonged labour who have been given opioids are particularly at risk because they have the added danger of gastric stasis.

Acid Aspiration Syndrome (Mendelson's Syndrome)

In 1946 Mendelson, a New York obstetrician, described an asthma-like syndrome associated with a mottled appearance on the chest X-ray which he considered was caused by the inhalation of liquid acid gastric contents with a pH of <2.5. This hypothesis is now widely accepted and the clinical picture is referred to as 'Mendelson's syndrome'. The syndrome varies greatly in severity but can be fatal. It does not, of course, supplant the possibility of acute asphyxia caused by inhalation of solid or semi-solid gastric contents.

The logical prophylactic measure is to reduce the amount of acid production by administering H_2 blockers such as ranitidine and raise the pH of the gastric contents by administering an alkali before anaesthesia. For elective Caesarean section, it is common practice to administer ranitidine 150 mg orally the night before and on the morning of surgery and 30 ml of 0.3 M sodium citrate immediately before induction of anaesthesia. Sodium citrate is non-granular but has a very short duration of action. For emergency Caesarean sections, oral ranitidine should be administered as soon as decision to perform surgery is taken; in extreme urgency, it can be administered intravenously in a dose of 50 mg slowly.

It is sometimes thought that Mendelson's syndrome occurs only in obstetrics. This is not so. The term may be applied to acid aspiration occurring in any branch of anaesthesia, and the prophylactic use of H_2 blockers and alkali is common in other conditions where patients are at risk from aspiration.

Nevertheless, all obstetric patients who are over about 20 weeks pregnant, whether for elective or emergency procedures, should be anaesthetised with a rapid sequence induction technique. This should include pre-oxygenation, a rapid intravenous induction immediately followed by suxamethonium and regurgitation prevented by pressure backwards on a previously identified cricoid cartilage until a tracheal tube is passed and its cuff inflated.

Treatment. This will consist (depending on severity) of parenteral steroids, bronchodilators, for example, salbutamol (Ventolin), antibiotics and symptomatic treatment of the respiratory state (again depending on severity) up to ventilation with 100% oxygen and positive end-expiratory pressure in the most serious cases.

Difficult and Failed Intubation

It is known that there is about an eight-fold increase in incidence of failure to intubate the trachea of a pregnant patient at term when compared with a non-pregnant patient. Several factors are responsible for this including the fact that the upper airway is oedematous due to retention of fluid and the enlarged breasts and the tilt required to prevent venacaval compression make it awkward to perform laryngoscopy. These problems occur more frequently during emergency general anaesthesia where the stress and hurry associated with the procedure is also responsible for this increased incidence. The decline in maternal mortality from hypoxia due to failed intubation since the mid-1980s has been largely due to increased consultant input and better training, improvement in monitoring and assistance for the anaesthetist and the increased use of regional anaesthesia even for emergency Caesarean section. However, failed intubation still occurs and each unit should have guidelines for the management of a patient in whom failed intubation has occurred. This should include the provision of adequate equipment and assistance. The 'drill' should be familiar to all and practised at regular intervals.

Haemorrhage

Because of the nature of parturition, haemorrhage is an ever-present risk and remains one of the commonest causes of maternal mortality. When the placenta separates from the wall of the uterus in the third stage of labour, a raw and very vascular surface is exposed. Fortunately, the same contraction of the uterus that shears off the placenta also clamps down on the branches of the uterine artery which supply it by passing through the criss-cross syncytial arrangement of uterine muscle fibres. This arrests the haemorrhage and the retraction down of the uterus prevents further bleeding into its cavity.

Any anaesthetic agent that prevents the uterus from contracting down is likely to increase the incidence and severity of post-partum haemorrhage. Historically two agents, chloroform and diethyl ether, were considered particularly to blame in this respect. However, these agents were always given in high concentrations with spontaneous respiration anaesthesia, and likewise the more modern, powerful volatile agents, for example, halothane, enflurane and isoflurane, given in high concentrations may prevent uterine contraction. Fortunately these agents do not cause significant uterine relaxation in the low concentrations in which they are used as adjuvants to nitrous oxide, oxygen and muscle-relaxant anaesthesia. Because of the low percentage of elective Caesarean sections requiring preoperative transfusion, routine cross-matching of blood has been abandoned in many units. Instead, a recent 'antibody screen' is carried out and provided this is negative, routine blood cross-matching is not required. Routine cross-matching is reserved for special cases, for example, those with known placenta praevia or a low haemoglobin or in whom antibodies have been detected. In an emergency it is considered very safe to use uncross-matched group O Rhesus-negative, Kell-negative blood in patients known to be Rhesus negative, and for patients known to be Rhesus positive, group O Rhesus-positive, Kell-negative blood while blood is being cross-matched.

Each area where obstetric procedures are performed should have a 'haemorrhage trolley' equipped with all the necessary equipment for dealing with a major blood loss.

Inferior Venacaval Compression Syndrome (Aortocaval Occlusion; Supine Hypotension)

It has been known for 30 years that some women feel faint when lying on their backs in the last few weeks of pregnancy. It was thought that in this small group of women (about 5% of pregnant women) the inferior vena cava was being occluded by compression between the gravid uterus and the vertebral column. The heart, deprived of the major part of its venous return, could not maintain an adequate output, the blood pressure fell and the woman felt faint. More recently it has been shown that the inferior vena cava is almost completely occluded in all women in the last weeks of pregnancy when they are supine (Fig. 38.1). Venous return from the lower part of the body then reaches the heart by a collateral system of veins in the paravertebral region and in the epidural space. If this alternative pathway for the blood is well developed, the woman lying supine behaves as if she had a patent inferior vena cava. If the collateral circulation is poor, the supine patient may feel faint within minutes. If the adequacy of the collateral system lies between these two extremes, the woman may be able to maintain her blood pressure, but only by compensatory vasoconstriction under the influence of the sympathetic nervous system. She is then particularly susceptible to the vasodilatation associated with both general anaesthesia and spinal or epidural analgesia, and should never be left lying on her back. A rubber or inflatable wedge placed under one hip (usually the right) will usually suffice to roll the uterus off the vena cava and restore the venous return. Alternatively some anaesthetists prefer to tilt the table to the left by about 15°.

It should be realised that with moderate degrees of venacaval occlusion, where the mother is maintaining her blood pressure at a reasonable level by vasoconstriction, the fetus may be adversely affected by the constriction in the blood vessels supplying the placenta.

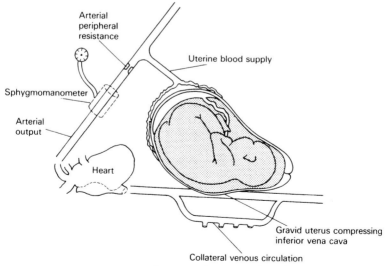

Figure 38.1 Mechanism of venacaval occlusion.

The alternative term 'aortocaval occlusion' is sometimes used and is justified in that at times, especially if the blood pressure falls, the aorta may also be compressed by the gravid uterus.

The older name 'supine hypotension syndrome' should be reserved for severe degrees of venacaval occlusion where the blood pressure actually falls.

● CAESAREAN SECTION UNDER GENERAL ANAESTHESIA

There is no doubt about the increased risks of aspiration and failed intubation during general anaesthesia for Caesarean section especially in an emergency. One of the approaches to reduce the number of deaths due to general anaesthesia has been to promote the use of regional anaesthetic techniques. Recent surveys of obstetric practice have shown that although the percentage of Caesarean sections done under general anaesthesia has decreased, the absolute numbers of general anaesthetics given has remained the same because of the increase in the number of Caesarean sections performed. It is thought that the greater input of consultants in maternity units and better training together with improved monitoring and assistance for the anaesthetist have been more important.

The need for general anaesthesia is unlikely to disappear altogether. There are patients in whom regional anaesthesia is contraindicated (e.g. clotting problems, blood loss, local infection). General anaesthesia is also most reliable when the baby has to be delivered at once. It is therefore important that the current trend in improved training in general anaesthesia for obstetrics is continued.

● AWAKE CAESAREAN SECTION

Women are increasingly requesting to be awake for the delivery of their babies by Caesarean section. Anaesthetists are keen whenever possible to accede to this request, because in addition to the obvious pleasure it gives to so many women, it also avoids the risks of aspiration of gastric contents, difficult and failed intubation, and the condition of the newborn baby is usually excellent.

Caesarean section is the most major operation routinely carried out under regional anaesthesia in the UK. Unlike non-obstetric procedures, it is not combined with light general anaesthesia or preoperative and intraoperative sedation. It therefore presents the anaesthetist with a considerable challenge, the main problems being the provision of good analgesia and the avoidance of hypotension.

Lumbar epidural, spinal or combined spinal–epidural (CSE) block are used. Reference to Chapter 41 will reveal that a block up to T5 is required to prevent pain impulses travelling along the sympathetic nerves and even then vagal sensation and pain fibres from the lower surface of the diaphragm running to the cervical nerves will be unaffected. With gentle and careful surgical technique no pain may be initiated in either of these unblocked areas, but it does mean that perfect analgesia cannot be guaranteed. CSE block has become increasingly popular for Caesarean section, because not only does it provide the best possible analgesia but, if facilities are available, the use of the epidural catheter to provide postoperative pain relief is particularly valuable to a woman wishing to care for her new baby.

Hypotension is avoided or minimised by adequate preloading with intravenous fluids, by careful attention to maternal posture (to avoid aortocaval occlusion) and the use of a vasopressor, ephedrine being the one usually preferred.

For these operations the highest standards of anaesthetic technique and nursing care in the anaesthetic room and theatre are required. The partner usually expects to come into the theatre to accompany the woman. If it can be arranged, a preoperative visit by the anaesthetic nurse as well as by the anaesthetist is invaluable.

● PAIN RELIEF IN OBSTETRICS

It is not necessary for the anaesthetic assistant to have a wide knowledge of this subject. The methods available are summarised briefly below.

Psychological

In its simplest form this includes the reassurance that can be given to the woman (especially the primiparous) by explaining the process of labour, the nature, origin and purpose of the pain she is likely to feel and the types of pain relief which will be available to her. More complex techniques include the teaching of special methods of breathing which the patient practises antenatally and then performs in response to the pains of labour. This is a form of conditioned response to the pain and acts largely by distraction.

TENS (Transcutaneous Electrical Nerve Stimulation)

This is described in Chapter 43. Whether its effect is greater than a placebo is uncertain, but it has become popular because it is non-invasive, non-toxic and portable. It is mainly used in the early stages of labour.

Parenteral Methods

Many drugs have been used in labour – the commonest by far, in the UK, being pethidine. This has the advantage that it requires no complicated apparatus and (with certain provisos) may be given by unsupervised mid-wives. Its disadvantages are that it is not always effective, it makes some patients nauseated and slows the gastric emptying; if given in the period leading up to delivery it may depress the newborn baby so that it has difficulty in establishing respiration. It has become less popular in recent years in units which have a wide choice of alternative methods.

Other opioids such as meptazinol (Meptid) are used in the belief that fewer side-effects are seen, although this is not always true.

Inhalational Methods

The only inhalational technique now approved by the United Kingdom Central Council for Nursing, Midwifery and Health Visiting in the UK for use by unsupervised midwives is the administration of Entonox (British Oxygen Company (BOC)), a premixed combination of nitrous oxide 50% and oxygen 50% available in one cylinder or piped to the labour ward (Chapter 6). Although very popular as a method of analgesia, disadvantages include the difficulty in maintaining the technique for long periods, the fact that the patient needs practice to obtain maximum benefit, and that the women sometimes become drowsy and uncooperative, despite the short action of nitrous oxide.

Regional Techniques

Complete pain relief in the first stage of labour may be obtained by bilateral blockade of the 11th and 12th thoracic and first lumbar nerves. In the second stage of labour, additional analgesia is required of the second to fourth sacral nerves. Blockade of all these nerves by one injection can be obtained only by one of the central nerve blocks. These consist of lumbar or sacral epidural (caudal) analgesia and spinal analgesia. More peripheral blocks have to be bilateral and usually multiple.

The great advantage of the central blocks, especially continuous lumbar epidural analgesia by means of an epidural catheter, is that they can give many hours of complete pain relief, adding a new dimension to analgesia in labour. Additionally, the epidural can be easily topped up to provide anaesthesia for instrumental or operative delivery in an emergency.

The main disadvantages of these blocks are that they require skill and experience to perform, they are potentially dangerous if not properly supervised on account of their detrimental effect on venacaval occlusion (see above) and they have a tendency to increase the forceps rate by obtunding the bearing-down reflex. However, with the advent of a more enlightened and less aggressive approach to the conduct of the second stage of labour in many centres, the incidence of forceps deliveries has returned to a level similar to that without the use of epidural analgesia. It has become increasingly popular in obstetric epidural analgesia to add an opiate, for example, fentanyl 2 μg/ml, to the local anaesthetic (Chapter 39). This makes it possible to achieve an approximately equivalent efficacy and duration of pain relief using half the concentration of local anaesthetic drug. The benefit gained is a lesser degree of motor block in the lower limbs which can even make it possible with some regimens for the woman to walk during labour – a 'walking' or 'mobile' epidural.

There has also been increased use of CSE techniques (Chapter 41) in labour. The use of intrathecal opioid and/or local anaesthetic by this method has advantages both for initiating 'walking' epidurals or for rapid onset of relief when pain has been allowed to become severe.

Hypnosis and Acupuncture

These are mentioned only for completeness. While hypnosis, in particular, has been reported at times to be effective, both techniques tend not to be universally applicable or effective, may be time-consuming and require skills possessed by few practitioners. It is difficult to envisage their use becoming widespread for relieving pain in childbirth in the foreseeable future.

Water-bath Births

While not strictly a method of obstetric analgesia, some women find it comforting and relaxing to spend part of their labour in a bath or pool. The safety to the baby of actual delivery in the bath has been questioned, and more research is awaited on this aspect of 'water-bath births'.

● THE OBSTETRIC FLYING SQUADS

Although there has been a great decline in domiciliary midwifery in recent years, it is still possible that an obstetric emergency may arise in a patient's home or in general practitioner units which lack the obstetric and anaesthetic expertise to deal with a serious emergency. The choice then is between resuscitating the patient and always transferring her to the base hospital for definitive treatment, and despatching a skilled team with portable anaesthetic and obstetric equipment from the base hospital to treat the emergency where she lies.

Over the past 10–15 years, there has been a steady decrease in the number of obstetric flying squads which are accompanied by an anaesthetist with portable anaesthetic equipment. At least part of the reason for this has been the increasingly high standards of monitoring recommended for use during anaesthesia in the UK. Flying squads now usually only fulfil a resuscitatory role. Paradoxically, this reduction in flying squad services has coincided with a government recommendation that women should be allowed greater freedom of choice of their place of delivery, which is likely to result in an increase in the number of women delivering in locations lacking effective resuscitation facilities.

39

Local Analgesic Drugs

•History •Definition •Pharmacology •Individual local analgesic agents

● HISTORY

For centuries the natives of Peru and Bolivia had chewed the leaves of a shrub, *Erythroxylum coca*, which lessened fatigue and appetite and numbed the tongue. These effects were due to the principal alkaloid, cocaine, contained in the plant.

In 1860 cocaine was isolated by Niemann and in 1884 Karl Kohler, a Viennese physician, noted its analgesic effect in the eye and published his results. Thereafter the use of local analgesia in its various forms developed quickly.

Dates of introduction of other particularly useful local analgesic drugs include: 1905 – procaine; 1925 – cinchocaine; 1948 – lignocaine; 1963 – bupivacaine; 1997 – ropivacaine; 1998 – levobupivacaine.

● DEFINITION

Local analgesics are drugs which block conduction when applied locally to nerve tissue. The block produced is completely reversible with no damage to nerve cells.

● PHARMACOLOGY

Properties Desirable in a Local Analgesic

These are as follows:

1. They should have a rapid onset of action. The desired duration of action varies with the indication, for example, a very long action would be ideal for postoperative pain relief, but a jaw made numb for many hours after a simple dental procedure would be tedious and inconvenient.

2. The systemic toxicity should be low.
3. They should be non-addictive, non-antigenic, non-irritant to tissues and should not interfere with wound healing.
4. They should be effective topically as well as when injected, although such versatility is not essential.
5. They should be soluble in water, stable in solution, and autoclavable at least once without loss of potency.

Sites of Application of Local Analgesic Drugs

Starting centrally and working peripherally, local analgesic solutions may produce the following types of analgesia:

- *Spinal block* – where the injection is into the subarachnoid space.
- *Epidural block* – where the injection is into the epidural space.
- *Nerve plexus block* – where the injection is made into a nerve plexus, for example, brachial plexus block.
- *Nerve block* – where the injection is into a single nerve trunk, for example, femoral nerve block, ulnar nerve block.
- *Local infiltration* – where the injection is into the tissues, for example, subcutaneous infiltration.
- *Intravenous regional (IVRA, Bier's block)* – where the injection is made into a vein of a limb whose circulation is occluded by a tourniquet.
- *Topical* – where the drug is applied to skin or mucous membrane.

Details of some of the local analgesic nerve blocks are given in Chapter 40.

Mode of Action

In its resting state, the outside of the cell membrane of a nerve fibre is positively charged relative to the inside. When a nerve impulse is propagated along the nerve fibre, there is a sudden increase in the permeability of the cell membrane to sodium ions, which then flow into the interior of the nerve fibre and reverse the electrical polarity across the cell membrane so that the inside becomes positively charged with reference to the outside.

This phenomenon is called 'depolarisation' and is fundamental to the transmission of the nerve impulse. It is this sudden increase in permeability of the cell membrane to sodium ions which in some way is interfered with by local analgesic drugs so that depolarisation is prevented and nerve fibre block occurs. The exact mode of action is unknown.

Chemistry

All local analgesic drugs of clinical interest belong to one main group, which has the following basic formula:

Aromatic group – intermediate chain – amino group

This main group of local analgesic drugs is divided into two subgroups depending on the method of linkage between the aromatic group and the intermediate chain. If this is an ester (–COO–) linkage the local analgesic belongs to the 'ester' group and if the linkage is an amide (–HN.CO–) linkage the drug belongs to the 'amide' group. Examples are illustrated below.

Most of the older analgesic drugs, for example, procaine, cocaine and amethocaine, belong to the ester group. Most of the newer agents, for example, lignocaine, prilocaine, bupivacaine and ropivacaine, belong to the amide group.

Metabolism and Excretion

The ester group of local analgesic drugs are hydrolysed in the plasma by the enzyme pseudocholinesterase (also involved in the breakdown of suxamethonium). Some of the breakdown products are metabolised further; some are excreted in the urine. The exception in this group is cocaine, which is largely detoxified in the liver, a small proportion being excreted unchanged in the urine. The amide group of agents are largely broken down in the liver, only a small fraction being excreted unchanged in the urine.

Toxicity

Toxicity means general systemic toxicity when absorbed into the circulation. In this, local analgesic agents differ from most drugs where toxicity is an exaggeration of their therapeutic effect. In the case of local analgesics, which are usually chosen for their local effect, the general toxic effects appear in other systems and do not have an obvious relationship to the local effect.

With the exception of those produced by cocaine, the toxic effects are similar for all local analgesic agents. They are mainly on the central nervous system, with secondary effects on other systems.

It has been customary to describe the central nervous system effects as stimulation first and then depression. It is now believed that the effect is purely depressant, the apparent stimulation being due to depression of inhibitory fibres revealing excitatory effects.

Clinically, the first sign is often numbness of the tongue and circum-oral region. There may also be light headedness, dizziness and tinnitus. Anxiety and muscular twitching progress to generalised tonic and clonic convulsions as the stimulatory effects on the higher centres escalate. As the depressant effects follow, the patient becomes unconscious, while depression of the medullary vital centres leads to cardiovascular collapse and respiratory arrest. The cardiac effects may be augmented by direct depression of the myocardium by high blood concentrations of local analgesic drug.

It should be noted that the milder, premonitory excitatory signs are by no means always seen with the amide group of local analgesic agents. With lignocaine, in particular, the first sign of systemic absorption is often drowsiness, and this may be quite marked in old people.

Factors Affecting Toxicity

Systemic toxic effects appear when the concentration of local analgesic drug in the blood rises above a certain level, which varies for different agents. Thus most factors affecting toxicity do so by increasing the rate of absorption into the bloodstream, or sometimes by reducing the removal of the agent from it.

General Factors

Age. It is a wise rule always to be particularly careful when giving any drug to the very old or the very young. Whether very young patients are particularly susceptible to the toxic effects of analgesic drugs is doubtful, but care must be taken on a dose/weight ratio. A technique for operating on congenital pyloric stenosis under local analgesia recommended a dose of 14 ml 0.25% lignocaine as the safe upper limit! Elderly patients are more liable to toxic effects than their body weight might indicate.

Sex. With the exception of the effect of body weight there is probably no difference between the sexes in their response to local analgesics. In the later months of pregnancy, however, smaller volumes of local analgesic drugs are required than are usual for the performance of spinal or epidural analgesia.

Body weight. Blood levels of drug reached are approximately inversely proportional to body weight. Toxic doses, as usually recommended, apply to an average 70 kg person and should be adjusted accordingly.

General condition. The acutely ill or chronically debilitated patient is more susceptible to the toxic effects of local analgesic drugs.

Liver function. Most modern (amide) local analgesics are metabolised in the liver. The state of liver function will have no effect on the acute toxicity produced by a single, excessive administration of drug, but may affect the gradual build-up to toxic blood levels produced by repeated doses of the drug, as in a continuous epidural technique.

Local Factors

Site of injection. Injection into particularly vascular areas is likely to lead to rapid absorption and high blood levels. Such areas include the head, neck and pelvic floor. Two other areas from which absorption can be alarmingly rapid are the upper respiratory tract and an inflamed urethra – when topical application is used.

Concentration of drug. This is a debatable factor, but it is suggested that absorption down a concentration gradient will be faster from a more concentrated solution.

Use of vasoconstrictor agents. The addition to local analgesic injections of agents such as adrenaline, noradrenaline or octapressin slows their absorption from the site of injection and reduces the blood level achieved. As a result, the maximum safe dose of the analgesic agent may be increased, and its action is usually prolonged.

Use of hyaluronidase. This enzyme breaks down intercellular cement and increases the spread of injected fluid through tissues. It increases the area for, and therefore the rate of, absorption of injected local analgesic drugs, and so makes toxic effects more likely.

Regional techniques that require very large and potentially toxic doses of local analgesic drug, for example, regional block for thoracoplasty, have now gone out of fashion. Toxic reactions simply due to a single overdose should no longer happen. The commonest cause today of toxic reactions is the inadvertent intravascular administration of the drug.

Also potentially dangerous is the progressive increase in blood levels that may accompany repeated increments of an agent – as in a continuous epidural technique.

Treatment of Toxic Effects

If administration of the drug is continuing, it may be sufficient to stop, give the patient oxygen and watch carefully for any sign of worsening of the effects. If signs of excitation are more marked, it has been customary to recommend giving thiopentone slowly to prevent or abolish convulsions. However, it must be remembered that the condition is basically one of central nervous system depression, and that depressant drugs must be given with the utmost caution. Probably diazepam given slowly intravenously is less depressant, and therefore a better choice than thiopentone.

For established convulsions, suxamethonium will abolish the muscular aspect of the convulsion and allow intubation and ventilation with air or oxygen. If fits recur when the suxamethonium wears off, diazepam may be given. Cardiovascular collapse requires appropriate symptomatic treatment, which might include raising the legs, intravenous fluids and possibly a vasopressor. If cardiac arrest occurs, treatment is as described in Chapter 23.

Other Uses of Local Analgesic Drugs

Anti-arrhythmic Effect

The effect produced by local analgesic drugs on the cell membranes of nerve fibres whereby depolarisation is slowed or stopped also occurs at other cell membranes, notably those of cardiac muscle fibres. In this way, lignocaine may be particularly effective in preventing the abnormal contraction of ventricular muscle tissue seen in ventricular dysrhythmias, especially ventricular extrasystoles. If these are considered dangerous, a bolus injection of 1 mg/kg plain lignocaine is given, followed usually by an intravenous drip of lignocaine at a rate adjusted to suppress the ectopic beats.

Preventing the Pressure Response to Intubation

Laryngoscopy and intubation can cause a rise in pulse rate and blood pressure. This may be harmful particularly in patients with increased intracranial or intraocular pressure. This pressure response to intubation is prevented by prior intravenous injection of 1–1.5 mg/kg of lignocaine 2–3 min before intubation.

Anti-convulsant Action

At lower blood levels than those required to produce convulsions, some local analgesic drugs have an anti-convulsant action. Few would advocate their use for this purpose nowadays as other agents are safer and more effective.

Toxicity of Vasoconstrictor Agents

Confusion may arise from the statement that addition of a potentially dangerous agent like adrenaline makes local analgesics safer. This fact is entirely due to the slower absorption of the analgesic into the systemic circulation which occurs when a vasoconstrictor is added.

However, adrenaline is potentially toxic, and a maximum dose of 500 μg (0.5 ml 1 : 1000) adrenaline HCl injected subcutaneously is usually recommended in a 70 kg man. This will normally produce minimal effect on the cardiovascular system. If inadvertently given intravenously, the patient will probably suffer palpitations, a feeling of anxiety and possibly retrosternal discomfort. An electrocardiogram (ECG) might show a ventricular arrhythmia, but a fit patient would be unlikely to come to serious harm. An adrenaline concentration of 1 : 100 000 need never be exceeded for local infiltration and 1 : 400 000 gives excellent vasoconstriction. The systemic effects of adrenaline may be potentiated in patients on tricyclic antidepressants and its use should be avoided.

Local analgesic agents are commercially available with adrenaline, usually in a concentration of 1 : 100 000 or 1 : 200 000. These are frequently used by surgeons (e.g. in plastic surgery and gynaecology) to reduce bleeding at operations under general anaesthesia. The presence of the local analgesic in these cases is usually unnecessary, and a cheaper alternative is to dilute the contents of an adrenaline ampoule in saline.

Noradrenaline is a safer alternative to adrenaline as it has less of adrenaline's powerful and stimulant effects on the myocardium. Its lack of popularity probably arises from its reputedly less powerful effect and risk of producing local sloughing of tissue.

Felypressin (octapressin) is a synthetic octapeptide with little cardiac effect. It has not gained popularity except in dentistry, where it is available in some cartridges of local analgesic.

It must be realised that a solution of local analgesic drug containing adrenaline may be toxic from the point of view of the local analgesic or the adrenaline, but the safety point may not necessarily be the same for each.

● INDIVIDUAL LOCAL ANALGESIC AGENTS

Many drugs have been tried since cocaine was introduced. Of those still available commercially, the choice differs somewhat from country to country. Only six will be discussed here:

1. Cocaine because of its unique properties and side-effects.
2. Lignocaine because it has become the classic agent against which new agents are compared.
3. Bupivacaine because it remains the most reliable of the agents with a longer action than lignocaine.
4. Ropivacaine and levobupivacaine for their safety profile.
5. Prilocaine for its unique ability to produce methaemoglobinaemia.

Cocaine

One of the ester group of drugs, cocaine is unique in several ways. It is the only naturally occurring local analgesic substance still in clinical use. It produces excitation of the central nervous system in low concentrations – the stimulatory effect on the higher centres being responsible for its addictive properties.

It is the only local analgesic agent which is a powerful vasoconstrictor, this action being the result of its potentiation of catecholamines. Its sympathomimetic action on the heart may cause ventricular fibrillation before the central nervous system effects can manifest themselves as convulsions. Although belonging to the ester group, it is mainly detoxified in the liver, the remainder being excreted almost unchanged by the kidneys.

It retains a place as a topical analgesic agent, mostly for producing topical anaesthesia and vasoconstriction in the nasal cavity for awake fibre-optic intubation and in ear, nose and throat (ENT) work. While potentially a very toxic agent, its powerful vasoconstrictor action prevents it from being absorbed rapidly and the maximum safe dose used in this manner is about 150 mg in a 70 kg adult. A 5% solution (50 mg/ml) is an adequate strength to use.

Lignocaine

Synthesised in Sweden in 1943, lignocaine (Xylocaine) was first used clinically in 1948. It has a rapid onset and good penetration in the tissues and can be used by any method of application. It causes tachyphylaxis – more frequent and increasing doses are required with repeated use. It is stable in solution and can be autoclaved more than once without losing potency. It belongs to the amide group.

Lignocaine has some local vasodilatory effect, while most other local analgesic drugs (apart from cocaine) have little or no effect. The maximum dose for a 70 kg man is 200 mg of the plain solution and 500 mg with adrenaline. Its use in the treatment of ventricular arrhythmias has already been discussed. The toxic blood level is about 5 μg/ml.

Bupivacaine

Synthesised in 1957 and first used clinically in 1963, bupivacaine (Marcain) also belongs to the amide group. Early claims for a duration of action of 5–12 h seem to be justified for peripheral nerve block and plexus blocks but not for epidural analgesia, where its action is usually about 2 h. However, this is longer than can be reliably expected from lignocaine, and as blood levels in mother and fetus are also slower to rise than with lignocaine, it has become the agent of choice for continuous epidural block in labour.

Adrenaline has much less effect in prolonging the action of bupivacaine or in lowering the blood levels after injection than is the case with most local analgesic agents. The reason is not clear, but it is known that at some concentrations bupivacaine has some vasoconstrictor action of its own. Consequently the safe dose is taken to be the same whether given with or without adrenaline – 150 mg in a 70 kg adult.

Cases have been reported where the first sign of bupivacaine toxicity has been cardiac arrest due to ventricular fibrillation, which has proved particularly resistant to treatment. Study of the case reports indicates that probably all these cases resulted from direct intravascular injection rather than from slower absorption from more peripheral tissues. However, this has led to a reappraisal of its use in circumstances where high blood levels might be expected, especially during Bier's block, for which as a result prilocaine and lignocaine are now the agents of choice.

Since its introduction, bupivacaine has steadily developed into one of the most popular local anaesthetic agents in clinical practice.

Ropivacaine

This is a new amide local analgesic which has been extensively evaluated by Astra Ltd and was marketed in 1997. It is similar to bupivacaine (a propyl group replacing the butyl group in bupivacaine) but its low lipid solubility results in less severe central nervous system and cardiovascular toxicity. Its motor sparing effect is now thought to be due to its low potency compared to bupivacaine. It has vasoconstrictor properties similar to bupivacaine and hence addition of adrenaline does not produce prolongation of effect. A safe maximum dose is 250 mg in a 70 kg patient (3.5 mg/kg).

Levobupivacaine

The original preparation of bupivacaine is a racemic mixture of *l*- and *d*-isomers. Levobupivacaine is a preparation of the single isomer *l*-bupivacaine and was introduced in 1998. Its efficacy is equivalent to that of bupivacaine and so in clinical practice a simple substitution for the same concentration and dose of bupivacaine is all that is required. Although the central nervous system and cardiac toxicity is similar to that seen with bupivacaine, a much larger dose is required to produce these effects. Currently a safe maximum dose of 150 mg in a 70 kg patient is recommended.

Prilocaine

Another of the amide group, prilocaine (Citanest) was first used in 1959. It is claimed to be less toxic than lignocaine (maximum dose 300 mg plain, 600 mg with adrenaline in a 70 kg adult), to which it is similar.

Unfortunately it was found that during its metabolism prilocaine produced a metabolite – o-toluidine – which caused the conversion of haemoglobin to methaemoglobin, a form which takes no part in oxygen transport. While this tended to occur only when about 600 mg prilocaine had been used, these amounts could quite easily be used in continuous epidural analgesia in obstetrics, where the baby could also be adversely affected.

Because of this tendency to cause methaemoglobinaemia, this agent has largely disappeared from many areas of regional anaesthetic practice, but remains popular for Bier's block and in dentistry.

Amethocaine Gel (Ametop) (see also Chapter 14)

Amethocaine 4% gel is an effective topical local analgesic commonly used prior to venepuncture. It should not be used for topical application over mucous membranes, for which lignocaine is safer.

EMLA (see also Chapter 14)

EMLA cream 5% is an eutectic mixture of lignocaine and prilocaine which is effective as a topical analgesic when applied to the skin under an occlusive dressing. It is very useful before venepuncture in children and can also be used as anaesthesia for split skin grafting.

40

Local Analgesic Nerve Blocks

•Principles of local analgesic nerve blocks •Types of nerve block
•Nerve stimulators

Both somatic and sympathetic nerves can be blocked by a variety of techniques. Certain nerve blocks can produce sufficient analgesia to be used as the sole anaesthetic. Often nerve blocks are performed in combination with general anaesthesia to supplement pain relief during and after operations. Nerve blocks are also useful for other acute (e.g. fractured ribs) and chronic painful conditions.

Sympathetic nerve blocks have been performed in a great many conditions with varying success (see below).

● PRINCIPLES OF LOCAL ANALGESIC NERVE BLOCKS

No attempt will be made here to list the vast number of local analgesic nerve blocks. Instead, some of the principles of local analgesic technique are discussed and some examples given of the commoner blocks.

Somatic nerves contain both motor fibres to skeletal muscle and sensory fibres carrying the sensations of pain, temperature, touch, position and proprioception. The sympathetic and parasympathetic nerves carry fibres to and from thoracic and abdominal viscera (e.g. the heart and bowel). Sympathetic fibres also pass to the sweat glands, to the erector pilae muscles affecting the skin hairs and, probably most important of all, to arterioles and venules throughout the body. The somatic motor fibres, which run from the spinal cord as the anterior nerve roots are found at all levels of the spinal cord, as are the somatic sensory fibres which are attached to the spinal cord by the posterior nerve roots.

The sympathetic nerve fibres do not arise at all levels, but only in the thoracic and upper lumbar levels (Figs 40.1 and 30.2). They leave the spinal cord in the anterior nerve roots in company with the motor fibres, and pass out of an intervertebral foramen with the anterior primary ramus of the spinal nerve. The sympathetic fibres soon leave the anterior primary ramus as a white ramus communicans and after a few centimetres join

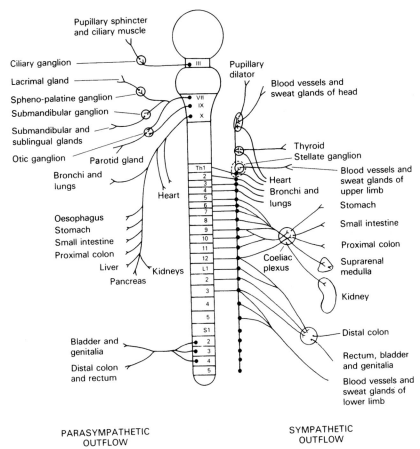

Figure 40.1 Sympathetic and parasympathetic nervous systems.

a sympathetic ganglion. These ganglia, of which there are some 24 on each side, lie anterolateral to the vertebral column and are joined by sympathetic fibres to form the sympathetic chain. Despite the limited outflow from the spinal cord, the sympathetic fibres are distributed to all parts of the body. The sympathetic ganglia are the sites where the preganglionic fibres from the spinal cord form synapses with postganglionic fibres. Most of the postganglionic fibres destined to supply vasoconstrictor fibres to limb blood vessels return to the spinal nerves via grey rami communicantes.

Parasympathetic fibres (both efferent and afferent) are carried only in the vagus and second, third and fourth sacral nerves (Chapter 30). It follows, therefore, that both spinal and epidural anaesthesia tend to block both the somatic and sympathetic nerve fibres. By carefully introducing a needle to the region of the sympathetic chain or ganglia, however, it is possible to produce a purely sympathetic block. It is not possible to produce the converse effect, i.e. a purely somatic block, by injecting more peripherally, as the sympathetic fibres to the blood vessels are distributed with the somatic fibres along the main nerve trunks. However, by common usage, these more peripheral blocks are often referred to as somatic nerve blocks.

● TYPES OF NERVE BLOCK

The following are some common examples of the different types of nerve block.

Somatic Nerve Blocks

Blockade of a nerve or group of nerves can be produced by injection of local anaesthetic at different levels in its anatomical distribution. The term central neural blockade is commonly used when these injections are performed near the spinal cord as in spinal and epidural anaesthesia (see Chapter 41). Peripheral nerve blocks are of two types: plexus blocks, when a group of nerves are blocked in a plexus, and single nerve block, when only one nerve is blocked. The following discussion on analgesia of the upper limb is used to demonstrate some of the plexus and single nerve blocks for local anaesthesia of the upper limb.

Upper Limb Blocks

The upper limb is supplied by the brachial plexus which arises from the fifth, sixth, seventh and eighth cervical and the first thoracic nerve roots. Although some of the branches supplying the upper limb skin, muscles and other tissues arise from these nerve roots, most of the nerve supply is via the three cords which eventually branch out as peripheral nerves, the common ones being the musculocutaneous, radial, median and ulnar nerves. The latter three end as digital nerves supplying the digits of the hands.

The branches of the plexus can be blocked by injecting local anesthetic solution in the facial compartment surrounding the plexus (brachial plexus block) or individual nerves (single nerve block) more peripherally as described below.

Brachial Plexus Block

This is the commonest of the nerve plexus blocks, although the multiplicity of techniques which have been described indicate that no method is perfect. Some of the advantages and disadvantages of three of the approaches which have achieved most popularity will be presented.

The interscalene approach. The injection is made into the plexus between the scalene muscles in the neck at the level of the sixth cervical vertebra. Advantages are that the method may be easier than others in obese patients, that it is effective for shoulder manipulations and surgery and it avoids the risk of a pneumothorax. Disadvantages include the possible injection into the subarachnoid or epidural spaces or into the vertebral artery, and phrenic nerve block causing diaphragmatic paralysis may occur. The ulnar nerve is relatively difficult to block with this high approach.

The supraclavicular approach. The injection is made from above the clavicle down onto the plexus as it crosses the upper surface of the first rib. This approach has declined in popularity, because although it also gives analgesia for shoulder manipulation, it is the technique most likely to produce a pneumothorax. Spread to other nerves – phrenic, vagus, recurrent laryngeal and sympathetic – can also occur.

The axillary approach. The injection is made into the axillary sheath round the brachial plexus by inserting the needle close to the axillary artery as high up as it can be felt in the axilla. The main advantages are that many of the complications of the other methods are avoided, for example, the risk of pneumothorax, or subarachnoid or extradural injection, or spread to other nerves. Disadvantages are the difficulty of the technique in obese patients, its impossibility if the arm cannot be abducted, the failure to produce analgesia for shoulder operations and at times the failure of the block to include the musculocutaneous nerve.

For brachial plexus block suitable local anaesthetic solutions are 1% lignocaine in 1 : 200 000 adrenaline or 0.25% bupivacaine plain or in 1 : 200 000 adrenaline.

Single Nerve Blocks

Ulnar Nerve Block

This is included as an example of a single nerve block. The ulnar nerve can easily be rolled over the posterior surface of the medial epicondyle of the humerus with the forefinger. This produces the familiar pain shooting down the inner aspect of the arm into the little finger and this part of the elbow is colloquially referred to as the 'funny-bone': 2–5 ml local anaesthetic injected here will produce analgesia of the little finger and the ulnar border of the ring finger. The preferred local anaesthetics are 2% lignocaine or 0.5% bupivacaine plain or with adrenaline.

Digital Nerve Block

The nerve supply to each finger runs as a pair of digital nerves along each side of the digit. Excellent analgesia for operations on the distal part of the digit may be obtained by injecting a few millilitres of local anaesthetic at each side of the base of the finger. The special consideration of this block is that the sole blood supply to the digit runs beside these nerves and if vasoconstrictor solutions are used gangrene of the finger or toe may occur.

Sympathetic Nerve Blocks

Sympathetic nerve blocks have been performed in a great many conditions with varying success. Vascular conditions probably provide the biggest group of indications. Damage to, thrombosis of, or embolism of a major vessel is associated with intense spasm in surrounding blood vessels which might provide a collateral circulation past the damaged vessel. Sympathetic block relieves this spasm and helps to restore arterial or venous circulation. Phenol may be used to produce a more prolonged block in more chronic vascular disease, for example, where rest pain or incipient gangrene is associated with these conditions. A sympathetic block may also be used before amputation to improve the blood supply to the amputation site. Other indications include causalgia and phantom limb pain.

Stellate Ganglion Block

The cervical sympathetic chain normally consists of three ganglia – the superior, middle and inferior cervical ganglia. The inferior cervical ganglion is often fused with the first thoracic ganglion and in this case the combined ganglion is called the 'stellate ganglion'. Through this ganglion runs the entire sympathetic nerve supply to the head, neck and upper limb on that side. Stellate ganglion block may be useful in arterial and venous injuries to the upper limb, in arterial and venous thrombosis and of prognostic value before considering operation for the treatment of Raynaud's disease of the upper limb. It may also be of use in causalgia and Miniere's disease. Its use in strokes and in central retinal artery thrombosis has been abandoned because sympathetic block does not produce vasodilatation of the cerebral blood vessels.

Lumbar Sympathetic Chain Block

As there is no sympathetic outflow below the second lumbar segment, blockade of the sympathetic chain below this level affects the entire sympathetic nerve supply to the pelvis and lower limbs. Apart from its use in vascular conditions, causalgia, phantom limb pain, etc., as already described, lumbar sympathetic chain block has been used in renal colic and obstetric pain. However, it is not usually regarded as a continuous catheter technique and this fact limits its usefulness in these latter types of pain. For longer term effect in intractable conditions, aqueous phenol solution may be used instead of local analgesic.

Intravenous Regional Analgesia (Bier's Block)

This technique was first described by August Bier in 1908 using procaine, and is often referred to by his name. It was reintroduced using lignocaine by Holmes in 1963 while he was working in Oxford. It has gained considerable popularity because very little skill is required, and little of the knowledge of anatomy needed for many other analgesic blocks.

After inserting a needle or cannula, usually in the back of the hand or forearm, the limb is exsanguinated using an Esmarch's bandage or, in the presence of a painful lesion, simply by raising the limb while compressing the brachial artery. A pneumatic tourniquet which has been applied on the proximal part of the limb is then inflated to about 100 mmHg above arterial blood pressure, and after removing the Esmarch's bandage local analgesic solution is injected via the indwelling needle into the exsanguinated limb. Many solutions have been used but the most popular is plain 0.5% prilocaine. About 40 ml solution is adequate for a man's forearm with proportionately less being used for a woman or child's upper limb. Analgesia begins quickly but may not be complete for up to 20 min. It begins proximally and works distally. Occasionally it may not extend to the fingers, but analgesia may be completed by injecting a few additional millilitres of local anaesthetic solution before removing the indwelling needle.

At the end of the operation the tourniquet is released and a considerable proportion of the local anaesthetic solution rapidly returns to the systemic circulation. The blood levels obtained may be high and toxic reactions have been reported. The proportion of local analgesic entering the circulation quickly is highest if the block has been maintained for a short time, and it is probably unwise to remove the tourniquet in under 20 min. The patient should be watched carefully for evidence of toxic effects, for example, bradycardia or arrhythmias. Probably the commonest toxic symptoms are auditory, either tinnitus or transient deafness. It has been suggested that toxic effects are less likely if the tourniquet is released and reinflated to slow the release of analgesic solution into the systemic circulation. Thus the tourniquet may be released for 5 s every 30 s for 5 min.

In view of the possibility of a toxic reaction, it is always a wise precaution to have an indwelling needle or cannula present in the other upper limb. It is also very important to test the apparatus for leaks before use.

Sooner or later most patients find the discomfort of the tourniquet intolerable. For this reason it is recommended that a second tourniquet be applied distal to the first tourniquet, it therefore being placed on analgesic skin. It can then be inflated to the same pressure as the proximal cuff,

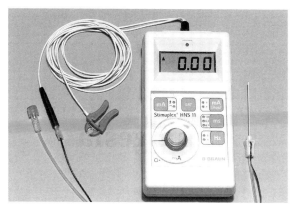

Figure 40.2 Nerve stimulator with insulated nerve block needle.

which is then released. Special double-cuff tourniquets have been designed for this purpose. Even with a second cuff, tourniquet pain is eventually felt, but tourniquet time in any case should not exceed normal orthopaedic limits of 60–90 min.

Intravenous regional analgesia (IVRA) may also be used in the leg, but even with a below-knee tourniquet the volume of solution required is greater and hence the risk of toxic reactions on release of the tourniquet more likely.

● NERVE STIMULATORS (Fig. 40.2)

Nerve stimulators similar to those used to assess neuromuscular block (Chapter 20) may be used to aid accuracy of needle placement for nerve block. The principle is that a current passed through the exploring needle (insulated except for the tip) produces a twitch in the associated muscle when the nerve being sought is approached. A 1 mA current is usually applied at a frequency of 1–2 Hz which is insufficient to cause sensory pain. An injection port attached to the needle allows the injection of local anaesthetic as soon as the nerve is located.

41

Spinal and Epidural Analgesia

•History •Anatomy •Factors affecting spread of solutions in the subarachnoid space •Factors affecting spread of solutions in the epidural space •Complications of spinal analgesia •Complications of epidural analgesia •Uses of spinal and epidural analgesia •Contraindications to spinal and epidural analgesia •Intrathecal and epidural opioids and other agents •Drugs and equipment •Combined spinal–epidural (CSE) anaesthesia •Continuous spinal anaesthesia

● HISTORY

Spinals

1885   Corning of New York accidentally performed the first spinal while experimenting with cocaine on a dog.

1899   The first spinal for a surgical operation was carried out by August Bier of Germany.

1907   Barker of London described the importance of the curves of the vertebral column and the use of gravity in the spread of spinal solutions.

1940   Lemmon described continuous spinal analgesia via a needle.

1945   Tuohy performed continuous spinal analgesia via a needle and ureteric catheter.

Epidurals

1901   Sicard and Cathelin of France independently performed the first epidurals by the sacral (caudal) approach.

1913   Heile of Germany tried epidural blocks via a lateral approach through the intervertebral foramina.

1921	Pagés of Spain was the first to use the midline lumbar approach, relying on his sense of touch to detect the passage from ligamentum flavum to the epidural space.
1941	Hingson and Southworth of the USA performed the first continuous lumbar epidural using a needle.
1942	Manalan of the USA performed the first continuous caudal using a catheter.
1942	Hingson and Southworth performed the first continuous caudal using a needle.
1949	Curbelo of Havana described continuous lumbar epidural block using a Tuohy needle and ureteric catheter.

● ANATOMY

Bony anatomy

There are 33 vertebrae grouped according to regions into seven cervical, twelve thoracic, five lumbar, five sacral (fused in the adult to form the sacrum) and four coccygeal (fused to form the coccyx).

A typical vertebra (Fig. 41.1a–c) consists of two main parts: (a) the weight-bearing vertebral body in front, attached to those above and below by intervertebral discs; and (b) the vertebral arch posteriorly, made up of the pedicles and laminae. The spinous, transverse and superior and inferior articular processes project from the arch. The lower and upper borders of the pedicles, helped by the adjacent bodies and disc and the superior and inferior articular processes, form the boundaries of the intervertebral foramina, through which the segmental nerves pass from the spinal cord.

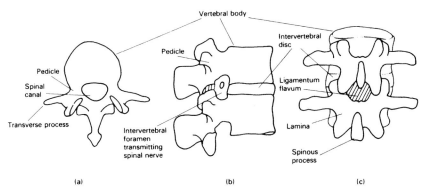

Figure 41.1 Lumbar vertebrae (a) from above, (b) from the side, (c) from behind.

Each lamina is joined to the one above and below by the fibro-elastic ligamenta flava. The vertebral foramen is formed by the vertebral arch and the posterior surface of the body. When the vertebrae are placed on top of one another the vertebral foramina become the vertebral canal, which houses and protects the spinal cord and membranes. At its upper end, the canal meets the skull at the foramen magnum and at its lower end it continues down into the body of the sacrum as the sacral canal and ends at the sacral hiatus.

The bodies, arches and processes have distinguishing features in the different regions of the vertebral column. One of the most important from the anaesthetist's point of view is the varying obliquity of the spinous processes in the thoracic and lumbar regions.

Spinal Cord and Spinal Nerves

The spinal cord begins at the level of the foramen magnum as the continuation of the medulla oblongata of the brain. It usually ends at the level of the upper part of the second lumbar vertebra, although in the newborn, and in some adults, it extends to the third lumbar vertebra. It gives off 31 pairs of nerves – eight cervical, twelve thoracic, five lumbar, five sacral and one coccygeal. The grey matter of the spinal cord is roughly H-shaped (Fig. 41.2). It contains the nuclei of the nerve cells, the anterior horns of the H containing the nuclei from which the motor fibres arise and the posterior horns containing the nuclei on which most of the sensory fibres end. In the thoracic and upper two or three lumbar segments there are also small lateral horns in which sympathetic fibres arise.

Each spinal nerve is made up of an anterior root containing motor fibres derived from the anterior horns (and at some levels sympathetic fibres derived from the lateral horns) and a posterior root containing sensory fibres passing inwards to the posterior horn.

A ganglion on the posterior root near the intervertebral foramen contains the nuclei of the sensory nerves. Just lateral to the ganglion the anterior and posterior roots fuse and their fibres intermingle to form a spinal nerve. Almost at once the nerve divides into the larger anterior primary ramus and smaller posterior primary ramus for distribution throughout the body.

The spinal nerves escape from the bony vertebral column through the appropriate intervertebral foramina, or in the case of the sacral and coccygeal nerves, through the anterior and posterior sacral foramina or sacral hiatus. The spinal cord having ended at L2, the nerve roots, especially the lower ones, have to pass downwards from their spinal cord origin to the point of emergence from their bony protection. The lower lumbar, sacral and coccygeal nerves thus form a bundle running vertically downwards in the

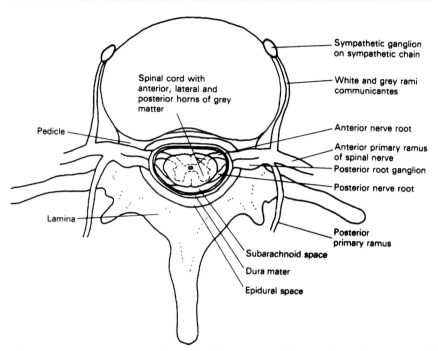

Figure 41.2 Cross-section at the level of the upper lumbar vertebrae showing spinal cord, subarachnoid and epidural spaces.

subarachnoid space named, from its resemblance to a horse's tail, the 'cauda equina' (Fig. 41.3).

Subarachnoid Space

There are three fibrous membranes which surround the spinal cord. They are named from within outwards the pia mater, arachnoid mater and dura mater. The pia mater closely invests the spinal cord. The blood vessels ramify in this membrane before entering the cord. The arachnoid mater is separated from the pia mater by the subarachnoid space containing the cerebrospinal fluid (CSF). It is a delicate layer closely applied to the inner surface of the thick, fibrous dura mater. Usually when a needle pierces the dura mater it also passes through the arachnoid into the subarachnoid space, although injection into the subdural space is possible.

The spinal subarachnoid space (which has a volume of about 25 ml) is in direct communication through the foramen magnum with the cranial subarachnoid space containing the CSF bathing the surface of the brain.

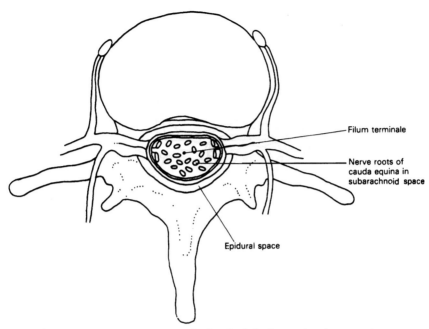

Filum terminale

Nerve roots of
cauda equina in
subarachnoid space

Epidural space

Figure 41.3 Cross-section at the level of the lower lumbar vertebrae.

It is therefore possible for solutions injected into the spinal subarachnoid space to gain access to the cranial nerves. The spinal subarachnoid space also communicates, though rather less freely, with the fourth ventricle of the brain by three openings in its roof. By this route it is possible for spinal solutions to reach the vital centres in the medulla.

Inferiorly the spinal subarachnoid space ends at the level of the second sacral vertebra (Fig. 41.4), where it is within easy reach of a marauding caudal needle!

Epidural Space

The remaining space between the dura mater and the walls of the vertebral canal is the epidural space. It is traversed by the spinal nerves in their dural coverings, but apart from these, epidural veins and a variable amount of fat, it is largely a potential space which can be opened up by air or liquid. Its outer boundary is made up of the periosteum lining the bony parts of the vertebral canal with the ligamenta flava filling in the gaps posteriorly between the laminae. Superiorly the epidural space is limited by the attachment of both the periosteum lining the vertebral canal and the dura mater to the margin of the foramen magnum. (This periosteum and the spinal

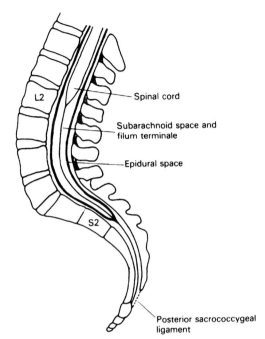

Figure 41.4 Structures at the lower end of the vertebral column.

dura mater correspond to the two layers of intracranial dura mater.) This lifts the upward spread of solutions injected into the epidural space.

Laterally, the epidural space is continuous with the paravertebral spaces which lie between the heads of the ribs in the thoracic region. As the pleura is one boundary of the paravertebral space, intrapleural pressure changes are transmitted to the epidural space.

Inferiorly, the epidural space ends where the posterior sacrococcygeal ligament roofs over the sacral hiatus (see Fig. 41.4). This is the point of entry for a needle when performing a sacral or caudal.

The anterior (consisting of motor and, at some levels, sympathetic fibres) and the posterior (sensory) nerve roots of all the spinal nerves have to traverse both the subarachnoid and epidural spaces. Local analgesic solution injected into either of these spaces therefore produces a type of nerve block. In the case of the former space it is called a 'subarachnoid', 'intrathecal' or 'spinal' block and in the case of the latter is called an 'epidural', 'extradural' or 'peridural' block.

After the injection of solutions into the subarachnoid or epidural spaces, various factors affect the extent of their distribution and they differ in importance between the two spaces.

● FACTORS AFFECTING SPREAD OF SOLUTIONS IN THE SUBARACHNOID SPACE

Specific Gravity and Posture

These two factors are considered together because they are interdependent. Different liquids have different densities, i.e. weight per unit volume. The specific gravity (SG) of a liquid is its density at any given temperature relative to the density of water at 4°C. When two liquids are mixed, the one with the higher SG sinks to the bottom of the container.

CSF has an SG very similar to that of water. The simple salts of local analgesic solutions have specific gravities not usually very different from that of CSF but can be made heavier or lighter than CSF; heavier usually by adding dextrose to the solution, lighter usually by warming. A local analgesic solution with an SG higher than that of CSF is called 'hyperbaric'; if the SG is the same as CSF it is 'isobaric' and if lighter, 'hypobaric'. Traditionally, the great majority of spinal blocks have been carried out using hyperbaric solutions and the following comments on factors affecting the spread of solutions in the subarachnoid space refer to these solutions.

If a hyperbaric solution is injected into the subarachnoid space, it rapidly sinks in the CSF. With the patient in the lateral recumbent position, the vertebral canal is practically horizontal, and little movement of the injected solution occurs. However, if the patient is turned on his back, the effect which the curvatures of the spine will have on the injected solution becomes apparent. It is found that there is a cervical convexity forwards, a deep thoracic concavity forwards, a lumbar convexity forwards again and a small sacral concavity. The injection is usually made at the L2–3 or L3–4 interspaces, which are about the summit of the lumbar convexity. The injected solution thus divides into a portion which runs towards the sacrum and a part which runs down into the thoracic concavity. The first portion does nothing which has not already been done by the injected bolus spreading across the cauda equina. The upper portion, having reached the lowest part of the thoracic concavity (the mid-thoracic region), is prevented from spreading further cephalad by the slope leading up out of the cervical end of that concavity. This represents a built-in safety factor in spinal analgesia in that it is virtually impossible for a normal volume of spinal analgesic solution to spread much higher than the mid-thoracic level of the spinal cord unless the patient is left at all head-down on his side, or with the head much too far down in the supine position.

The other common posture for administering spinal analgesia is the sitting position. The patient may then be immediately laid down, or more commonly left in the sitting position for some minutes. With this latter technique, there is almost no analgesia above the level of insertion of the needle.

Indeed, if the injection is made slowly enough, the analgesic solution may not even cut right across the cauda equina but, trickling down, anaesthetises only the lower sacral and coccygeal nerves. Because of the area rendered analgesic, this is termed 'saddle-block' analgesia, and provides excellent analgesia for operations on the urethra, anus and other perineal structures.

Volume/Mass

Mass, i.e. the weight of solution, is more important than volume. Ten milligrams of drug, for example, will spread as far whether contained in 1 ml of 1% solution or 2 ml of 0.5% solution. However, since spinal solutions, at least in the UK, are invariably supplied as solutions rather than crystals which have to be dissolved, most anaesthetists tend to think in terms of volume.

It is now believed that within certain limits, volume/mass of a hyperbaric solution has little effect on spread. This is because posture/SG has such a dominant effect that either a small amount of local anaesthetic can be made to extend over many segments, or a large amount confined to a small area by appropriate posturing. The volume/mass of drug has more effect on the duration of action.

It was formerly believed that the volume/mass of drug did have an important effect on spread of spinal solutions, as it was thought uptake by fatty nerve tissue limited the spread. This is now considered an ineffective and unreliable factor in controlling the spread of hyperbaric solutions.

The spread of plain local anaesthetic solutions (which are all approximately isobaric) is more directly related to a volume/mass of drug.

Rate of Injection

If the injection is made quickly, there is a tendency for turbulent currents to be set up in the CSF, and these spread the local analgesic more extensively. This factor has less influence on the spread of spinal solutions since the almost universal adoption of small-bore spinal needles, which make very rapid injection impossible.

Barbotage

This technique is a more elaborate way of setting up turbulent currents. After injection of some or all the contents of the syringe, aspiration is rapidly carried out and followed by forceful reinjection. This manoeuvre may be repeated several times. The result tends to be a more widespread, but thinner distribution of the local analgesic. It is again difficult to make effective use of this factor with small-bore needles.

There is no single technique for producing spinal analgesia to a particular level. Various combinations of posturing the patient before and after the injection and (particularly in the earlier days of spinal analgesia) different amounts of barbotage can produce identical results with different volumes of solution. Any individual anaesthetist will use a combination of these factors which experience has shown him will produce consistent results.

● FACTORS AFFECTING SPREAD OF SOLUTIONS IN THE EPIDURAL SPACE

The site of action of local analgesic drugs injected into the epidural space is not known for certain, and it is possible that multiple sites are involved. From a clinical viewpoint, however, it is acceptable to consider that the local analgesic acts on the nerve roots in the epidural space in an area centred on the site of injection. This gives a segmental band of analgesia with epidural blocks, as opposed to the complete analgesia below the site of injection which occurs with spinal blocks because injection is into the cauda equina.

Volume

This is by far the most important factor affecting the spread of epidural solutions. Spread tends to occur up and down the space from the site of injection, the degree of spread being proportional to the volume.

Gravity

The epidural space is filled primarily with semi-liquid fatty connective tissue, but this is not true liquid like CSF. Thus SG has no effect on the spread of epidural solutions and no attempt is made to alter their baricity by adding dextrose. Gravity itself, however, tends to have some effect on the spread of epidural solutions, but to nothing like the same extent as intrathecal injections.

Site of Injection

While most epidurals are carried out in the lumbar region, the intention is to stop the needle well short of the spinal cord and it is accepted technique to carry out epidural block at any level. This has considerable advantages over the spinal technique if some high but restricted area of analgesia is required, for example, to relieve the pain of fractured ribs.

Rate of Injection

Rapid injection may spread epidural solutions further, but again this is much less so than with spinal injections. In addition, many epidural injections are made through a catheter, which makes rapid injection impossible.

Concentration

It has been shown that a given volume of a more concentrated solution spreads further than the same volume of a lower concentration of the same drug. This is not a pronounced effect.

● COMPLICATIONS OF SPINAL ANALGESIA

Effects on Cardiovascular System

The preganglionic sympathetic nerve fibres arise from the spinal cord between the first thoracic and second or third lumbar segments. Blockade of these nerves leads to dilatation of the resistance and capacitance vessels. The reduction of peripheral resistance tends to cause a fall in blood pressure and the venous pooling to a fall in venous return, a reduction in cardiac output and further lowering of the blood pressure. With less extensive blocks, the blood pressure tends to be maintained by compensatory vasoconstriction in unaffected segments, but in general the reduction in blood pressure tends to be proportional to the height of the block.

A block to T1–4 involves the cardio-accelerator sympathetic fibres which may cause bradycardia and further depression of the blood pressure. Intravenous atropine will cure the bradycardia and help to restore the blood pressure.

Effects on Respiratory System

Most spinal solutions are powerful enough to produce at least partial motor paralysis in the nerve segments affected. Thus as the block spreads upwards, the intercostal muscles may be progressively affected, but the diaphragm with its C3, 4 and 5 innervation is unaffected until the block reaches the mid-cervical level. Fortunately, the spread of local analgesic solution to these higher levels is usually so thin that it is not strong enough to block the motor fibres. If the block is intense in the thoracic and cervical regions, all respiration may cease.

Respiration will also cease if local analgesic solution spreads up to the fourth ventricle where the respiratory centre may be affected directly.

Nausea and Vomiting

These distressing symptoms are often associated with restlessness and of course are seen only when supplementary anaesthesia has not been used with the spinal or epidural block. There are two main causes – hypotension and traction on hollow viscera. The latter causes pain and nausea because most intra-abdominal structures have some nerve supply from the vagus, which does not run in the vertebral canal and is therefore unaffected by spinals and epidurals. It is essential to diagnose the cause of the patient's symptoms before administering depressant sedative drugs.

Headache

Headache is never caused by a correctly performed epidural, but it is one of the commonest side-effects of spinal analgesia, or more simply of lumbar puncture. There are three possible causes.

Leakage of CSF (Post-spinal or Post-dural Puncture Headache)

There is normally a pressure of some 80–150 mmH$_2$O in the subarachnoid space and a slightly negative pressure in the epidural space. This causes the CSF to leak through the dural hole caused by the needle and it will continue to do so until the hole heals over. It is thought that the loss of fluid allows movement of the brain within the skull and causes headache by traction on pain-sensitive structures in the basal blood vessels and dura mater. The incidence of this type of headache, and its severity and duration, are thus directly related to the bore of needle used. Spinal needles used today are usually small bore and have special points (see below) so that severe headache is unusual. The worst headaches tend to result from inadvertent dural puncture by a wide-bore epidural needle.

Post-spinal or post-dural puncture headache (PDPH) is classically retro-orbital or may spread over the top of the head into the neck. It is worse when the patient is upright and nearly always disappears when lying flat or head-down. There may be associated symptoms, for example, nausea, vomiting, vertigo, tinnitus and even deafness. While it is no longer believed that after dural puncture the incidence of PDPH is reduced by a period of recumbency, if PDPH does develop, then conservative treatment consists of lying the patient down for 24 h and ensuring adequate hydration to replace lost CSF. A variety of other treatments has been tried, but none has been conclusively shown to produce permanent cure. These include abdominal binders, epidural boluses or infusions of crystalloid and intravenous caffeine or theophylline.

The most effective treatment is to perform an 'epidural blood patch'. This involves the epidural injection at the believed level of the dural puncture (or lower) of up to 20 ml of the patient's own blood, removed under sterile conditions from any accessible vein. This is believed literally to 'patch' the dural hole until the patient's own healing processes can effect a permanent repair. While remarkably effective in many cases, argument still continues as to the ideal time to perform the patch and how much blood should be used.

Meningitis

By definition, infection of the meninges is meningitis. With modern equipment and methods of sterilisation this most serious complication should not occur.

Meningism

This may mimic meningitis, but is an aseptic irritant reaction caused probably by blood in the CSF or antiseptic from the skin. Before the advent of modern pharmaceutical techniques, it was also caused by impurities in the local analgesic solutions.

Cranial Nerve Palsies

These are rare and like spinal headaches are probably caused by stretching of the cranial nerves by movement of the brain within the skull due to leakage of CSF, and so may occur after simple lumbar puncture. Most of the cranial nerves have been reported as being affected, but the commonest is the sixth cranial nerve (the abducens nerve) which supplies the lateral rectus muscle in the eye, paralysis of this muscle causing diplopia. These cranial nerve palsies usually recover spontaneously.

Other Neurological Lesions

A great variety of permanent lesions affecting the nerve roots, spinal cord or even brain have been reported following spinal analgesia. However, it has not been proved that these are caused by the local analgesic agent. Other possible explanations include contaminants of the local analgesic solution, a virus or other infection introduced by the needle, ischaemia of the spinal cord due to hypotension (especially if a vasoconstrictor is added to the spinal solution), or some unidentified coincidental cause (as these lesions may occur without lumbar puncture or spinal analgesia). Certainly, with modern analgesic solutions, series of many thousands of cases have been collected without any neurological sequelae, and when used by anaesthetists who are familiar with the technique and in suitable cases, spinal analgesia must compare favourably for safety with general anaesthesia.

The 'Total' Spinal

If local analgesic solution reaches as high as the cranial subarachnoid space, not only are the respiratory muscles paralysed, but the patient also loses the use of the cranial nerves, so that apnoea occurs, there is profound hypotension and the patient becomes unconscious. The solution may also enter the fourth ventricle where it may directly paralyse the respiratory and vasomotor centres. The treatment involves ventilation, maintaining the blood pressure by raising the legs, administering intravenous fluids and probably using vasopressors. Provided that this is carried out, the condition is self-limiting as the local analgesic loses its effect.

With the small volumes of local analgesic used as hyperbaric solutions, this complication is seen only if the patient is left steeply head-down. It is more likely to occur if the needle pierces the dura mater unnoticed while attempting epidural analgesia and a larger (epidural) volume of solution is injected intrathecally.

● COMPLICATIONS OF EPIDURAL ANALGESIA

Effects on Cardiovascular System

These are similar to those seen with spinal analgesia and are again caused by, and proportional to, the extent of sympathetic blockade. They may be less severe because of the slower onset.

Effects on Respiratory System

Nerve fibres are blocked by local analgesic solutions with a readiness which depends on their diameter. The fine sympathetic fibres are most easily blocked, pain and other sensations next and motor nerve fibres, which are the thickest, are the most difficult to block. Most local analgesic solutions in common use for epidural analgesia produce only partial motor block, so that a 'differential block' is achieved. Thus, even with a high block respiration may be only slightly affected.

Backache

Some tenderness over the injection site for about 48 h is common after epidural analgesia due to the relatively large bore of the needle. There is as yet no evidence from prospective studies that epidurals cause backache.

Haematoma

It is not unusual when performing an epidural to cause some bleeding into the epidural space by damaging an epidural vein. This seldom causes any problem, but theoretically could produce pressure on nerve roots and require laminectomy.

Epidural Abscess

This could result from faulty technique or as a result of infection of an epidural haematoma by blood-borne bacteria. It is a serious complication usually requiring immediate laminectomy.

Retention of Urine

When an epidural catheter is inserted to produce prolonged analgesia, retention of urine may occur because of loss of bladder sensation.

Breakage of Catheter

This is most likely to happen by the shearing-off of the distal portion of the catheter on the bevel of the Tuohy needle, if an attempt is made to withdraw the catheter through the needle. It might also happen on forcibly removing a 'trapped' catheter, which could stretch and ultimately break.

Neurological Lesions

Slight motor or sensory weakness (usually a numb patch on one thigh) occasionally persists for days or weeks after epidural analgesia, especially where a catheter technique has been used to 'soak' the nerve roots repeatedly. Spontaneous recovery is the rule. More serious and prolonged neurological complications are even more rare than after spinal analgesia, many thousands of cases having been collected without serious nerve lesions. When they occur, they are usually of the anterior spinal artery syndrome type, and are probably the result of a period of hypotension.

Toxicity of Local Analgesic Solution

The possibility of exceeding the safe dose of local analgesic solution must be kept in mind when any nerve block is carried out. There is a reasonable margin of error with most epidural blocks, but there is danger of accumulation to toxic doses when repeated increments are given through an epidural catheter, especially during obstetric analgesia, or when an obstetric epidural is 'extended' for Caesarean section.

Summary

This list of complications of spinal and epidural blocks may look formidable, but close scrutiny will show that most of them are either minor or short term, and the more serious and longer term ones can be almost completely avoided by scrupulous attention to technique and to sterility of equipment.

● USES OF SPINAL AND EPIDURAL ANALGESIA

Operative

Both types of block may be used as the sole method of analgesia for surgical operations. This is particularly applicable to operations below the diaphragm, although vagus blocks may need to be added for some intra-abdominal procedures. The number of occasions on which these blocks are the technique of choice either alone or in conjunction with general anaesthesia was drastically reduced by the advent of muscle relaxants. The extent to which they are used as the sole anaesthetic depends largely on public expectation. In the UK, most patients having surgery expect to be put to sleep, but this is by no means so in all countries.

There undoubtedly remain some operations where spinal or epidural analgesia is the method of choice. These consist of operations on the perineal structures or legs, especially in patients with severe cardiovascular, respiratory or metabolic disease. A 'saddle-block' spinal or caudal epidural has no adverse effect whatsoever on any of these systems. However, Caesarean section has now become easily the most major abdominal procedure routinely carried out under regional anaesthesia (see Chapter 38).

Therapeutic

This group of indications consists of conditions where a longer duration of effect is usually required than can be obtained from a single dose of local analgesic agent. This means that a catheter technique is required for additional injections and in the majority of cases an epidural catheter is used.

Analgesia for Pain Relief in Labour

Numerically this is the commonest indication for epidural analgesia in the UK.

Postoperative Pain Relief

Superb pain relief may be obtained but hypotension has to be looked out for when local analgesic solutions are used.

Chest Injuries

Again, excellent analgesia is obtained, and without affecting the level of consciousness. This may be particularly useful if there is an associated head injury.

Renal and Biliary Colic

These agonising types of pain can readily be abolished by a few millilitres of epidural local analgesic solution.

Back Pain

Epidural injection of local analgesic solution, usually with an injectable steroid (Depo-Medrone), has been used for many years to treat low back pain.

Hypotensive Anaesthesia

Both spinal and epidural analgesia may be used to produce deliberate hypotension and reduce bleeding at certain operations. This indication has been less common since the introduction of pharmacological agents that produce more flexible control of blood pressure.

Acute Arterial or Venous Thromboembolic Conditions

Epidural analgesia may be used to produce vasodilatation of the collateral circulation which tends to go into spasm when there is acute thrombosis or embolism of major arterial or venous channels.

Intractable Pain

Intractable pain may be relieved by the injection of neurolytic solutions into the subarachnoid or epidural spaces. Spinal injections (e.g. 5% phenol in glycerine) are more effective than epidural injections for this purpose.

● CONTRAINDICATIONS TO SPINAL AND EPIDURAL ANALGESIA

Bleeding Tendency

A haemorrhagic tendency due to either disease or anticoagulant therapy may result in an extensive epidural haematoma if an epidural vein is damaged by a needle or catheter.

Skin Sepsis

Skin sepsis near the injection site is an absolute contraindication to spinal or epidural block.

Shock

Any patient whose circulating blood volume is depleted for any reason (e.g. haemorrhage, vomiting or diarrhoea) attempts to maintain his blood pressure by peripheral vasoconstriction. This attempt at compensation is impaired by a spinal or epidural block affecting the sympathetic outflow from the spinal cord, and a profound fall in blood pressure may result.

Absence of Patient's Consent

Although there are certain circumstances in which an anaesthetist may feel that a spinal or epidural block is in the patient's (or, in obstetrics, the baby's) best interests, it must never be performed if the patient refuses consent.

Demyelinating Conditions of the Spinal Cord

These conditions (e.g. multiple sclerosis) have been regarded as relative contraindications because the block may be blamed if there is a subsequent exacerbation of the condition. However, there is no evidence that spinal or epidural block produces such an effect and many anaesthetists perform these types of block after obtaining informed consent.

Chronic Back Problems

These may also be considered as relative contraindications but, as indicated above, as these cases have often been treated by epidural injections it is reasonable to perform these techniques on a consenting patient.

● INTRATHECAL AND EPIDURAL OPIOIDS AND OTHER AGENTS

The discovery 25 years ago of specific opiate receptors in the brain and in the substantia gelatinosa of the spinal cord led to much speculation and investigation into the possible uses of intrathecal and epidural opioids. The potential advantages of opioids used in this way are that they might relieve pain without the complications of motor block, sympathetic block or even of numbness. Since then, a number of other receptors have been found in the spinal cord, the stimulation of which by certain drugs may relieve pain. Of these other drugs, at present the most investigated and effective is the α-adrenergic-stimulating agent clonidine.

All these agents may be given intrathecally or epidurally. Investigations continue, but certain general conclusions can be reached. Agents used in this way are more effective in relieving some kinds of pain than others. They are more effective intrathecally than epidurally (probably because of their injection in closer proximity to the spinal cord). They are not always fully effective (except in high concentrations) when used alone. There are side-effects, some of them potentially serious. In the case of the opioids, the serious effect is the possibility of respiratory depression, which may be delayed for hours. Less serious, but at times important, are nausea, vomiting, pruritus and retention of urine. The rate of onset of pain relief (and side-effects) is quicker with highly fat-soluble opiates (e.g. fentanyl) than with less fat-soluble opiates (e.g. morphine). However, duration of action is inversely proportional to fat solubility, being short with fentanyl and longer with morphine.

One of the most important discoveries has been the finding of synergism between many of these drugs, especially between the opioid and local analgesics. This has considerable benefit in reducing the likelihood of toxicity and side-effects of both drugs. For example, the addition of fentanyl in a dose of 2 μg/ml to bupivacaine makes it possible approximately to halve the concentration of bupivacaine for the same efficacy and duration of pain relief. Apart from the reduction in the side-effects, the reduction in the loss of motor power in the lower limbs allows greater mobility – especially beneficial for postoperative pain relief or in labour.

Opioids may also be added to subarachnoid or epidural local anaesthetic solutions to improve the quality of analgesia during awake surgery, for example, fentanyl may be added in a dose of 10 μg intrathecally or 100 μg epidurally to the local anaesthetic solution used at Caesarean section.

● DRUGS AND EQUIPMENT

These will be mentioned only briefly as they are best learned in the anaesthetic room or classroom.

Drugs

While the standard solution of 0.5% plain bupivacaine has been quite extensively used as a spinal solution (it acts as an isobaric or marginally hypobaric solution), there is now only one solution in the UK specifically manufactured for spinal use and approved by the Committee on Safety of Medicines. That is 0.5% bupivacaine in 8% dextrose marketed by Astra Pharmaceuticals Ltd as Marcain Heavy.

A wider range of epidural solutions is available. These include:

- 0.25% and 0.5% plain bupivacaine
- 0.25% and 0.5% bupivacaine in 1 : 200 000 adrenaline
- 0.75% plain bupivacaine
- 1% and 2% plain lignocaine
- 1% lignocaine in 1 : 200 000 adrenaline
- 0.25%, 0.5% and 0.75% plain ropivacaine
- 0.25% and 0.5% levobupivacaine.

It should be remembered that the toxic dose of 1.5% plain lignocaine is only 13–14 ml in a person of 70 kg.

Needles

Many different spinal needles have been designed but have now been largely replaced by a smaller range of disposable needles. The other recent change is the return to popularity of 'pencil-point' or similarly tipped needles. First introduced in 1951, these needles, often called 'Whitacre' needles, have a conical tip with the orifice proximal to the tip, as opposed to the Quinke tip needles where the orifice is at the tip (Fig. 41.5). Their claimed (now confirmed) advantage is that as the point separates rather than cuts the fibres of the dura mater, there is less leakage of CSF after the needle is withdrawn and consequently less PDPH. This makes their use particularly appropriate in groups susceptible to PDPH, for example, women having spinal anaesthesia for obstetric procedures. Needles as fine as 29G are now available, and with all these smaller gauges of needle a transparent plastic hub greatly aids the early detection of CSF.

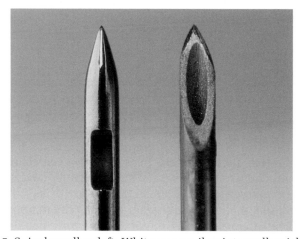

Figure 41.5 Spinal needles: left, Whitacre pencil-point needle; right, Quinke.

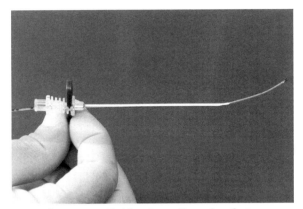

Figure 41.6 Epidural needle and catheter.

Disposable epidural needles are in common use. The most frequently used design of needle is the Tuohy needle which has its bevel pointing laterally to increase the ease of introduction of the plastic catheter (Fig. 41.6). The most common size used in the UK is 16G for adults, but 17G and 18G are also available. Whatever size is chosen, it is vital if a catheter is to be inserted that it will pass through the needle.

● COMBINED SPINAL–EPIDURAL (CSE) ANAESTHESIA

This technique (or techniques) has gained enormously in popularity in the past 10 years. As the name implies, it involves gaining access to the subarachnoid and epidural spaces in the same patient. While it may be achieved in several ways, including inserting an epidural needle and catheter at one lumbar interspace before performing a spinal injection at another, the most popular method is a needle-through-needle single interspace technique. For this, a normal length epidural needle is inserted into the epidural space in the usual way. A fine spinal needle, with a shaft long enough to protrude a few millimetres beyond the tip of the epidural needle (Fig. 41.7), is then introduced through it into the subarachnoid space. After injection of the spinal solution, the spinal needle is removed, and a catheter introduced into the epidural space before the epidural needle too is removed. The patient is then positioned appropriately for the spread of the spinal solution. Because of the popularity of this technique, all the major needle manufacturers now make packs separately for it, with spinal and epidural needles of appropriate lengths.

The advantages of the technique are that it provides the speed and reliability of the spinal technique, while the epidural catheter can be used to modify the extent of analgesia if the spinal technique is not perfect

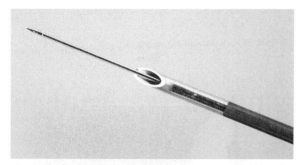

Figure 41.7 CSE, spinal needle protruding out of epidural needle.

and can also be used to provide postoperative pain relief. The epidural needle also acts as a guide, leading the fine spinal needle almost to the subarachnoid space.

● CONTINUOUS SPINAL ANAESTHESIA

This was suggested by Dean of London as long ago as 1907 by leaving a needle in place, long before Lemmon described a series of such cases in 1940. Tuohy was the first to use a flexible (ureteric) catheter for continuous spinal block, and over the next 45 years catheters of epidural size were occasionally used for continuous spinal block.

In 1989 Hurley and Lambert described an incredible 32G catheter which could be passed through a 26G needle. These tiny catheters were expensive and technically very difficult to use, so that they were already being replaced by 28G catheters which could be passed through 22G or 23G needles, when all catheters <27G were banned for spinal use in the USA following a number of cases of cauda equina syndrome.

While small-bore catheters for continuous spinal anaesthesia are still available in the UK and some European countries, they do not enjoy widespread popularity.

42

Postoperative Analgesia

The most important aim of postoperative analgesic therapy is to provide satisfactory pain relief, without nausea, vomiting or significant sedation during the postoperative period. The method used should be free as far as possible from peaks and troughs to allow the patients to feel comfortable and confident at all times. It is possible that an element of euphoria is a good idea, particularly where inoperable or only partially successful surgery has occurred. In addition, there should be an absence of respiratory depression, particularly important with thoraco-abdominal surgery. There should be no effect on gastrointestinal motility or absorption and the sphincter of Oddi (at the lower end of the common bile duct) should remain patent (opiate-induced spasm causes jaundice).

● DRUGS AVAILABLE

Parenteral Opiates

Opiates can be administered either intermittently or continuously. The parenteral routes are more suitable for postoperative use since most patients are unable to take oral medication either because of nausea or because of the nature of the surgery.

Parenteral opiate administration can be intermittent using either intramuscular injections or patient-controlled analgesia (PCA) where the drug is self-administered at preset doses and time intervals, initiated by demand from the patient. Continuous opiate administration can either be intravenous, using an infusion pump, or subcutaneous, where the drip rate is inevitably slow. Intravenous administration is very popular in intensive care, where doses can be continuously monitored, varied and assessed.

The disadvantages of these methods are largely common to all routes of opiate administration and include:

- increased incidence of nausea and vomiting
- reduced gastrointestinal motility, reduced gastric emptying, constipation

- cough suppression
- sedation and drowsiness
- hypoventilation
- euphoria
- dependence and addiction, although this should not be a problem with relatively short-term use.

It is important to remember that the effects of intravenous opiates are almost immediate and more profound than an equivalent dose administered intramuscularly. While this is ideal for rapid-onset analgesia, particularly in the recovery room when a waking patient is in severe pain, the accompanying respiratory depression will be equally rapid in onset and intensity. Pethidine, in particular, should not be given in as large a dose intravenously as intramuscularly, since it has myocardial depressant activity.

Oral Opiates

Sustained release oral (MST) morphine is an excellent analgesic, but its use postoperatively is inappropriate unless the patient is taking orally. Indeed, severe respiratory depression has occurred in patients given repeated large doses of oral morphine in this situation. Its use is normally limited to patients with chronic pain, usually due to neoplastic disease, in whom opiate addiction is not a problem. Similar disadvantages occur with opiate-related oral analgesia, for example, codeine-containing compounds, since codeine is significantly metabolised to morphine.

Non-opiates/Synthetic Opioid Analgesics

These still have similar side-effects to the opiates, but are said to be non-addictive and not to produce as much nausea and vomiting.

Pentazocine (Fortral) is an analgesic derived from nalorphine, which can be administered both orally and intravenously. It does produce respiratory depression, although this is not nearly as marked as with true opiates. It is less effective than morphine, and disorientation is relatively common since it is a potent hallucinogen, as well as possessing mild addictive properties. It also raises pulmonary artery pressure and so should not be used in patients following acute myocardial infarction.

Nalbuphine (Nubain) is a similar drug to pentazocine, though said to produce less disorientation. It has been suggested as being appropriate for administration by PCA and may be useful if sufficiently strong.

Buprenorphine (Temgesic) is again similar to pentazocine, though much longer acting. It can usefully be given by the sublingual route which allows its use postoperatively in patients who are unable or not permitted to swallow. Like pentazocine it can produce disorientation, confusion and hallucinations.

Tramadol (Zydol) produces analgesia both by an opioid effect and by enhancement of serotonin and adrenergic nerve pathways. It is said to have fewer of the typical opioid side-effects listed above.

Non-steroidal Anti-inflammatory Drugs

Diclofenac (Voltarol) and ketorolac (Toradol) are very useful adjuncts to opiate analgesia and do not produce any central nervous disturbance, sedation or stimulation of the chemoreceptor trigger zone (CTZ), adjacent to the vomiting centre. They are moderate analgesics with a significant anti-inflammatory action and, as prostaglandin inhibitors, may induce bleeding through coagulation abnormalities. Diclofenac is painful intra-muscularly, but a suitable suppository preparation is widely used. They may also precipitate renal failure in susceptible patients, particularly the elderly and patients with pre-existing disease or those whose kidneys are impaired due to hypoperfusion, hypoxia or aminoglycoside antibiotics.

Oral Non-opiate Agents

These include codydramol, dihydrocodeine, paracetamol and aspirin, either singly or in a variety of combinations, for example, codeine and paracetamol (Co-codamol). Codeine-containing compounds are powerful analgesics and are metabolised in part to morphine. Codeine phosphate and dihydrocodeine (DF118) can be administered intramuscularly as well as orally and are particularly suitable in the post-neurosurgical patient, although they still have the potential to cause respiratory depression. Like morphine, codeine-containing compounds frequently cause constipation. Gastrointestinal irritation is another significant problem, particularly with aspirin-containing compounds and non-steroidal anti-inflammatory drugs (NSAIDs).

● METHODS AVAILABLE

Local Analgesic (Anaesthetic) Techniques

The injection of local anaesthetic solution can produce very satisfactory postoperative analgesia in a number of ways:

1. Direct local infiltration of the wound will only anaesthetise the skin and subcutaneous tissues and deep pain may still be present. Nevertheless, it is often the cutaneous pain which is the most severe.
2. Specific nerve blocks which supply the operation site, for example, intercostal, ulnar and digital nerve blocks. Any nerve which is closely

related to a bony landmark can easily be blocked, providing anaesthesia of the operation site.
3. Specific local blocks of a small region, for example, ilio-inguinal field block (hernia block) and penile block.

In all cases, these blocks will only last for a few hours. Bupivacaine will produce anaesthesia for about 6 h, although its ability to attenuate pain may be much longer. In many relatively minor operations, this may be quite sufficient to cover the acute postoperative pain, which rapidly becomes controllable over a few hours. The addition of adrenaline to the local anaesthetic does not consistently prolong the block.

Regional Anaesthetic Blocks

These include epidurals and spinals (Chapter 41), together with paravertebral and intrapleural blocks. In most cases the solution used is a dilute mixture of 0.167% bupivacaine with 5–10 mg of diamorphine or 100 µg fentanyl in 60 ml. All these methods provide excellent analgesia and enable coughing, deep breathing and movement in a patient immediately after major surgery.

Epidural anaesthesia in particular, has the great benefit that the use of a catheter technique will permit continuous infusion and therefore a relatively unlimited duration of analgesia for many days. This is virtually the only technique which offers complete analgesia and is particularly suitable after major thoracic and abdominal surgery.

Epidurals do, however, need careful monitoring since many of the side-effects of epidural anaesthesia can still occur, for example, hypotension, respiratory inefficiency, nausea, vomiting, itching and urinary retention. Although many patients are now nursed on surgical wards with continuous thoracic and lumbar epidural anaesthesia running, it is vital that the nursing and medical staff are aware of the potential problems and how to treat them. Significant hypotension and respiratory insufficiency are the two main problems. The use of specifically designed postoperative analgesic observation charts and a firm commitment to nurse education have made this very valuable technique available to many more patients than previously. Patients are also occasionally somewhat hyperaesthetic when the block wears off, which may be worse than not to have had a block in the first place. However, this usually only occurs after single rather than prolonged blocks.

Some are now using patient-controlled epidural anaesthesia to good effect, though again this needs careful monitoring.

Patient-controlled Analgesia

This is another very popular technique which allows intermittent intravenous analgesic administration under the control of the patient. A purpose-built programmable infusion pump, calibrated for a particular type and size of syringe, allows on-demand drug delivery. The drug concentration, individual dose and lock-out time (i.e. the interval between doses) are all preset, together if desired with a total dose limit and a background infusion, although this is not frequently used. The pump is connected to the side arm of an intravenous infusion and the patient supplied with a push-button switch. The patient needs careful instruction to give sufficient confidence to cope with the device. The drugs used are normally opiates and this can present a problem due to the associated nausea and vomiting. The patient will not press the switch because it makes them feel sick. The addition of anti-emetics to the analgesic solution has only met with limited success. PCA is an excellent technique, but the ideal drug to use has yet to be found.

The 'Acute Pain Team'

Many hospitals now have acute pain teams, led by an anaesthetist and, most importantly, a dedicated senior nurse. It is crucial that all postoperative analgesia and, in particular, complex techniques such as epidurals and PCA have clearly defined protocols. These should address all the important areas such as dose limits, methods of administration, prescribing, syringe changing and when to summon assistance. It is also important to maintain uniformity and to keep individual variations and idiosyncrasies to a minimum to avoid prescribing and administration errors.

Postoperative analgesic techniques set up by the anaesthetic staff are communicated to the team, usually via a notice board, and the patients are then regularly visited to ensure adequacy of the technique, absence of side-effects and general satisfaction for both the patient and the ward staff. The ability to call a dedicated expert has relieved a considerable amount of anxiety on the part of the ward staff who are otherwise left to deal with what to them is a potentially dangerous technique. The pain team also plays a vital role in the teaching and communication of these techniques to new nurses, junior medical staff and the paramedical specialities, though to a chest physiotherapist, a thoracic epidural is often like 'manna from heaven'!

43

Treatment of Chronic Pain

•Assessment of patient •Methods of pain relief •Treatment of back pain
•Spinal and extradural techniques – analgesics, opioids, neurolytics
•Counter-irritation •Central nervous modification of chronic pain

With the establishment of pain clinics the relief of chronic pain has become an important sub-speciality of anaesthesia. A great many patients suffer varying degrees of chronic pain, which may be caused in several ways, for example, postoperatively, post-traumatically, from neoplastic disease, from spinal disorders and from infections such as herpes zoster (shingles). Although many patients with chronic pain may accurately describe both the nature and site of their pain, the fact that they have borne it for some time often means that a considerable psychological overlay is involved, and it is important to consider this aspect of pain relief as well as the more definitive use of analgesic techniques.

● ASSESSMENT OF PATIENT

In ideal circumstances, considerable time needs to be taken to assess the patients adequately and if necessary to admit them to hospital for further examination and tests. Those with disabilities and severe pain may take a long time to undress, and a busy out-patient clinic is not the place to examine them. It is necessary to obtain a detailed history of the factors causing the pain and those which aggravate it, together with its frequency, duration, nature and the mechanical factors or drugs which relieve it.

Much chronic pain results from previous treatment, either surgical or medical, so detailed knowledge of operations performed and treatment attempted is also important, together with the results of previous physical examination. Current drug therapy and possible allergies to analgesics and other agents employed in the past must also be sought, together with an evaluation of the underlying psychological influences in each particular case. These may include family pressures and, in some cases, the fact that litigation by the patient is in process as the result of an accident.

Examination of the patient may show the degree of physical impairment, and particularly what movements or activities cause the pain. Trigger areas and other sensitive spots which spark off cyclical pain may also be sought. It may be possible to evaluate the degree of the patient's over-reaction or under-reaction to their particular pain, which may help in future treatment, although accurate measurement of pain is at present unavailable and one has to rely on qualitative impressions.

Sometimes patients will present to a pain clinic having not been investigated before or examined for the existence of underlying pathology which may cause their particular pain. Laboratory tests, X-ray examinations and electrocardiograms (ECGs) may be necessary to exclude underlying treatable conditions as a cause of the pain, and it is important not to overlook these by attempting simply to provide analgesia.

● METHODS OF PAIN RELIEF

Since there are so many factors both producing and influencing chronic pain, many different methods of relief may be employed. These range from locally applied techniques such as heat, massage, physiotherapy, ultrasound and counter-irritation, to local analgesic techniques either alone or combined with anti-inflammatory agents – and finally to specific neurolytic techniques designed to destroy nerves. Chronic pain is a vicious circle which if interrupted may result in permanent pain relief. The central nervous factors modifying the degree and nature of the pain are often amenable to treatment with sedatives and antidepressants.

Mechanical Methods of Pain Relief

Many patients in chronic pain benefit considerably from physiotherapy, which may include the use of heat, cold or vibration to modify pain and to restore mobility to painful joints. To produce good results it is essential that there is a close liaison between physiotherapists and anaesthetists treating patients in chronic pain. It is also important, before referring the patient to the physiotherapy department, to have adequate radiological and clinical evidence of the patient's lesion.

Local Nerve Blocks

The use of local anaesthetic techniques is an essential part of treatment within a pain clinic. Since local anaesthetics work only for a relatively short time, it is often possible to use them for diagnostic as well as therapeutic benefit. Painful or tender areas, as well as trigger points which may precipitate pain over a more diffuse region, are all amenable to injections of local anaesthetics; if this achieves satisfactory analgesia, then either a repeat block or the use of a neurolytic agent where a specific nerve is involved may have a more permanent effect. Pain in the distribution of a particular cutaneous nerve is relatively easy to treat, provided that the nerve is accessible to local anaesthesia. However, referred pain (e.g. shoulder tip pain from diaphragmatic irritation) should not be forgotten. Disseminated cancer may also produce specific nerve pain, which is treatable by local anaesthesia.

In some patients it may be necessary to anaesthetise the nerve as it leaves the spinal cord, either by injecting local anaesthetic into the cerebrospinal fluid (CSF) (spinal block) or by an extradural technique. If local nerve block is successful, in most cases this can be followed by treatment designed to produce permanent nerve damage. Nerves may be destroyed either by injection of neurolytic substances (e.g. phenol, chlorocresol and alcohol) or by using heat (diathermy), cold (cryosurgery), or by permanent surgical section. Local injection of neurolytic agents is usually a less complicated procedure more applicable to out-patient treatment, although diathermy and cryosurgery are both widely used. If the nerve is attacked in its course along a limb, these locally applied neurolytic techniques do not destroy the cell body but merely the axon of the nerve, and regeneration is sometimes possible. This may result merely in a return of the pain, or may sometimes produce hypersensitivity of the area worse than the original pain. Some types of pain are more suitable for local nerve blocks than others, and this must be considered when the method of pain relief is being contemplated.

Sympathetic Nerve Blocks

Deep-seated burning pain, phantom limb pain and areas of hypersensitivity are all often resistant to conventional nerve blocks, and sympathetic blockade is sometimes necessary to produce relief. The sympathetic nerves, which supply the leg, leave the spinal cord and join the sympathetic chain lying along the anterolateral borders of the vertebral bodies. Local injections in this region may produce sympathetic nerve block, which can also be achieved by intravenous injection of a dilute solution of guanethidine into an isolated limb, in a similar way to Bier's block (Chapter 40). Sympathetic blockade of the arm is best produced by stellate ganglion block.

● TREATMENT OF BACK PAIN

Many patients present to a pain clinic with low back pain. Most have already received specialist investigation and treatment in other units, particularly orthopaedic and neurosurgical, and therefore come to the clinic as a last resort. By this stage many already have considerable psychological overlay and any planned course of treatment must take this into account. In some cases specific nerve involvement can be demonstrated and may be treatable locally, particularly by injection of individual lumbar or sacral nerves as they leave the spinal cord, but many patients may be suffering from a more diffuse pain which is difficult to treat. This may arise from the sacro-iliac or intervertebral facet joints and recent methods of treatment of low back pain have concentrated on this. Lumbar extradural anaesthesia with local anaesthetic mixed with long-acting steroids may also be successful in breaking down adhesions in the extradural space which give rise to pain. Nevertheless, the treatment of chronic low back pain is often laborious and sometimes unsuccessful. Most pain clinics have a back pain programme to assess all the components of pain and then to link pharmacological or invasive treatment with physiotherapy and appropriate psychological support.

● SPINAL AND EXTRADURAL TECHNIQUES – ANALGESICS, OPIOIDS, NEUROLYTICS

If local anaesthetics, administered either extradurally or spinally, provide satisfactory but temporary analgesia, it may then be necessary to use a more prolonged technique. This would be either intermittent or continuous infusion of opioids or a neurolytic technique.

Opioids administered either spinally or extradurally are popular in the treatment of some forms of back pain, although the analgesia produced is usually not as profound as that achieved with local anaesthetics. Long-term infusion techniques using tunnelled spinal or extradural catheters have been developed to provide a continuous infusion over a prolonged period.

Most of the neurolytic techniques require precise application of the agent to the affected nerve root and therefore are unsatisfactory when used extradurally. Specific intrathecal (spinal) nerve blocks are more commonly employed. Hyperbaric solutions of phenol or chlorocresol are used and after lumbar puncture the patient is positioned so that a small puddle of the neurolytic agent lies over the nerve to be destroyed. This technique is particularly useful with severe lesions resulting from spread of cancer, when the results are often excellent and the occasional loss of accompanying motor function or bladder control is less important to patients with only a short life expectancy.

● COUNTER-IRRITATION

Counter-irritation is used every day to alleviate pain, for example, when rubbing a child's limb to remove the pain from a bruise, or applying local heat or cold to relieve backache. Transcutaneous nerve stimulation is an alternative method of producing pain relief, by counter-irritation of the skin overlying the painful area. Counter-irritant creams or lotions, and acupuncture, may also help to alleviate pain in this way and it is important to explore every avenue of possible relief in patients suffering chronic pain.

● CENTRAL NERVOUS MODIFICATION OF CHRONIC PAIN

Some psychological factors influence the degree and duration of pain. Anxiety and depression not only occur as a result of prolonged intractable pain, but may also influence the success of treatment such as nerve block. Many patients benefit from simultaneous analgesia and sedation or anti-depressant therapy, and sometimes from such drugs alone. Diazepam and lorazepam in relatively small doses may be of benefit to patients in helping them to tolerate severe pain, the intensity of which depends on its interpretation. Some patients get severely depressed during long illnesses and the use of tricyclic antidepressants (e.g. amitriptyline or imipramine) may be of considerable help. In many cases a single dose of antidepressant at night ensures a good night's rest and, as the effect is long lasting, continues into the following day without causing drowsiness.

Adequate and caring conversations with the doctors and nurses concerned may also help. Patients who feel that they have been sympathetically treated often improve considerably by comparison with patients who become antagonistic towards the staff looking after them, implying that no one is doing any good for them and no one really cares about their pain either. Unfortunately this is not infrequent in patients suffering from chronic pain, and must be guarded against if treatment is to be successful.

44

Principles of Intensive Care and Parenteral Nutrition

Almost all hospitals in the UK, with any responsibility for acute medical care, contain an intensive care unit, although many such units are conversions of existing wards rather than purpose-built units. These hospitals usually also contain a coronary care unit which may be either part of the intensive care complex or separate. Although a mixture of coronary care and intensive care within the same unit is far from ideal, this may have advantages from the nursing, and particularly the teaching and training, point of view.

Intensive care itself is mainly concerned with the treatment of acute respiratory, cardiac and metabolic disorders, and the commonest types of case admitted to a general hospital intensive care unit are as follows:

1. General medical cases:
   (a) overdoses
   (b) respiratory failure
   (c) neurological
   (d) renal failure.
2. Major trauma.
3. General surgical cases (usually postoperative care):
   (a) vascular
   (b) massive haemorrhage
   (c) coagulation problems
   (d) airway and respiratory problems
   (e) endocrine
   (f) nutritional.

Other cases which may require intensive care depending on specialist surgery are: (a) cardiothoracic, (b) neurosurgical, (c) renal dialysis, and (d) burns.

● CONCEPTS OF INTENSIVE CARE

Seriously ill patients require intensive medical care, intensive nursing care and the use of specialist equipment for both monitoring and treatment. It is far more logical and economical to concentrate these facilities in one unit to which the patient is brought, rather than to nurse such patients in general medical and surgical wards, necessitating duplication of personnel and equipment. Much of the success in intensive care units is attributable to the accurate and scrupulous care of the patients made possible by a high nurse to patient ratio, in contrast to the routine care available in the general wards. At the same time it is important for the clinician running an intensive care unit to realise that it is impossible to be an expert in all aspects of intensive care. They must act as both decision-maker and coordinator, able to bring together skills necessary to treat a particular case.

● MONITORING TECHNIQUES

By concentrating all seriously ill patients in a single unit, more extensive monitoring of the patient is possible, from the point of view of both the skills of the staff and the equipment and time available. In general, all patients are monitored regularly and frequently in terms of blood pressure, electrocardiogram (ECG), oxygen saturation, end-tidal carbon dioxide, temperature, pulse rate and central venous pressure. It is essential that adequate and accurate records are kept, minute by minute if necessary, of the patient's condition, particularly in relation to when drugs are given, to assess the effects of both the drug and the dose on the patient concerned; this can be achieved only with adequate medical and nursing care. In addition, detailed intensive care charts allow accurate estimation of fluid input and output, which is often critical in seriously ill patients and in whom there is no room for inaccuracies or missing data – which inevitably occur on general wards. More extensive monitoring of the patients depends on the particular condition being treated, but may include monitoring of direct arterial blood pressure, pulmonary artery pressure, pulmonary capillary 'wedge' pressure (reflecting left atrial pressure), cardiac output and intracranial pressure. In addition, other advanced techniques such as electro-encephalography may be necessary and available.

Although the patients may be heavily sedated or apparently unconscious, it is important to remember that as they recover they require a great deal of encouragement and even orientation, many of them having been admitted to the unit as an emergency and waking up totally unaware of their surroundings. The importance of 'tender loving care' cannot be overemphasised in this often terrifying situation and indeed the patients' relatives may be subjected to far more stress and strain than the patients themselves, who may be largely unaware of what is going on or how seriously ill they are. It is necessary for the relatives to speak as frequently as they wish with members of both the medical and nursing staff. They should be kept fully informed of all events, and be free to come and go as often as they wish, provided that they do not interfere with intensive therapy.

● EQUIPMENT

The ideal number of beds for a general hospital intensive care unit is probably 1% of the total hospital bed complement, although this may need to be increased when specialist units, for example, cardiac and neurosurgery, are being considered. It is impossible to estimate the cost of intensive care but it is about ten times the cost of a normal hospital bed per day. The equipment that is available in intensive care units is both specialised and variable. The enormous expense of individual items of equipment is one of the basic reasons for concentrating intensive care on one site and bringing the patient to it, where both doctors and nurses have been specially trained in using the facilities available. Although the ECG is usually displayed at the bedside of each individual patient, remote display is often useful, particularly in coronary care where it is distressing for patients to be 'observed' continually. The unit should contain its own defibrillator together with other essential pieces of equipment such as ventilators, syringe pumps and multi-channel monitoring facilities. The use of special intensive care beds often allows both X-ray examination and weighing of the patient in bed, which may be a considerable advantage. Each bed station should have its own supply of piped oxygen, compressed air, nitrous oxide and suction, together with adequate electrical outlets. Most purpose-built intensive care units also contain their own facilities for blood-gas and electrolyte determinations together with haemoglobin and other essential investigations. This is important as these factors may need to be measured at frequent intervals during the day, making transport to routine laboratories impracticable.

● MEDICAL AND NURSING COMPLEMENT

An intensive care unit ideally requires one nurse continually assigned to each patient, together with one nurse per shift to carry out administrative and other duties, and any unit which possesses such a complement during the day and is reduced to ordinary ward staffing at night cannot be called an intensive care unit, as this requires 24-h patient care. A resident junior doctor, usually an anaesthetist or a physician, together with regular ward rounds and consultations with more senior members of the medical staff, are both essential to the intensive medical care necessary to improve the condition of patients and to enable the unit to run smoothly. Ideally, a busy intensive therapy unit requires a full-time consultant presence during normal working hours, in addition to out-of-hours availability.

● DAILY INTENSIVE CARE

The combination of general and specialised nursing care ranges from washing and turning the patient, to ventilator care, monitoring and recording, haemodialysis, etc. This daily nursing care must be accompanied and augmented by daily medical care, which consists of examination and investigation of the patient. It is important to do more than merely view the patient and the charts from the end of the bed, as investigations can only supplement clinical medical knowledge. The patients should be examined by the resident doctor as often as necessary, depending on their condition, and further specialist attention sought if needed. Detailed attention should be paid to both fluid and electrolyte balance, which are accurately charted on the input and output charts. Routine investigations include chest X-ray, ECG, haemoglobin, full blood count, urea and electrolytes, liver function tests, blood gases and specific microbiology. Other investigations, depending on the patients concerned, might include blood sugar, liver function tests, clotting factors and plasma cortisol, which may be done at intervals during the week rather than every day. Although patients in intensive care are looked after continuously and become familiar to the doctors and nurses, it must not be forgotten that unless the patients' condition improves and they make daily progress, they are not getting better.

● SEDATION IN INTENSIVE CARE

Intravenous sedative techniques are widely used in intensive care in both ventilated patients and those breathing spontaneously. It is important to assess the relative needs for sedation and analgesia, since opiate infusions may be required in addition to pure sedation. Benzodiazepines, particularly midazolam, are frequently used to provide continuous sedation, but unlike the short-acting intravenous induction agents, their action may be considerably prolonged following cessation of infusion. They provide good cardiovascular stability and anxiolysis and in addition are potent amnesics, which may be of considerable advantage in the intensive care situation.

Propofol infusion provides very controllable sedation with the ability to produce rapid changes in its level, for example, to assess the patient neurologically or to allow them to wake up and breathe spontaneously. Because of its hepatic metabolism, there are no prolonged effects of the drug, which is frequently very advantageous. Propofol infusion does produce hypotension in some patients, particularly those who are hypovolaemic or dehydrated.

Neuromuscular blockade may also be required in the restless head-injured or multiple trauma patient, but should only be given together with adequate sedation and analgesia. In patients with severe respiratory problems, in whom oxygen transfer is critically impaired, heavy sedation and neuromuscular blockade may be required to reduce oxygen consumption to a minimum.

● PROBLEMS IN INTENSIVE CARE

Most problems occurring in intensive care, apart from the initial pathology, concern three main systems: cardiovascular, respiratory and renal. Neurological and alimentary problems may also occur but are less common. Cardiovascular problems may involve hypotension together with reduced cardiac output and will require supportive drug therapy and other measures to improve the peripheral circulation. Respiratory problems are largely concerned with respiratory failure and may lead to a decision to employ artificial ventilation or other forms of respiratory assistance. These are often avoided by vigorous and regular physiotherapy, which is another benefit available in intensive care. Renal problems may necessitate fluid restriction, peritoneal or even haemodialysis, and siting an intensive care unit near the renal unit is logical. Many units are now equipped to carry out haemofiltration on site, thus avoiding the need for transfer of critically ill patients to a unit linked to a haemodialysis centre.

Alimentary problems are mainly concerned with malabsorption resulting from nasogastric feeding and other nutritional problems which may require temporary parenteral feeding. Many of the neurological problems which occur, such as confusion, are often minimised by adequate communication with the patient in ways other than verbally. Nevertheless, many patients become very agitated by their lack of ability to communicate with those looking after them. Specific neurological lesions due to pressure on nerves, or corneal abrasions, are not uncommon but are usually avoidable.

The coexistence of other diseases and previous drug treatment complicating the patient's condition must not be forgotten. This information is often not available when the patient is initially admitted and it is important to consult relatives or the patient's own general practitioner as soon as possible to ascertain any potentially complicating additional pathology.

Other problems that occur in intensive care include those of coagulation, particularly in relation to disseminated intravascular coagulation following massive haemorrhage, shock lung or fat embolism (Chapter 24). Many patients in intensive care receive long-term intravenous therapy necessitating the use of central venous catheters, which are best maintained in a sterile condition in intensive care (see below). Some patients may require tracheostomy if prolonged ventilation is contemplated, and although the enthusiasm for this fluctuates between hospitals and countries, it is still widely used, particularly the percutaneous, Seldinger, technique.

Finally, it should not be forgotten that patients who are admitted to intensive care as a result of trauma and who are apparently untreatable may still become potential organ donors, an important factor when one considers the benefits of transplantation to the remainder of the population.

● HIGH-DEPENDENCY CARE

Many postoperative patients, although not requiring intensive care and artificial ventilation still need a higher level of care than is available on a normal surgical ward. This is due both to the increasing complexity of operative treatment and to the increasing tendency to operate on more severely ill and elderly patients. In addition, the variety and complexity of postoperative analgesic techniques, for example, spinal, epidural and patient-controlled analgesia (PCA) (Chapter 42) and the use of more detailed and invasive monitoring, central venous pressure, intracranial pressure, direct arterial pressure, oxygen saturation, end-tidal carbon dioxide analysis, etc., all necessitate high levels of technical skills among the nursing staff.

With the advances in nurse education, less trained staff are available for routine work and resources must be concentrated where they are most needed. High-dependency care can relieve the ever increasing pressure on intensive care beds and forms the link in the progressive patient care chain between the intensive care unit and the wards. For some patients, it is a halfway house for non-ventilated patients, while for others a high-dependency unit is a long-stay recovery room. One of the other significant advantages is that high-dependency care is a far more economical use of a 'special' nurse who can be used to care for more than one patient in such a situation, where monitoring facilities are more intensive than on a routine ward.

● PARENTERAL NUTRITION

Parenteral nutrition is extensively used both in intensive care units and preoperatively in malnourished patients, although it is sometimes used in addition to oral feeding to increase calorie intake (hyperalimentation). It is important that parenteral feeding be considered as the sole source of the patient's calories and calculated accordingly.

A 70 kg man requires about 3000 cal/24 h, usually administered in 3000 ml intravenous fluid. As a general rule, 1 ml fluid must contain 1 cal. The normal diet is a balance of protein, fat and carbohydrate together with amino acids and electrolytes, which the body is able to conserve or excrete as necessary. A parenteral feeding regimen must aim to reproduce normal food intake, despite the fact that the gut is being bypassed. In general, parenteral feeding should only be employed in those patients with impaired intestinal absorption, nasogastric (enteral) feeding being preferable whenever possible. The individual requirements of an intravenous feeding regimen are best considered under their separate headings.

● PROTEIN

The daily protein requirement to balance urinary loss is about 1 g amino acid per kg body weight, containing the equivalent of 10–15 g nitrogen per day for a 70 kg person. In order that the amino acid supplied to the body may be fully incorporated into body protein, 200 cal in the form of carbohydrate is required for every 5 g nitrogen supplied. Although several amino acid solutions are available the most important are as follows.

Vamin

Vamin is either supplied as an amino acid solution alone containing 9 or 14 g nitrogen or combined with glucose which is added to provide the total daily requirement of amino acids, carbohydrate and electrolyte in one solution. The energy yield of Vamin Glucose is 650 cal/l.

Aminoplex/Aminosteril

These are produced either as 12, 14, 16 or 24 depending on the number of grams of utilisable nitrogen per litre. They provide a high level of nitrogen input as L-form amino acids in a low fluid volume. The calorie yields are low but the nitrogen content is about 12, 14, 16 and 24 g/l, respectively.

Synthamin 14

This is another amino acid solution containing a similar amount of nitrogen to Aminoplex 14, and the two solutions are used in similar circumstances.

Vitrimix KV

This is another complete feeding regimen, which combines Vamin 9 Glucose 750 ml with 250 ml Intralipid 20%. The two solutions are presented separately in a composite pack, for reconstitution prior to use.

● CARBOHYDRATE

The most widely used carbohydrate source in parenteral feeding is dextrose, in concentrations ranging from 10% to 50%. In normal circumstances carbohydrate metabolism yields about 4 cal/g (glucose), and therefore a litre of 20% dextrose, containing 200 g/l, will yield about 800 cal. For this reason, any dextrose concentration below 10% is inadequate, since the fluid volume required to yield adequate calories will be too large. Most pharmacies now stock litre bottles of glucose with added electrolytes similar to Glucoplex 1200 (30% glucose) or 1600 (40% glucose) which yield 1200 and 1600 cal/l, respectively.

It is now recognised that administering intravenous dextrose alone does not result in the sugar passing intracellularly where it is needed for metabolism. This function is insulin dependent, and patients being parenterally fed on dextrose usually need insulin added. This may be accomplished in three ways, either by using a sliding scale based usually on 4-hourly urine or blood sugar testing, or by adding insulin to the intravenous solution or by using a separate infusion of insulin. Insulin, however, is adsorbed on to the plastic of the intravenous solution container and giving set, and the amount reaching the patient therefore varies. Administration of glucose and insulin will also result in potassium passing intracellularly, and it is important not to allow the patient to become hypokalaemic.

Other carbohydrate source include fructose, which was popular for a time, largely in the belief that insulin was not required to help in the passage of fructose into cells. This has now been proved incorrect and the vogue for fructose is declining. It is still sometimes administered in conjunction with amino acid solutions, where it produces a similar calorie yield to other carbohydrate sources. Sorbitol was also used, but produced unacceptable degrees of metabolic acidosis.

Ethanol may be used and yields 7 cal/g as opposed to 4 cal/g for the other sugar solutions. The amount of ethanol which may be given daily is limited and it cannot therefore be used to supply the total carbohydrate requirements.

● FATS

Intralipid and Ivelip, as either a 10% or 20% solution, are the main fat sources used at present. Since fat yields 9 cal/g, Intralipid is a good source of energy, a litre of 10% yielding 1000 cal and 20% 2000 cal. When Intralipid was introduced certain problems were encountered with the high viscosity producing micro-aggregation in small vessels that was similar to fat embolism. This has now been overcome and fat should be considered an essential part of any intravenous feed regimen. It should be remembered, however, that blood samples should not be taken while fat emulsion is running because considerable inaccuracies may occur on auto-analysers used for electrolyte determination.

● VITAMINS

It is important that both the fat-soluble and water-soluble vitamins are administered regularly in the form of Multibionta, Solvito or Vitalipid. These can only be added to isotonic fluid solutions such as dextrose or saline in the case of water-soluble vitamin preparations, or to Intralipid for the fat-soluble vitamins.

● IONIC REQUIREMENTS

In addition to producing an adequate calorie intake, patients still require their normal intake of sodium, potassium and other trace elements such as magnesium, zinc and calcium. Some glucose- and protein-containing solutions contain various amounts of sodium and potassium and some of the trace elements, but it is important to determine the amount of sodium and other ions being administered to check that this is neither inadequate nor excessive. The specific requirements for fluid and electrolytes have already been discussed in Chapter 2. The overall daily requirements of individual ions are as follows:

Sodium	70–150 mmol/24 h
Potassium	60–80 mmol/24 h
Calcium	1000–1500 mg/24 h
Phosphate	1000 mg/24 h.

● SUGGESTED INTRAVENOUS FEEDING REGIMENS

Although it may appear convenient to administer intravenous feeding consecutively in bottles, this is far from the normal way in which we obtain food. Serious metabolic imbalance may result from administering protein for 4 h followed by dextrose for 4 h followed by fats for 4 h. Parenteral feeding is best accomplished by the simultaneous administration of two or more solutions through a central venous line, controlled by drip counters. Many hospital pharmacies have a sterile preparation area where a composite 24-h, 3 l bag can be made to match the requirements of a particular patient. These bags are sterile and, as with all parenteral feeding solutions, should not have anything added to them. If it is not possible to obtain a 3 l bag, most parenteral feeding solutions are obtainable in either 500 or 1000 ml bottles (Fig. 44.1) and a satisfactory fluid and calorie input which is versatile enough to allow addition of electrolytes and vitamins is best achieved as follows:

Line A
0–8 h 500 ml of Aminoplex 12
8–16 h 500 ml 20% Intralipid
16–24 h 500 ml of Aminoplex 12

Line B
500 ml 30% dextrose
500 ml 5% dextrose or normal saline
500 ml 30% dextrose.

Obviously this regimen can be adapted to suit individual requirements by substituting one bottle for another, depending on whether one wishes to include a high nitrogen, a high calorie or high electrolyte input. It has several important advantages.

First, dextrose, a carbohydrate source, is given simultaneously with the amino acid solution, the two being necessary for efficient utilisation of amino acids. Simultaneous administration of insulin will be necessary to permit glucose to pass intracellularly.

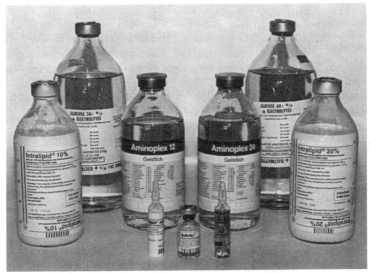

Figure 44.1 Balanced range of parenteral feeding solutions.

Secondly, the regimen may be adjusted so that Intralipid is not running in the morning when blood is taken for urea and electrolyte determinations.

Thirdly, a single bottle of isotonic 5% dextrose or normal saline allows addition of both vitamins and added electrolytes where these are needed. Although Aminoplex 12 contains a considerable amount of sodium and some potassium, it is often necessary to supplement the potassium intake in particular. Most pharmacies will make up isotonic electrolyte solutions containing trace elements if these are required for intravenous feeding. The overall regimen provides just under 3000 cal in 3 l of fluid, although this may be adjusted as necessary.

● PROBLEMS OF PARENTERAL NUTRITION

If intravenous feeding is used scientifically and early, it should considerably reduce morbidity from major surgery. Indeed, it is often now used preoperatively, particularly in patients who are malnourished as a result of their illness. Nevertheless, fluid overload may be a problem if one is particularly anxious to increase the calorie intake, although certain solutions such as 20% Intralipid go some way towards removing this risk. Some solutions, such as those containing amino acids, are irritant and certainly cannot be given through a peripheral drip. A central venous feeding line which is not used for aspirating blood or for giving other drugs is essential to maintain absolute sterility. These lines are best introduced either through the antecubital fossa or into the subclavian or internal jugular vein under strictly aseptic conditions. The use of triple-lumen central venous catheters has greatly facilitated the simultaneous administration of parenteral nutrition and drugs via a single catheter. Accurate monitoring of fluid and electrolyte balance is vital as these are difficult to correct if allowed to get out of control. Hypokalaemia may be a problem and since there is a limit to the amount of potassium which can safely be administered intravenously, even under ECG control, it is important to consider adequate potassium replacement early.

● ASSESSMENT OF PARENTERAL FEEDING

Although frequent measurements can be made of fluid and electrolyte balance, one of the most important indices of the adequacy of parenteral feeding is the nitrogen balance. This is not normally undertaken but is simple and revealing in some circumstances. By collecting all the urine which the patient passes during a 24-h period and measuring its volume and urea content, the overall urea output per 24 h can be measured. Then, as 100 mmol urea = 6 g urea = 3 g nitrogen = 20 g protein (normal nitrogen output 9/10 in the urine, 1/10 in the faeces), it is possible to assess both the daily protein output and whether this exceeds the daily protein intake. Protein intake is easily calculated when parenteral feeding alone is used, but when this is combined with nasogastric feeding, or indeed nasogastric feeding is used alone, it is important to know the protein content of the individual nasogastric feeds used such as Nutroxyl, Fresubin, Fresubin 750, Fortison and Nutrison. Simple calculations can therefore prevent patients getting into dangerously negative nitrogen balance.

45

Humidifiers and Nebulisers

•Effects of anaesthesia and intensive care •Methods of humidification •Nebulisers

● EFFECTS OF ANAESTHESIA AND INTENSIVE CARE

The most important function of the nose and upper respiratory tract is to warm and humidify inspired air or gases. It performs this task with remarkable efficiency considering that – assuming a minute volume of 8 l/min – an average person breathes in over 10 000 l of air in 24 h. Over a wide range of inspired air temperatures the nose is capable of raising the temperature of the inspired air to within <1°C of body temperature.

As regards humidification, the alveoli function best when the air presented to them is almost fully saturated. Here, an important physical principle is involved – namely, that the amount of water vapour required to saturate air or a gas mixture fully increases with the temperature. Thus the clear air of a warm day changes to mist or fog in the evening as the temperature falls and the air is unable to contain the water vapour which precipitates out. In the morning as the temperature rises, the air once again becomes clear as the amount of water vapour that it is able to contain increases.

For comfort, room air should only be about half-saturated with water vapour. However, even if fully saturated it contains only about 2 vol.% of water vapour, while at body temperature (37°C) air requires 6 vol.% of water vapour to be fully saturated. This task of adding large quantities of water vapour to the inspired air is remarkably well achieved by the nose and upper respiratory passages.

With most modern anaesthetic breathing systems (e.g. Magill and Bain systems, or a system with a non-rebreathing valve next to the face mask or tracheal tube) the patient receives at each inspiration an almost completely fresh supply of dry gases from the cylinders or pipeline. These gases may result in drying up of mucosal surfaces and increase the viscosity of respiratory secretions resulting in mucus plugs, collapse of alveoli and reduction in gas exchange and increased risk of infection.

When a face mask is used the nose can still perform its function adequately, but when an oropharyngeal airway is inserted a proportion of the inspired gases bypasses the nose so that warming and humidification are less effective. A tracheal tube completely bypasses the upper respiratory tract, so warming and humidification have to be achieved in the lower respiratory passages. It is becoming a common practice to attempt humidification during anaesthesia on a routine basis.

With a circle anaesthetic system, humidification is not quite so difficult because the patient does rebreathe his own expired gases to some extent. However, even in this arrangement the temperature of the expired gases rapidly falls to room temperature in the anaesthetic tubing so that much of the water vapour condenses out on the inside. On re-inspiration the air passages once again have to rewarm the gases to body temperature and resaturate them with water vapour at this higher temperature.

The problem of humidification is much more serious in intensive care, where spontaneous respiration or intermittent positive pressure ventilation (IPPV) may be carried out for days or even weeks through an endotracheal or tracheostomy tube. Some form of artificial humidification is necessary to prevent a serious or even fatal drying up and crusting of secretions. The various methods used are described below.

● METHODS OF HUMIDIFICATION

Direct Instillation of Water Droplets

This consists of the direct injection of water droplets into an endotracheal or tracheostomy tube. While simple, this method is rather crude and ineffective and at times may result in a picture similar to a mild degree of acid-aspiration syndrome. It should therefore have little place in modern intensive therapy.

Water Bath

In its simplest form this consists of bubbling the gases through water in a bottle, as shown in Figure 45.1. This is most inefficient for two reasons: first, the bubbles tend to be too large to become fully saturated with water vapour, and secondly, saturation at best occurs only at room temperature, which means only partial saturation when the gases are raised to body temperature. The system tends to be made even less efficient by the cooling effect produced by vaporising the water.

The efficiency of this type of humidifier is greatly increased by breaking up the big bubbles into smaller ones so that they are more readily saturated and by adding a heater to the water bath (Fig. 45.2). Because of the fall in temperature along the tube leading from the humidifier to the patient, for maximum efficiency the temperature of the water should be

Humidifiers

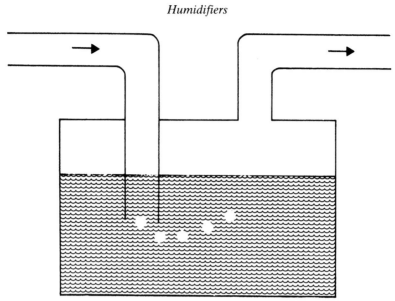

Figure 45.1 Water-bottle humidifier.

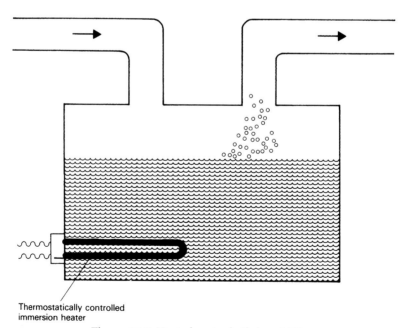

Thermostatically controlled
immersion heater

Figure 45.2 Heated water-bath humidifier.

kept at about 55°C. However, as air when fully saturated at body temperature contains less water vapour than when fully saturated at 55°C, some water vapour must condense out in the tube before it reaches the patient. Care must be taken either by positioning the humidifier below the patient or by using a water-trap to prevent pooling of water, which might spill into the patient's respiratory tract.

If the water temperature is kept near 60°C, sterility of the humidifier is maintained by a prolonged pasteurisation effect. This type of humidifier should have a thermostat as well as a thermometer and an automatic cut-out in case the temperature exceeds its setting. In some of these humidifiers it is also possible to override the thermostat so that the apparatus can be fully sterilised by boiling before being used in another patient.

These water-bath humidifiers are usually placed on the inspiratory side of a ventilatory system. Others – usually referred to as blower humidifiers – are intended for use when the patient is breathing spontaneously. In these circumstances the humidified air is blown past a T-piece inserted into the patient's tracheostomy or endotracheal tube.

Condenser Humidifiers, Heat and Moisture Exchangers

These lightweight pieces of apparatus are designed to fit onto a standard catheter mount of a tracheal or tracheostomy tube and are the most commonly used type of humidifier in everyday anaesthetic practice. The apparatus consists of a compact plastic casing which is filled with a variety of condensation materials, for example, foam or mesh, with a large surface area covered with a hygroscopic material such as paper coated calcium chloride or glass fibre. The moisture from the expired air condenses on the mesh material as it cools. This warms the mesh as the cooling moiture emits latent heat of vaporisation. As gas is inhaled it is therefore both humidified and warmed and hence the name heat and moisture exchangers (HMEs). The pore size is small enough ($0.2\,\mu$m) so that the mesh acts as a bacterial filter as well. HMEs are single-use disposable, lightweight and inexpensive, as well as relatively efficient (Fig. 45.3).

● NEBULISERS

Nebulisers are not synonymous with humidifiers because they deposit water droplets to the inspired gases rather than water vapour as humidifiers do. When they are used as humidifiers there is a danger of fluid overload occurring because of deposition of water droplets in the alveoli or large airways, depending on the size. A more useful function of nebulisers therefore is to deposit drugs such as bronchodilators and local anaesthetics in the respiratory tract.

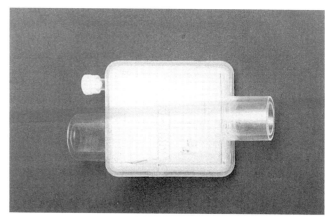

Figure 45.3 Heat and moisture exchanger.

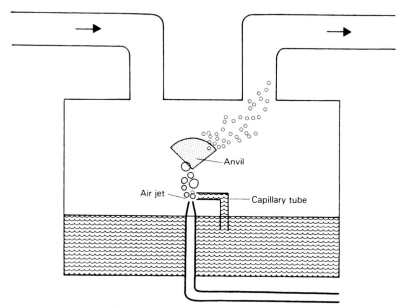

Figure 45.4 Gas-driven nebuliser.

Gas Driven

Most examples of this type of nebuliser (Fig. 45.4) depend on the Bernouilli effect whereby gas blown at high pressure through an orifice causes a fall in pressure around the orifice. Fluid is drawn up a capillary tube to the area of the orifice where the fluid is vaporised by the gas jet. The larger droplets can be filtered off by striking an 'anvil' or metal plate.

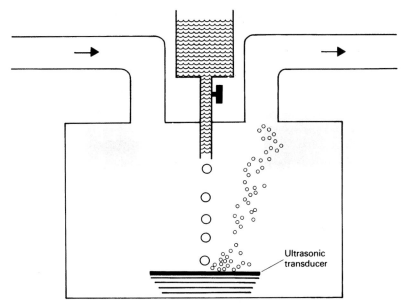

Figure 45.5 Ultrasonic nebuliser with water dropping on to the transducer head.

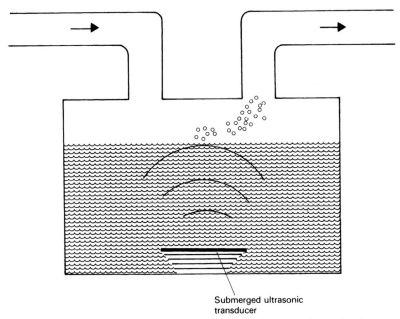

Figure 45.6 Ultrasonic nebuliser with submerged transducer head.

The efficiency of this type of nebuliser can be increased by heating the liquid in the container.

Spinning Disc Nebulisers

A rotating disc is mounted on a hollow shaft up which the liquid is drawn. As the liquid touches the disc it is thrown out by centrifugal force in a variety of droplet sizes.

Ultrasonic Nebulisers

In these nebulisers either liquid is dropped on to a transducer which vibrates at ultrasonic speed (Fig. 45.5), or liquid in a container covers the head of a transducer which vibrates at an ultrasonic frequency (Fig. 45.6). The size of the droplets depends on the speed of vibration.

With nebulisers of all types, the size of the droplets is important. If these are $>20\,\mu$m diameter they tend to condense out in the tubing of the apparatus or in the upper respiratory tract and are merely a nuisance. Droplets of 5–$15\,\mu$m size deposit mostly in the trachea and larger bronchi which they help to keep moist. Droplets of $1\,\mu$m diameter pass on to the alveoli where they are deposited. Droplets of $<1\,\mu$m diameter tend to be remarkably stable, passing into alveoli and out again. They may escape into the atmosphere, where they become an infection risk.

The droplets produced by the ultrasonic nebulisers tend to be largely in the $1\,\mu$m range so that, while they tend to be extremely efficient as humidifiers, overhydration of the patient is a possibility, especially in children.

46

Sterilisation of Anaesthetic Equipment

In recent years two developments have tended to reduce the extent to which anaesthetic nurses, operating department assistants (ODAs) and other theatre staff have been directly involved in maintaining and sterilising anaesthetic equipment. The first of these has been the introduction of theatre sterile supply departments (TSSUs) and central sterile supply departments (CSSDs). The second factor is the ever-expanding use of disposable equipment. While this originally applied mainly to simple items of equipment such as syringes and needles, now quite complicated packs (e.g. for setting up central venous lines or performing epidural blocks) may be entirely disposable.

Economic considerations make it impossible to provide fully sterilised anaesthetic apparatus in every case, even in those parts of the system through which rebreathing has occurred. Fortunately, although cross-infection between patients can occur by means of contaminated anaesthetic apparatus, it seems to be unusual except in the case of ventilators. The risk of this has been further reduced by the use of disposable breathing filters (heat and moisture exchangers, HMEs) on the anaesthetic circuitry used for each new patient. Economy also leads to a tendency to try to reuse or resterilise equipment which is meant to be disposable, although this practice is now declining. This should be done only with the utmost caution because certain materials, especially plastic and rubber, tend to deteriorate rapidly with repeated sterilisation.

Thus, although the standards of sterility in anaesthesia tend to be a compromise between what is desirable and what is economically practicable, it is essential that all those working with anaesthetic equipment should not only understand what standards of cleanliness and sterilisation are acceptable in everyday practice, but also have some knowledge of the methods of sterilising such equipment.

● DEFINITIONS

Sterilisation

The process by which all micro-organisms, including bacterial spores, are destroyed.

Disinfection

The process by which the vegetative forms of micro-organisms are destroyed, but not usually bacterial spores.

Pasteurisation

A process of disinfection by heat at temperatures of about 60–80°C.

Disinfectant

An agent, usually a chemical solution, used for disinfection. Sometimes heat is employed (see above).

Antisepsis

A process by which micro-organisms are destroyed on the surface of living tissues. Spores are not usually killed and, while some vegetative forms may also survive, they are usually reduced to low levels not normally harmful to health.

Antiseptic

A chemical agent, usually weaker than a disinfectant, used in antisepsis. It must be non-toxic and non-corrosive.

Fumigation

This is also a method of disinfection, but by exposure to the fumes of a vaporised disinfectant (e.g. formaldehyde).

Pyrogen

Organic protein matter which is capable of producing fever and is sometimes found in sterile infusion fluids. It is produced by bacteria entering the fluid during distillation and storage. The bacteria are killed during sterilisation but the pyrogenic particles of protein are left behind.

● METHODS OF STERILISATION

Heat Sterilisation

Moist Heat: Autoclaving

The autoclave is a special sterilising container from which the air is first removed and replaced by steam under pressure. As the pressure is increased, the temperature of the steam rises and the length of exposure required for sterilisation is reduced. For example, at a temperature of 134°C a period of 3 min is satisfactory, and at a temperature of 147°C only 30 s is required for sterilisation. Of course, the full autoclaving cycle takes longer than this.

The method is effective against spores as well as vegetative bacteria, provided that the items to be sterilised are packed in such a way that the steam can gain access to them. The steam penetrates paper, cardboard and fabrics, but unfortunately tends to dull sharp edges slightly and speeds the deterioration of rubber and plastic.

Dry Heat

Theoretically, dry heat in hot air ovens is a simple method of sterilisation, and sealed containers may be used. However, a long period of exposure is required (e.g. 160°C for 1 h) and it is difficult to ensure that all parts of the load have been held at the full temperature for the necessary time.

Gas Sterilisation

Two methods are available.

Ethylene Oxide

This colourless gas is effective against both vegetative bacteria and spores. It has excellent powers of penetration, leaves most materials undamaged, and is useful for sterilising heat-sensitive materials and ventilator circuits, where a closed-circuit technique is used. Its disadvantages are that it is toxic to inhale, it is explosive, slow (up to 8 h) and needs considerable skill for correct use. It is also difficult to eradicate all traces of ethylene oxide from materials like rubber and plastics.

Low-temperature Steam Plus Formaldehyde

In normal autoclaving, the pressure is raised above atmospheric to produce steam at temperatures above 100°C. In this technique a sub-atmospheric pressure is produced in a purpose-built autoclave, and formaldehyde and then steam at 73°C are added and the temperature is held steady for 2 h. This method is faster and cheaper than ethylene oxide and the formaldehyde is easier to get rid of at the end of the process.

Sterilisation by Irradiation

Gamma Rays

Gamma rays from a radioactive source, usually cobalt-60 in a dose of 2.5 Mrad, are used. This method gives good penetration of closed packs and is commonly used for disposable equipment. Glass tends to turn brown and may be damaged. Also damaged are some types of rubber and, if irradiated more than once, many other materials including metals, polyvinyl chloride (PVC), nylon, paper, wool and cotton.

Ultraviolet Light

This method has only a limited application as it is effective only on the surface area exposed.

● STERILISATION INDICATORS

Sterilisation indicators are important, since without them it is impossible to be sure which packs have been sterilised. Some of the commoner indicators are listed below.

Autoclave Tape

This adhesive tape incorporates a heat-sensitive stripe which turns dark brown when exposed to normal autoclave conditions. Two such types of tape are approved by the Department of Health and Social Security (DHSS) for the Bowie Dick Autoclave Test, in which the autoclave tape is buried inside a stack of towels and then examined for uniformity of colour change after autoclaving.

Sterilisation Indicator Panels

These panels are found on sterilisation bags and contain a stripe similar to autoclave tape.

Browne's Tubes

Various tubes are available for different sterilisation processes, for example, autoclaving and hot air sterilisation. The liquid changes from red to green when sterilisation is complete.

Irradiation Labels

These are small adhesive discs which change from yellow to red when irradiation has taken place.

● METHODS OF DISINFECTION

Disinfection by Heat (Pasteurisation)

Traditionally this term was used for the process of raising the temperature of a liquid (commonly milk, whose proteins would be denatured by boiling) to temperatures between 60 and 80°C for periods of between a few seconds and about an hour. This treatment is sufficient to kill most bacteria and viruses, but not spores.

In hospital, pasteurisation is carried out by either hot water or steam.

Hot Water Pasteurisation

This is usually carried out in tank pasteurisers or washer pasteurisers. The former usually have a preset process timer. The washer pasteurisers are useful for simultaneously cleaning and pasteurising anaesthetic equipment, some being fitted with long metal spouts upon which tubing is mounted. The Scott's washer is an example.

Note: Boiling, now seldom used in hospitals, is only a method of disinfection, not sterilisation, as it cannot be guaranteed to be sporicidal.

Steam Pasteurisation

This is carried out in the special autoclaves constructed for sterilisation with low-temperature steam plus formaldehyde (described above), but in this technique the formaldehyde is omitted. This method has become more popular with the increased use of materials damaged or destroyed by higher temperatures.

Chemical Disinfection and Sterilisation

A wide variety of chemical disinfectants is marketed, one of the most commonly used being 2% glutaraldehyde (Cidex). The makers claim that after careful cleaning, immersed instruments are disinfected in 10 min and sterilised in 10 h.

● FILTRATION

Bacterial filters for use on the inspiratory side of ventilators used in intensive therapy units have been available for some time. Some of these are combined with heat and moisture exchangers (Chapter 45) and are now frequently used in anaesthesia. Epidural filters remove particles down to a diameter of 0.5 μm and are routinely used. Bacterial filters are also available for use with intravenous infusions.

● CLEANING AND STERILISING ANAESTHETIC EQUIPMENT

Face Masks

These are usually made of antistatic rubber which may be boiled or autoclaved. However, both methods cause rapid deterioration of the rubber, and it is accepted practice simply to wash the mask with soap or cetrimide and rinse thoroughly.

Airways and Endotracheal Tubes

The disposable varieties are commonly used, including double-lumen and armoured tube. If reusable versions are employed, it is important that they be thoroughly cleaned inside with a suitable brush. Sterilisation is most commonly achieved by autoclaving, but this hastens the deterioration of plastic and rubber, the former becoming discoloured and harder, while the latter becomes softer.

Laryngoscope Blades

After removal, laryngoscope blades may be boiled or autoclaved. It is common practice simply to scrub laryngoscope blades with soap and water between cases. It is likely that disposable laryngoscope blades will become mandatory for use in patients undergoing tonsillectomy, as part of the preventive measures against bovine spongiform encephalopathy (BSE).

Corrugated Tubing and Reservoir Bags

These are usually made of antistatic rubber, which deteriorates rapidly on boiling or autoclaving. These items of equipment should be thoroughly washed and rinsed after every use, but in many hospitals are only cleaned at the end of every list. If a greater degree of sterility is required, then pasteurisation is usually carried out in low-temperature steam or a washer pasteuriser.

Most of the tubing used now is disposable, although reservoir bags of antistatic rubber are still sometimes used.

Ventilators

Various methods have been described for sterilising ventilators. Most are rather specialised, some are expensive and none is entirely satisfactory. They include the use of formaldehyde vapour, ethylene oxide, ultrasonic alcohol and ultrasonic hydrogen peroxide. The best solution is to design ventilators with patient circuits which are fully autoclavable.

Syringes and Needles

Reusable syringes and needles are much less used nowadays, except for specific procedures and situations, for example, phenol injections. Syringes are sterilised by autoclaving with the plunger removed from the barrel. Needles must be carefully washed through with a detergent and rinsed in water or in an ultrasonic washer. Finally they are blown through with high-pressure air before autoclaving.

Fibreoptic Laryngoscope/Bronchoscope

After use, this is thoroughly washed with soapy water and then kept in a chemical disinfectant, for example, Cidex, for 10–20 min, after which it is again washed with clean water and the channel sucked through with water and air to remove all the Cidex.

● HEPATITIS B AND C ANTIGENS

Hepatitis B is the antigen (HBAg, Australia antigen) carried by the dangerous virus which can cause serum hepatitis and ultimately irreversible liver damage. It is highly infectious and is transmitted in the blood or secretions of patients who either have active hepatitis or are symptom-free (or healthy) carriers (Chapter 15). All hospitals must have a detailed policy for dealing with such patients requiring operation. Hepatitis C can cause similar problems, although potential carriers are not routinely identified, as there is no specific immunisation programme available.

The virus is readily killed by autoclaving and the general policy with potentially contaminated instruments and materials is to autoclave or incinerate them. Of the chemical agents, hypochlorite is the most effective.

● ACQUIRED IMMUNE DEFICIENCY SYNDROME (AIDS)

As in the case of serum hepatitis, the causative organism of AIDS is a virus. This has been given a number of different names, of which the commonest is HIV or human immunodeficiency virus. Not surprisingly, therefore, the Microbiology Advisory Committee to the DHSS, in a report which has also been approved by the Expert Advisory Group on AIDS (EAGA), recommended that whenever practicable the same procedures are used in HIV as in hepatitis B contamination.

While these precautions should be adequate to prevent contamination with the AIDS virus, it must be realised that patients with established AIDS may be suffering from opportunistic infection by a wide variety of potentially pathogenic bacteria, against which more elaborate precautions may be required.

47

Pollution and Electrical Safety

•Possible hazards •Anaesthetic scavenging systems •Summary •Electrical safety •Abnormal electric currents •Prevention of explosions

It is only in recent years (as indeed is the case with more general environmental and atmospheric pollution) that serious consideration has been given to the possible hazards of pollution of the operating theatre atmosphere by gaseous anaesthetics. As soon as the problem was identified a great deal of evidence was accumulated, much of it conflicting and none of it conclusive. This chapter indicates some of the possible hazards, and what methods should be used to reduce the severity of pollution in the operating theatre.

● POSSIBLE HAZARDS

Spontaneous Abortion

An increased incidence of spontaneous abortion among females working in operating theatres is the possible hazard for which there is the most convincing evidence, but even this is not certain. The evidence merely relates to their exposure to a theatre environment, the inference being that anaesthetics are responsible.

Effect on Fetal Development and Infertility

Some surveys indicate an increased incidence of fetal abnormalities of a minor nature and an increased tendency towards involuntary infertility in women working in operating theatres. The evidence is not clear, but merits further investigation. The supposed increased incidence of female children born to practising anaesthetists is also not statistically proven.

Cancer and Other Tumours

It has been suggested that anaesthetists have an increased tendency to develop neoplasms. One study from the USA indicated an increased incidence of tumours of the lymphoid and reticulo-endothelial systems (e.g. lymphosarcoma, Hodgkin's disease) among anaesthetists. However, this was not confirmed in a second, similar study.

It has also been suggested that there is an increased incidence of cancer in female anaesthetists, but again evidence is unconvincing.

Impaired Mental Performance

Another possible hazard among operating theatre staff is impairment of their mental function by traces of gaseous anaesthetics. While the concentrations of nitrous oxide and halothane in unscavenged operating theatres are not considered high enough to affect mental performance in other theatre staff, anaesthetists using unscavenged anaesthetic circuits may be exposed to high enough concentrations of these agents to be affected in this way.

Even in the case of the spontaneous abortion question there is no justification for assuming a cause-and-effect relationship with trace concentrations of gaseous anaesthetics in the operating theatre atmosphere. It may well be that the special physical and emotional effort required in operating theatre work may be the true cause of the increased tendency to abortion. Indeed, in one Scandinavian survey the nurses exposed to the highest concentrations of anaesthetic vapours were not those with the highest incidence of abortion, the rate being highest in scrub nurses, next intensive therapy unit nurses, and finally anaesthetic nurses.

Although there is a lack of convincing evidence that atmospheric pollution by traces of anaesthetic agents has any serious effects on theatre staff, it is just as difficult to prove that it has not. For this reason, because unscavenged systems at times expose anaesthetists to quite high concentrations of anaesthetic vapours, and because traces of gaseous anaesthetics may summate with other adverse factors (e.g. impaired physical health, fatigue or other poor environmental conditions) to reduce mental performance, it is wise to minimise the amount of such vapours inhaled by staff working in these areas. The Association of Anaesthetists of Great Britain and Ireland (AAGBI) has recommended the use of scavenging devices whenever they are available and the Department of Health and Social Security (DHSS) has issued a circular to the same effect.

● ANAESTHETIC SCAVENGING SYSTEMS

These may be passive or active.

Passive Systems

In these systems the gases are driven away by the patient's own expiratory effort. This adds to the expiratory resistance, the extent depending in particular upon the length and diameter of the tubing and the number of acute bends it contains. More severe obstruction may occur if there is kinking of the tubing.

The system may vent either directly to the atmosphere via an external wall or roof, or into the hospital ventilation system. If the outlet is to the atmosphere, variations in pressure, either positive or negative, caused by variations in the strength or direction of the wind must be checked by ventilation engineers. It is also important that the outlet be fitted with an insect-proof wire mesh cover. If the system vents into the hospital ventilation, again it is necessary for engineers to test for the variations in pressure occurring at the outlet point. Other theoretical risks include the transfer of flammable anaesthetic gases into the ventilation systems and the possible deleterious effect of some anaesthetic vapours on lubricants used in that system.

The Cardiff Aldasorber is another type of passive scavenging system. The patient's expired gases pass through activated charcoal which adsorbs volatile agents like halothane and ether, but not, unfortunately, nitrous oxide.

Active Systems

In these systems the expired gases are carried away by active suction provided by a pump, fan or ejector. It is important that this suction is not applied directly to the patient's airway. If the hospital piped suction is used, the negative pressure supplied is about 1000 times too high! In addition, there are again potential hazards of flammable vapours in the main hospital suction pump and of those vapours on pump lubricants. For these reasons it is better to have a separate extraction system tailor-made for scavenging anaesthetic gases. For example, Penlon Ltd and the British Oxygen Company provide a variety of active and passive systems (Figs 47.1–47.3).

● SUMMARY

At present the literature on the occupational hazards of anaesthesia provides reasonably convincing evidence only of an increased risk of spontaneous abortion among females working in operating theatres. Even then, there is no particular reason to believe that this is caused by trace quantities of anaesthetic gases. There is no convincing evidence of any other hazard. Nevertheless, it is now accepted that attempts should be made to

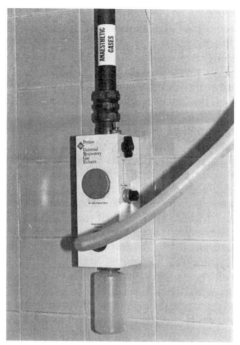

Figure 47.1 Penlon Universal active/passive gas exhaust system.

reduce atmospheric pollution in operating theatres because it is also difficult to refute an association between atmospheric pollution and some adverse effects. All theatres and anaesthetic rooms should now be fully equipped with an approved and functioning scavenging system.

However, it should be realised that while these attempts to reduce pollution may lead to increased safety for the operating theatre staff, none of the methods does anything to add to patient safety. Some of the potential dangers of the various scavenging systems have already been mentioned. In addition, both active and passive systems increase the dangers of disconnection, misconnection and infection of the tubing. Also, the muffling effect of the lengths of expiratory tubing required reduces the anaesthetist's ability to hear when something is amiss with the anaesthetic – a useful safety bonus with old, noisy valves like the Heidbrink.

Finally, there are areas other than operating theatres where pollution may occur with anaesthetic gases and vapours and, in some of these, scavenging arrangements may be even more difficult to introduce. These include obstetric units (where patients may exhale large volumes of nitrous oxide), surgeries where dental anaesthetics are given, and particularly recovery rooms. Here the patients inevitably exhale significant quantities of

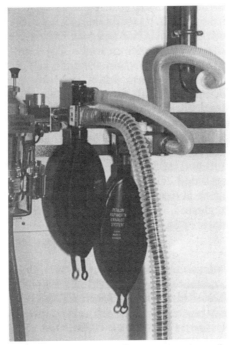

Figure 47.2 Penlon Papworth active gas exhaust system attached to a Lack co-axial circuit.

anaesthetic gases and vapours, which are impossible to extract. Although the quantities involved rapidly decrease, recovery staff are theoretically more exposed than their theatre-based colleagues, which may be a particular risk during the first trimester of pregnancy.

● ELECTRICAL SAFETY

Several individual gases and anaesthetic agents are potentially inflammable. Although their use in the UK is rapidly declining, in some centres particularly in the developing world, ether, for example, is still used extensively. In this situation, it is essential that potential sources of ignition, usually electric sparks, be minimised in operating theatres. Inflammable agents include ether and cyclopropane, both of which are potentially explosive when combined with oxygen. Since neither agent is now used in the UK, electrical safety is to a certain extent neglected. Electric sparks not only cause ignition of inflammable gas mixtures either inside or outside the body, but may also produce burns.

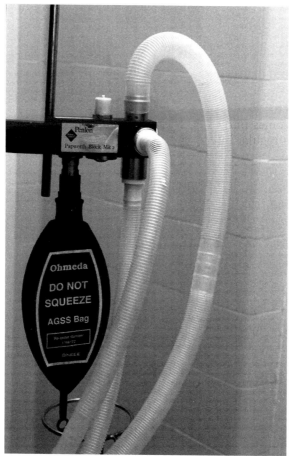

Figure 47.3 Penlon Papworth active gas exhaust system attached to a circle system with carbon dioxide absorption.

● ABNORMAL ELECTRIC CURRENTS

Abnormal electric currents may arise in four important ways.

Static Electricity

Static electricity builds up when two dissimilar materials in contact with one another are pulled apart, for example, a nylon shirt next to the skin. It commonly occurs when one substance which does not conduct electricity is in contact with one that does. Important non-conductors include rubber, plastic, wool, cotton and nylon. To allow the flow of static electricity to earth it is important that all rubber on anaesthetic and operating equipment (e.g. anaesthetic circuits, trolley tyres, operating table and stool tops) should be made of conducting rubber with antistatic properties. Such rubber is widely used in theatres and is black due to the inclusion of conducting carbon. All routinely used rubber anaesthetic equipment is antistatic. It is also important that the floor of the operating theatre be a good conductor so that static electricity will flow away when conductive equipment comes into contact with it, and for this reason, copper strips are placed at regular intervals between the terazzo tiles.

Electric Current

Normal flow of electricity occurs intra-operatively, both intentionally – when diathermy is used to produce coagulation or cutting – and unintentionally – due to faulty electrical equipment such as X-ray machines or electric motors producing sparks. Surgical diathermy is a low-voltage, high-frequency current which produces heat and therefore coagulation at the tip of the diathermy forceps. With unipolar diathermy, it is essential that the current should be conducted away from the patient through a large earth electrode, thereby reducing the intensity of the current and preventing burns occurring under the electrode. If the earth is not attached to the patient, current will be conducted through the patient's body, passing into whatever conductive surface he or she is touching. If this area of contact is small, high current density may result in electrical burns. It is also possible for other electrical equipment (e.g. electrocardiogram (ECG) leads) to act as an earth in the absence of a normal diathermy earth, and this is dangerous. Bipolar diathermy removes this risk, since the two diathermy electrodes are contained within the hand-held device, for example, forceps or diathermy blade.

It is essential that all electrical apparatus in theatre should be frequently inspected for poor connections and other faults. All monitoring apparatus is now patient isolated, which means that leads from the patient do not come into direct contact with the electronic circuitry within the machine, thereby minimising risks of abnormal currents flowing.

Diathermy and Pacemakers

Permanent indwelling cardiac pacemakers are usually inserted in patients with heart block (Chapter 15). They are of the 'demand' type, only 'cutting in' if the heart rate falls below a predetermined level. Although in theory, diathermy current may trigger the pacemaker and may even 'trip' it into a faster mode, this is not usually a problem provided that the diathermy earth plate is correctly applied and is as remote as possible from the pacemaker site.

Temporary transvenous pacemakers are potentially more of a problem, since the pacemaker box is a separate item of electrical equipment like any other in the theatre and as such is subject to electrical interference. The most important rule, apart from siting the diathermy earth as far away from the pacemaker electrodes (i.e. the heart) as possible, is to place the pacemaker box itself at a distance from the diathermy apparatus, usually on the anaesthetic machine.

Heat

If intense enough, heat produced by hot surfaces or wires (e.g. resectoscopes and endoscope bulbs) is also a potential source of ignition of inflammable gases.

● PREVENTION OF EXPLOSIONS

Apart from minimising the ignition risk in operating theatres and avoiding the use of inflammable anaesthetic agents whenever possible, several methods for minimising the explosion risk in theatre are essential.

1. The use of antistatic materials, in clothing, blankets, anaesthetic and surgical equipment and the soles of footwear to prevent the generation of electrostatic sparks.
2. The provision of an adequately conductive theatre floor.
3. Maintenance of a humid atmosphere within the theatre, as static sparks occur much more commonly in a dry atmosphere. Relative theatre humidity should not fall below 50%.
4. Ensuring that diathermy equipment is safe and that the earth electrode is correctly applied.
5. The avoidance of the use of diathermy when inflammable gases such as ether are being used.
6. If explosive anaesthetics are essential, their administration should be stopped 5 min before diathermy is to be used.

Other electrical equipment should not be used within 25 cm of apparatus containing an inflammable gas. Cardiac pacemakers and ECG machines are often inadvertently kept in close proximity to the anaesthetic machine.

With modern equipment, explosions in theatres are rare, but their effects, particularly when occurring close to or even in the airway of a patient, may be severe or even fatal. Ether is still used as the agent of choice in certain circumstances, particularly in children or in patients suffering severe bronchospasm, and great care is essential whenever this agent is being employed, particularly if an ether/oxygen mixture is used rather than ether/air, the former being considerably more explosive.

Recommended Reading

Association of Anaesthetists of Great Britain and Ireland, London. www.AAGBI.org
Anaphylactic Reactions Associated with Anaesthesia (1990)
Assistance for the Anaesthetist (1990)
Checklist for Anaesthetic Apparatus (1997)
Guidelines for Management of a Malignant Hyperthermia Crisis
HIV and other Blood Borne Viruses (1996)
Immediate Post Anaesthetic Recovery (1993)
Management of Anaesthesia for Jehovah's Witnesses
Recommendations for Standards of Monitoring during Anaesthesia and Recovery (2000).
Aitkinhead A.R. (1998). *Textbook of Anaesthesia*. Edinburgh: Chuchill Livingstone.
Atkinson R.S., Boulton T.B. (1989). *The History of Anaesthesia*. London: Royal Society of Medicine and Parthenon Publishing.
Boulton T.B., Blogg C.E. (1989). *Ostlere and Bryce-Smith's Anaesthetics for Medical Students*, 10th edn. London: Churchill Livingstone.
Brown D.L. (1996). *Regional Anaesthesia and Analgesia*. Philadelphia, PA: W.B. Saunders.
Caldicott L., Lumb A., McCoy D. (1999). *Vascular Anaesthesia. A Practical Handbook*. Oxford: Butterworth-Heinemann.
Cousins M.J., Bridenbaugh P.O. (1998). *Neural Blockade in Clinical Anaesthesia and Management of Pain*, 3rd edn. Philadelphia, PA: Lippincott-Raven.
Craft T.M., Upton P.M. (1992). *Key Topics in Anaesthesia*. Oxford: Bios Scientific.
Davenport H.T. (1986). *Anaesthesia in the Elderly*. London: Heinemann Medical.
Davey A., Moyle J.T.B., Ward C.S. (1992). *Ward's Anaesthetic Equipment*, 3rd edn. London: Saunders.
Davis P.D., Parbrook G.D., Kenny G.N.C. (1995). *Basic Physics and Measurement in Anaesthesia*, 4th edn. Oxford: Butterworth-Heinemann.
Dobson M.B. (1988). *Anaesthesia at the District Hospital*. Geneva: World Health Organization.
Dorsch J.A., Dorsch S.E. (1994). *Understanding Anaesthesia Equipment*, 3rd edn. Baltimore, MD: Williams & Wilkins.

Ellis H.E., Feldman S. (1988). *Anatomy for Anaesthetists*. Oxford: Blackwell Science.

Ganong W.F. (1999). *Review of Medical Physiology*, 19th edn. Stamford, CT: Appleton and Lange.

Ghosh S., Latimer R. (1999). *Thoracic Anaesthesia. Principles and Practice*. Oxford: Butterworth-Heinemann.

Hutton P., Prys-Roberts C. (1994). *Monitoring in Anaesthesia and Intensive Care*. London: W.B. Saunders.

Katz J., Benumof J.L., Kadis L.B. (1990). *Anaesthesia and Uncommon Disease*, 3rd edn. Philadelphia, PA: W.B. Saunders.

Latto I.P., Vaughan R. (1997). *Difficulties in Tracheal Intubation*, 2nd edn. W.B. Saunders.

Latto I.P., Ng W.S., Jones P.L., Jenkins B.L. (2000). *Manual of Central Venous Catheterisation*, 3rd edn. W.B. Saunders.

Lumb A.B.J.F. (2000). *Nunn's Applied Respiratory Physiology*, 5th edn. Oxford: Butterworth-Heinemann.

Macintosh R., Mushin W.W., Epstein H.G. (1987). *Physics for the Anaesthetist*, 4th edn. Oxford: Blackwell Science.

Mather S.J., Hughes D.J. (1996). *A Handbook of Paediatric Anaesthesia*, 2nd edn. Oxford: Oxford University Press.

Millar J.M., Rudkin G.E., Hitchcock M. (1998). *Practical Anaesthesia and Analgesia for Day Surgery*. Oxford: Bios.

Mollison P.L. (1987). *Blood Transfusion in Clinical Medicine*, 8th edn. Oxford: Blackwell Science.

Nimmo W.S., Rowbotham D., Smith G. (eds) (1994). *Anaesthesia*, 2nd edn. Oxford: Blackwell Science.

Popat M. (2001). *Practical Fibreoptic Intubation*. Oxford: Butterworth-Heinemann.

Rendell-Baker L., Thompson P.W., Mapleson W.W. (1980). *Automatic Ventilation of the Lungs*, 3rd edn. Oxford: Blackwell Science.

Resuscitation Council (UK). *Guidelines for Resuscitation*. www.resus.org.uk

Rushman G.B., Davies N.J.H., Cashman J.N. (1999). *Lee's Synopsis of Anaesthesia*, 12th edn. Oxford: Butterworth-Heinemann.

Russell R. (2000). *Anaesthesia for Obstetrics and Gynecology*. London: BMJ Publishing Group.

Russell R., Scrutton M., Porter J. (1997). *Pain Relief in Labour*. London: BMJ Publishing Group.

Scurr C., Feldman S., Soni N. (1990). *Scientific Foundations of Anaesthesia*. 4th edn. Oxford: Butterworth-Heinemann.

Sumner E., Hatch D.J. (1999). *Paediatric Anaesthesia*. London: Arnold.

Sykes M.K., Vickers M.D., Hull C.J. (1981). *Principles of Clinical Measurement*, 2nd edn. Oxford: Blackwell Science.

Vickers M.D. (1978). *Medicine for Anaesthetists*, 2nd edn. Oxford: Blackwell Science.

Vickers M.D., Morgan M., Spencer P.S.J., Read M.S. (1991). *Drugs in Anaesthetic and Intensive Care Practice*, 8th edn. Oxford: Butterworth-Heinemann.

Walters F.J.M., Ingram S.G., Jenkinson J.L. (1994). *Anaesthesia and Intensive Care for the Neurosurgical Patient*, 2nd edn. Oxford: Blackwell Science.

Wildsmith J.A.W., Armitage E.N. (1987). *Principles and Practice of Regional Anaesthesia*. London: Churchill Livingstone.

Yentis S.M., Hirsch, Smith G.B. (2000). *Anaesthesia and Intensive Care. A to Z*, 2nd edn. Oxford: Butterworth-Heinemann.

Yentis S.M., Brighouse D., May A., Bogod D., Elton C. (2000). *Analgesia, Anaesthesia and Pregnancy: A Practical Guide*. Philadelphia, PA: W.B. Saunders.

Index